CBT + DBT + ACT

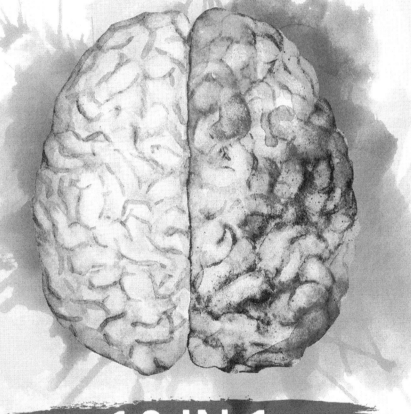

10 IN 1

COGNITIVE BEHAVIORAL THERAPY, DIALECTICAL BEHAVIOR THERAPY, ACCEPTANCE AND COMMITMENT THERAPY, VAGUS NERVE, POLYVAGAL THEORY, ANXIETY IN RELATIONSHIPS & DEPRESSION CURE

JOSEPH OWENS

TABLE OF CONTENTS

COGNITIVE BEHAVIOR THERAPY

DIALECTICAL BEHAVIOR THERAPY

ACCEPTANCE AND COMMITMENT THERAPY

HIGHLY SENSITIVE EMPATH

VAGUS NERVE

COGNITIVE BEHAVIOR THERAPY

INTRODUCTION

"It is a great life if one can be moderate and content. The wise man has anticipated the risks; he neither rushes headlong into the thick of the fray nor turns his back upon it."
-Seneca

Cognitive Behavior Therapy (CBT) is a type of psychotherapy that helps individuals understand their thoughts, beliefs, and behaviors to try to change them. It helps people learn how these thought patterns impact their emotions and how they react to certain events or situations. These skills can be used to manage stress and depression symptoms. Initially, the client is taught to identify self-defeating thoughts that lead to negative feelings. Patients are also taught behavioral techniques such as problem-solving, goal setting, and relaxation. For example, when someone's anxiety causes him to fall apart -- the therapist might teach him how to take a deep breath and count slowly from 1 to 5, then repeat this exercise a few times before returning to work or school. The goal is for the patient to learn strategies he can use in daily situations. This intervention could help him become more aware of his thought processes and, therefore, better able to control or change them.

"The relationship between thinking (cognition) and behavior represents a fundamental aspect of human existence. Since the 1960s, there has been a growing interest in consciousness and cognition related to behavior change. Cognitive therapy (C.T.) is one of the earliest and most extensively studied forms of cognitive behavior therapy and aims to use cognition to modify maladaptive patterns of behaviors associated with emotional distress and life difficulties."

CBT therapy is usually an individualized approach; each person's situation is different and thus may require a different type of intervention instead of using styles or techniques taken from other therapies. CBT is based on the belief that how we perceive and interpret things, our actions, responses to events, and interpersonal relationships, can influence how we feel. The CBT therapist will help the patient examine negative thought patterns to replace them with more realistic and healthy thoughts.

CBT has been proven more effective than placebos in treating anxiety disorders and depression. It has also been shown to be an effective treatment for substance abuse, eating disorders, psychosis, personality disorders, and even schizophrenia. This type of therapy works best when the client is highly motivated; these techniques are often difficult to apply consistently at first – but with practice comes success.

The American Psychological Association (APA) describes Cognitive Behavioral Therapy (CBT) as short-term psychotherapy supported by research as an effective treatment for many mental health concerns. CBT is goal-oriented and focuses on the present while considering past experiences. Unlike psychoanalysis, which takes place over five to six years or longer, CBT can last only a few months. People with a past episode of depression often can benefit from CBT, as it is geared towards treating immediate situations that might trigger future problems.

"Cognitive-behavioral therapy is a form of psychotherapy (treatment or cure) that works to change how your mind and body interact to improve your ability to manage your moods and anxiety." CBT is used in many hospitals and medical centers throughout the United States and offers effective treatment for patients with various mental health concerns. CBT focuses on the present moment and addresses how thoughts are ultimately processed into behaviors.

Guided by the belief that our thoughts cause our feelings and behaviors -- not external circumstances -- cognitive therapists focus on making patients aware of these thoughts to change thinking patterns and behaviors. In some cases, patients are directly asked to challenge their ideas by looking for evidence that contradicts these thoughts. Patients are encouraged to become aware of negative self-talk by keeping a daily journal.

The cognitive therapist helps patients examine the relationship between their thoughts and feelings. For example, suppose a patient believes he is unpopular because people dislike him. In that case, the therapist may ask him to take time each day to write down his negative automatic thoughts about others. The therapist also may have the patient observe his behavior in social situations, especially when talking with others. The goal is to help patients understand how their perception of themselves affects their thoughts and feelings and how those beliefs affect how they react in certain situations.

Behavior Therapy is "applied behavior analysis," a class of techniques and principles of learning used to improve human functioning. The methods derived in large part from the work of B.F. Skinner is heavily used by behavior analysts as well as other types of therapists (e.g., cognitive therapists).

In systematic desensitization, a person is exposed to stimuli that provoke anxiety, usually in a controlled setting. The person is asked to repeat the desensitizing stimuli repeatedly (think of this as the exposure-response) until they have become tolerant. If the feared stimulus causes fear and anxiety, or if the individual finds it too painful or frightening to do this at home in real life, numerous other techniques can be utilized to learn how to deal with the fear of such a stimulus (e.g., gradual exposure therapy). Once someone knows not to be afraid of certain situations (e.g., spiders), they can move on to confronting the fear in real-life situations.

A significant component of behavior therapy is reinforcement – giving a child or adult something he wants when he performs a specific action. Reinforcement is an essential part of achieving any goal. It can be very effective in modifying behaviors, especially those related to learning disabilities, mental illness, and addiction (smoking).

Some forms of behavior therapy are conducted by therapists who are not clinically licensed but receive training. This may be effective in cases where traditional psychotherapy has failed and patients cannot manage the stress that leads to addiction, depression, or other mental illnesses. Specific programs have been effective in treating drug addiction.

A "graded extinction" technique is used when a person fears certain situations or objects. For example, the therapist may ask the individual to either approach the feared object or not. Sometimes this can be done without exposing the person to the actual situation; for example, an individual may be asked to confront his fears through a program of careful desensitization. The idea is to teach people not to be afraid of certain situations and objects; this provides individuals with an experience they can use in real life as a coping skill (e.g., confronting a fear of heights by practicing on steps).

Cognitive-behavioral therapy or CBT is one of the licensed professionals' most common forms of treatment. Cognitive-behavioral therapists believe that a person's thoughts cause their feelings. By addressing these cognitions, the therapist can change a person's feelings and behaviors (or vice versa).

An example is escaping from a situation that triggers negative thoughts, leaving an inflexible environment, and finding healthier outlets for emotions. Rather than telling someone to "think positive," they recommend replacing negative thoughts with positive ones – replacing thinking that "I'm not good enough" with "I can do this."

Moreover, Cognitive Behavioral Therapy (CBT) is a form of psychotherapy or "talk therapy" which helps patients understand and change problematic patterns of thinking, feeling, and behaving. It became one of the most popular psychotherapeutic treatment methods in the 1970s because it addresses the cognitive and behavioral aspects of depression, substance abuse, and other disorders.

Processing, the second of the three main components of CBT, is how thoughts and feelings are recognized and changed. These cognitions are then used as a basis for changing behaviors. CBT uses a range of techniques, including relaxation, and the "ABC" model, such as recognizing the presence of a consequence and using behaviors to avoid it in the future. This can be achieved by self-monitoring and evaluating behavior.

Cognitive therapy is primarily used to help people with depression, anxiety, or related disorders. In some cases, people with severe anxiety may have nightmares associated with their anxiety that they believe prevent them from sleeping. Cognitive therapy also helps people work through their thoughts and feelings regarding a situation or event that has caused them to become anxious or depressed.

Cognitive therapists help people learn new ways to think about themselves and their lives concerning the world around them. This allows them to develop new coping skills to overcome anxiety or depression.

Some cognitive-behavioral therapies have been shown to treat depression, anxiety disorders, and some eating disorders. Cognitive Behavioral Therapy (CBT), developed by Aaron T. Beck, focuses on the interaction between one's thoughts, feelings, and behaviors. Another variant of CBT is Cognitive Therapy (C.T.), developed by Gerald C. Davison and John M. Neale in the 1970s due to a split between the founders of CBT at Beck's clinic at the University of Pennsylvania in Philadelphia. C.T. focuses more on the cognitive aspects of the disorder.

Cognitive behavior therapy is often used with other forms of therapy or treatment, such as psychodynamic therapy, psychopharmacology, interpersonal therapy, group therapy, and a host of others. A few people can be treated successfully with only cognitive-behavioral therapies; however, such cases are rare. Cognitive-behavioral therapies help people overcome fears, phobias, depression, delusions, obsessions, and compulsions. Cognitive behavioral therapy is usually used in conjunction with psychotherapy. Cognitive-behavioral therapy has been used successfully to treat people with a debilitating fear of heights and social phobia.

Cognitive behavioral therapy (CBT) is a type of cognitive therapy that focuses on how people think and how their thinking affects their feelings/behaviors/actions. This treatment approach also helps individuals identify, challenge, and change perceptions (the meaning attached to situations), beliefs (the importance of something in one's life), and urges or urges to act (e.g., "I could not sleep tonight because I am anxious").

Therefore, CBT is essential since it occurs when a person is consciously aware of these thoughts, feelings, and urges. This can be in the form of a conversation between the therapist and the client. A CBT therapist will help you deal with the stresses that lead to various behaviors. In some cases, CBT may have been effective because it enables individuals to recognize that they have control over how they act—not just how they feel—and to use this knowledge to develop healthy coping strategies.

Cognitive-behavioral therapy treats anxiety disorders, depression, phobias, and chronic pain effectively. Cognitive-behavioral therapy is a short-term, goal-oriented psychotherapy treatment that focuses on the here and now. CBT helps individuals change faulty patterns of thinking or behavior that have contributed to personal distress or difficulties in interpersonal relationships. CBT treats many problems, including depression, stress, anxiety disorders, low self-esteem, marital issues, and anger management. Cognitive behavioral therapy is effective in treating social phobia and specific phobias. For example, studies are mixed as to whether cognitive behavioral therapy works better than exposure alone for social phobia (social anxiety disorder).

CBT IS A POPULAR PSYCHOTHERAPY TREATMENT

As a popular psychotherapy treatment, CBT has significantly reduced symptoms of depression, general anxiety disorders, and other mental health problems.

Cognitive Behavior Therapy is a psychotherapeutic approach as well as a structured set of techniques in psychotherapy that seeks to identify cognitive and emotional factors that contribute to distress or disability and modify these factors with empirically supported therapies (i.e., specific treatment strategies identified through clinical trials), and promote behavioral changes that bring about lasting improvement. It should not be confused with "cognitive therapy," the broader term for rational emotive behavior therapy (REBT) within the larger group of cognitive behavioral therapies. The latter is not a therapy that treats mood disorders but is psychotherapy for treating conditions like depression and anxiety.

Cognitive Behavior Therapy (CBT) is a specific approach to psychotherapy. It relies on the idea that our thoughts, feelings, and behaviors all interact to create a feedback loop or "cycle" that can keep us stuck in specific ways of thinking and behaving. CBT aims to break the cycle by changing faulty beliefs to more realistic ones, coping skills to help deal with daily stressors, and behaviors like relaxation techniques or exposure therapy, so we change our reactions. The goal of CBT is not necessarily "feel good," but more "function well.

It is nowadays very common since it is a widely known and often applied form of treatment. Many practitioners offer this technique in different ways, aiming to reach the same goal: to help individuals with the symptoms of mental problems. Cognitive behavioral therapy (CBT) is a psychotherapy that uses behavioral techniques to teach patients to change how they think and behave. CBT is based on the work of Albert Ellis, who pioneered the application of cognitive psychology to the treatment of depression.

There are numerous ways for CBT to be delivered, which has led to a bewildering variety of names and terminologies in widespread media usage. However, one can identify what should be referred to as CBT as a structured set of techniques in psychotherapy that seeks to identify cognitive and emotional factors that contribute to distress or disability, modify these factors with empirically supported therapies (i.e., specific treatment strategies identified through clinical trials), and promote behavioral changes that bring about lasting improvement.

CBT is popular since it is a widely known and often applied form of treatment. Many practitioners offer this technique in different ways, aiming to reach the same goal: to help individuals with the symptoms of mental problems.

Cognitive Behavioral Therapy (CBT) is a psychotherapy modality that uses behavioral techniques to teach patients to change how they think and behave. Many therapies use behavior techniques, including "thought stopping," "cognitive restructuring," "exposure therapy," and "behavioral rehearsal." It is based on the work of Albert Ellis, who pioneered the application of cognitive psychology to the treatment of depression.

CBT considers that we have automatic thoughts and emotions that affect our thinking, feelings, and behavior in several ways. For example, we may react to a stressful event by having a negative thought like "I am not going well today," or we may see ourselves as generally incompetent. Hence, a minor mistake made us feel stressed out and overwhelmed. The goal of CBT is not necessarily "feel good" but more "function well.

In addition, CBT is commonly used since it is an effective treatment for many clinical problems, having been validated in more than 400 scientific studies on its efficacy.

Cognitive Behavioral Therapy is among the most widely used therapies for various psychological disorders and problems, including depression and anxiety, anger management issues, eating disorders, trauma, and even substance abuse.

Cognitive Behavior Therapy has been described as a structured set of techniques in psychotherapy that uses empirically supported therapies (specific treatment strategies identified through clinical trials) to promote behavioral changes that bring about lasting improvement. For CBT to be effective, the patient mustn't overestimate the effectiveness of the treatment. The ultimate goal of CBT is not necessarily "feel good," although it can help you feel better, but more "function well.

CBT techniques can be broadly divided into two categories: (1) cognitive and (2) behavioral.

- Cognitive techniques alter how a person thinks about an object or event to influence their emotional reaction. These include reframing, rational emotive therapy, thought stopping, thought challenging, relaxation training, and imaging tools (e.g., relaxing images).
- Behavioral techniques aim to alter a person's behavior through reinforcement or punishment to increase desirable behaviors and reduce undesirable behaviors. The behavioral component often includes exposure therapy, systematic desensitization, interoceptive exposure (venturing within a panic threshold), relaxation training, assertiveness training, and social skills training.

Cognitive Behavioral Therapy, in the abbreviated form of CBT, consists of a series of techniques designed to change how a person thinks and behaves. Similarly to the other therapies, patients are often asked to keep logs and detailed records for therapists and patients that reveal how much progress has been made so they can take stock of their progress.

The cognitive behavioral therapy treatment plan outlines how the patient's emotions and thoughts will differ after each session. The treatment plan is set out at the beginning of each appointment. Then, the patient is given several homework assignments between treatment sessions requiring some thought and effort.

The cognitive behavioral therapy plan is generic and can be used whether the patient has been referred by their GP or has come directly to the therapist. Using the SPIKES approach as part of an assessment plan for depression or anxiety is no longer considered necessary. However, it can still be used in specific situations to help patients better understand themselves.

Cognitive Behaviour Therapy (CBT) is a psychotherapy based on cognitive theories of mind and behavior. It aims to modify distorted thinking patterns using various techniques developed by Albert Ellis (1913–2007). Ellis originally called his therapy rational therapy, which became rational emotive behavior therapy (REBT). Today the term REBT is more often used for a specific form of CBT that does not include the original psychoanalytic techniques.

Many health care providers use cognitive behavioral therapy (CBT) as evidence-based psychotherapy. It holds that distress and impairment result from the interaction of maladaptive thoughts and behaviors, so they are best changed through cognitive and behavioral interventions. CBT has been proven effective in treating depression, anxiety disorders, eating disorders, addictions, and other problems. Therefore, Cognitive Behavioral Therapy (CBT) is a psychotherapy based on cognitive theories of mind and behavior.

Benefits that CBT has as a popular psychotherapy treatment

Cognitive Behavioral Therapy (CBT) is a relatively new approach compared to other psychotherapeutic treatment methods. However, since it has appeared on the psychological scene for about fifty years, it has considerably impacted psychotherapy and its usage by different practitioners. Just like everything else in life, things change, and change is good. This field of study is one of those that have changed the most throughout the years. It is still being altered to fit its usability with all age groups worldwide. To provide appropriate psycho-education, people need to understand how this relatively new therapy differs from other forms of treatment like behavior and cognitive therapies.

There are many different areas in which CBT differs from other forms of psychotherapy. One of the most important attributes involves several skills and techniques. This approach to therapy does not simply rely on one single type of therapy for each specific person but rather uses different forms of treatment for each client; how people view their experiences and thoughts impacts their life experiences, so it is also necessary to use this as a main aspect of CBT.

The brain processes information that is received through various senses. The person's ability to work without difficulty within this system depends on the mental and physical abilities developed throughout a person's lifetime. One of the most important factors related to the brain is the consistency of thought. If thoughts are consistent, individuals can make better decisions and use their skills more effectively to reach their goals.

A lot of focus is placed on one's thoughts and actions because they are interconnected. Whether it is a conscious or unconscious process, certain thoughts manage to stay on your mind even after you have moved on from the situation. The constant repetition of those thoughts makes them a significant part of one's life, so they become automatic thoughts. The individual may not be aware that they can control their thinking process.

Cognitive behavioral therapy has been a well-accepted treatment for the past fifty years. It has begun gaining research support and acceptance by society since many studies have been performed confirming its effectiveness and reliability. However, there are still many questions regarding its effectiveness and whether it is truly an effective treatment method for various problems. Since CBT is a relatively new approach alongside psychoanalytic and dialectical behavior therapy, there are still many unanswered questions regarding its effectiveness in treating people with various mental health issues.

Although there are several questions and concerns regarding the effectiveness of cognitive behavioral therapy, there is still a lot of support for using this form of treatment. Among the major people who support using CBT are those who have researched it. They have done a great deal in studying various aspects related to its effectiveness and reliability. A significant amount can be discovered due to their experience treating different types of patients with different mental health problems. Thus, they have been at the forefront as they contribute extensively to this field by providing new ways of looking at mental health issues and methods for treating them.

There are still several questions about the effectiveness of this therapy. Thus, it is necessary to assist these major concerns to be answered. To attempt to answer some of the more important concerns, more research needs to be done. A study will have to be done on people of different ages and socioeconomic levels to assess their effectiveness with each treatment method.

There are still many questions about their effectiveness and reliability when it comes down to treating specific types of mental health problems. This is because many aspects still need to be investigated, and the results will be considered valuable information. Thus, more and more research needs to be done to familiarize people with different issues and their particular treatment methods.

Despite all the questions about the effectiveness of cognitive behavioral therapy, there is still a lot of support for its use. For now, this may remain a popular form of psychotherapy in many mental health clinics worldwide. However, it will take some time before the support that it has now becomes sustainable enough for every person who wishes to receive psychotherapy treatment from undergoing it. For now, it will remain an important part of psychotherapy.

One of the primary indicators of using cognitive behavioral therapy is that it has been around for over fifty years. It is one type of treatment that has gained popularity in the last few decades and continues to be used by many health professionals to treat different mental health disorders. Although it has been used for the past several decades, there are still many unanswered questions about its effectiveness and reliability when treating numerous conditions that affect people around the globe.

Soon after beginning to use cognitive behavioral therapy, many people have reported great improvements in their lives and mental health issues. Thus, there is much resistance to changing this popular form of psychotherapy. However, there are still concerns about its effectiveness and how effective it can be when treating certain problems. Thus, more research needs to be done for the benefits of this approach to be more sustainable and begin to stand on a more solid foundation.

As mentioned earlier, cognitive behavioral therapy is one of the most commonly used forms of psychotherapy. There are many reasons why people choose cognitive behavioral therapy over other types of treatment. One reason for its popularity may be that it has proven effective and reliable in helping people with specific mental health disorders such as depression or anxiety.

Benefits of CBT include:

1. It focuses on the individual's thinking.

By this, CBT focuses on helping each person understand and analyze their thoughts and behavior. It also helps them reflect on their thinking patterns and how these thoughts affect the way that they react to situations in which they are usually triggered.

2. It helps people become aware of the emotions from their own life experiences.

CBT helps people realize the importance of managing their feelings, especially when an extreme emotion such as anger is triggered within them. This form of CBT centers around learning how to recognize and regulate different types of anxious and mixed feelings that people may experience during stressful times or whenever a typical negative thought enters their minds.

3. It helps people learn how to identify negative thought patterns and cognitive distortions.

CBT helps patients to be able to recognize their negative thoughts as well as the negative or distorted way, for example, that they interpret their experiences through visual images, false beliefs, or unreasonable fears and beliefs.

4. It teaches the most effective ways to communicate with others.

CBT teaches each person how to deal with communication difficulties that can occur within intimate relationships more effectively by teaching them how to understand their own emotions instead of reacting based on situations that seem threatening instead of realistic.

5.   It improves people's ability to control their emotions in stressful circumstances.

CBT helps individuals recognize the difference between an emotion and the action or behavior motivated by a feeling. For example, helping a person to understand the difference between feeling angry and acting aggressively towards others.

6.   It teaches each person how to accept constructive feedback from others.

It helps people recognize that as long as they maintain their self-esteem, it is important for them to be open-minded when receiving advice from loved ones who wish to help them improve their lives.

7.   It helps individuals resolve their problems instead of relying on other sources of support.

CBT helps each person to identify and resolve their problems instead of relying on other sources of support such as friends, family members, or therapists.

8.   It increases a healthy lifestyle within each individual.

CBT helps people to do activities that are beneficial to their physical health and well-being, such as exercise and drinking enough water.

9.   It improves interpersonal relationships in each person's life.

CBT helps individuals become more socially competent by engaging in conversations with others and learning how to communicate effectively with others in different situations.

10.   It helps individuals achieve higher self-esteem through praise or criticism but their efforts alone.

CBT strengthens self-esteem by helping people recognize how they can control negative self-talk.

As with any other form of psychotherapy, cognitive behavioral therapy has pros and cons. Cognitive behavioral therapy may be considered a more practical treatment because it does not require much time to implement. It does not require patients to spend extended time in sessions with a therapist. This may be appealing for some because it does not seem like such a long process or commitment as other types of psychotherapy may seem to some people. Another benefit of CBT is that it may be perceived as more helpful than other forms of psychotherapy because it can help people with issues such as depression or other mental health disorders. There are many different types of OCD which include the type that may have begun after a person was exposed to a traumatic event at an early age. There are different types of OCD which include OCD related to HIV, sexual obsessions, scrupulosity, and contamination. Therefore, CBT may be more effective as a treatment for these conditions because it helps people to focus on counteracting their negative thoughts instead of avoiding the situations that trigger them. As a result, CBT works well with highly structured forms of therapy, such as exposure-based therapies.

Finally, another positive aspect of CBT is that therapists and patients can focus less on past experiences than on the present when working together. This form of therapy has the potential to be successful because it helps individuals to recognize how certain triggers influence their current moods or behaviors in their lives. Therefore, they can more easily focus on the present situations they encounter throughout their lives versus dwelling on the past.

11.   It helps the person understand and to accept the severity of the condition or problem.

CBT can help individuals accept that they have a mental health problem or illness that may not have been caused by any form of trauma in their life. It can help them understand that there is no need to feel guilty due to their condition because it is not something they brought upon themselves. They may also learn how to deal with new situations that trigger an extreme emotion within them, such as anger, through CBT and learn how to avoid negative thinking patterns. This form of therapy explains how proper treatment for OCD will benefit them in the long run.

12. It teaches the patient to be more assertive and not introverted.

CBT can teach the patient what they can say to themselves before they speak when they feel uncomfortable in situations to be assertive. CBT can help the patient learn to recognize what is bothering them and avoid negative or extreme thoughts that may interfere with their life. For example, a person with a social anxiety disorder needs to understand that they worry needlessly about negative thoughts that tend to ruin their self-esteem. With CBT, therapists will try different ways. Hence, patients understand why it is helpful for them to communicate with others instead of being quiet in an attempt to avoid rejection or harsh criticism from others.

13. It helps the patient understand and modify unwanted behaviors.

CBT can help the patient learn how to identify what inappropriate thoughts are causing them to become anxious in certain situations. CBT gives them more information on identifying their unusual thoughts and how they can use it to help them avoid excessive worry about those negative thoughts.

14. It helps the patient learn how to manage stress and anxiety by learning that it is manageable with proper treatment.

The goal of CBT is for the person to be able to recognize when they become overly anxious or stressed, which is an underlying symptom of OCD, and work towards learning new strategies to cope with their adverse reactions to specific situations that trigger their extreme negative emotions. This form of therapy benefits the patient because it may alleviate their stress and anxiety. After all, they know they can rely on other forms of treatment to get better. If a person continues to engage in positive activities, they are more likely to be successful in managing their stress or anxiety as a result.

15. It helps individuals understand how thoughts influence emotions to alter them accordingly.

CBT enables the patient to become aware of how their feelings can be changed or influenced by certain events or thoughts. They can learn to recognize inappropriate thoughts that may negatively influence their emotions and change them immediately. CBT can help the patient to recognize which situations may make them angry or embarrassed because of their OCD. They can also learn how to use CBT techniques to minimize their negative feelings when triggered by certain situations that previously caused extreme emotion.

Many factors contribute to CBT's success as a form of psychotherapy. Through understanding the benefits, drawbacks, and possible ways that CBT helps people, clients may receive better results through this treatment instead of other forms of therapy. Suppose a person is struggling with OCD and may be at a socioeconomic disadvantage due to their finances. In that case, it may be difficult for them to receive treatment through Medicare. Therefore, patients need to recognize CBT's options and advantages over other forms of therapy, such as medication. Hopefully, this report can help individuals learn why CBT is a distinctive form of therapy that has helped people overcome many severe mental health disorders.

On the other hand, CBT is not always a perfect form of therapy. It may not be suitable for all people due to its inability to address the core motivations of particular beliefs and negative emotions. In some instances, careful analysis of core beliefs and how negative thinking patterns maintain them can help people achieve a better quality of life by assisting them in making more positive thinking choices. As previously mentioned, cognitive behavioral therapy does not address these core issues. In other words, it does not focus directly on identifying the most important factors influencing thoughts and actions. For example, a significant reason why some people struggle with their OCD is due to their irrational beliefs. This type of therapy does not necessarily address or modify these issues as effectively as CBT, so it may be necessary to engage an individual in other types of therapy, such as acceptance and commitment therapy.

Although recent research is sparse and not always methodologically sound, cognitive behavioral therapy has been widely studied. The effectiveness of CBT in treating anxiety disorders is supported by several randomized clinical trials, with the effect size being moderate to large and clinically significant. In general, the studies show that CBT increases anxiety disorder symptom reduction (that is, in general, decreases the amount of time that patients have severe anxiety). This effect has been found to persist for up to two years after treatment. Note that a similar effect has been found for medicated patients as well.

In addition, CBT is associated with lower relapse rates and recovery rates than other therapeutic approaches. For example, one study found that CBT was more effective for treatment-resistant depression than cognitive therapy or a combination of both.

However, several meta-analyses have suggested that there may be a point at which therapy stops working. Some meta-analyses, for example, suggest that the effect size of CBT decreases after six to eight months of treatment.

Therefore, there is a suggestion that further improvement may be small and not clinically significant. This is in line with findings that show a dose-response relationship between exposure and response to therapy, which has been observed mostly in studies with people who have not had previous exposure to CBT.

Another limitation of the research is that it primarily focuses on depression and anxiety disorders. Therefore, it is unclear how useful CBT would be for other diagnoses, such as specific phobias and eating disorders.

However, studies have shown that CBT is effective for OCD and social anxiety disorder, which have unique diagnoses. While more research is needed to understand the effectiveness of CBT for these diagnoses, it is clear that further research can help us to determine when further improvement has stopped and when further improvement may be achieved. A promising practice for understanding the effect of therapy on depression and anxiety disorders is propensity-score matching.

This approach performs a statistical analysis such that patients are assigned to the treatment groups at each baseline visit based on their smoking status (cognitive behavior model or active control) or their propensity score (CBT or active control). These methods allow for an unbiased comparison of the effect size between the active treatment (CBT) and the control condition and provide a much more accurate estimate of real-world effectiveness than a simple analysis of whether or not treatment was more effective than control. In addition, this matching technique allows for an unbiased estimate of how many patients would respond to a specific intervention. For example, it is unknown how many people who suffer from depression will benefit from CBT. The propensity score matching allows researchers to determine who is likely to benefit and then assign them to either CBT or inactive control conditions. The results show that when tending to depressed patients, 19–40% of people may benefit from CBT based on their propensity score.

This is a much more accurate estimate of the potential success of CBT in comparison to the previous studies, which looked at those who had already received treatment. In addition, while it may be true that CBT does not work for everyone, it can help millions of people worldwide due to its effectiveness and practicality.

Although CBT is a highly effective treatment for depression and anxiety disorders, it is important that, as a society, we recognize that CBT is not always the most effective approach to mental health disorders. As mentioned, this report heeds this fact to help individuals and other key stakeholders understand why CBT is easily the most effective approach for many people who suffer from anxiety and depression disorders.

Cognitive behavioral therapy is one of the most effective treatments in helping patients suffering from severe anxiety disorders such as generalized anxiety disorder, social phobia, panic disorder, post-traumatic stress disorder (PTSD), OCD, and depression.

CBT is used to treat psychotherapy since:

1. Clinically useful and well-established.

CBT is useful for adult patients who are suffering from severe anxiety disorders.

For this reason, CBT is used for the treatment of anxiety disorders and disorders related to learning disabilities which include:

* Attention Deficit Hyperactivity Disorder (ADHD)
* Autism spectrum disorder (ASD)
* Dyslexia
* Learning difficulties
* Mood Disorders such as Depression, Bipolar, and Severe Depression.

CBT has also been effective for anxiety disorders such as post-traumatic stress disorder, generalized anxiety disorder, panic attacks, phobias, obsessive-compulsive disorder, and night-time insomnia.

2. CBT has a high success rate.

The success rate of CBT ranges from 40-80% when treating anxiety disorders (this is the same success rate as medications).

There are different approaches in cognitive behavioral therapy based on the patient's clinical needs. Therefore, there are many variations in procedures and techniques used by therapists to treat anxiety disorders based on their needs.

This way, cognitive behavioral therapy is not just one treatment but can be tailored to suit each patient's needs. It can be an effective approach to mental health care for patients suffering from severe anxiety disorder and depression problems.

3. It's more cost-effective than other therapies.

The cost of CBT is much cheaper than other therapies used to treat severe anxiety disorders.

Because of this, it is highly recommended that people in psychotherapy consider using CBT if they can afford it, as it will prove to be more effective and cost-efficient.

4. Proven in helping patients who have not received treatment before.

CBT is effective for anxiety disorders such as post-traumatic stress disorder, generalized anxiety disorder, panic attacks, phobias, obsessive-compulsive disorder, and night-time insomnia.

This means that people who have not previously sought treatment for their mental illness problems can benefit from CBT due to its high success rate when treating severe anxiety disorders.

5. It can be used to treat depression and anxiety disorders in collaboration with medication.

Sometimes, therapy and medication may not be enough to treat severe anxiety disorders. Also, many people do not want to take any medications, as they may become dependent on them or do not think they will work effectively.

CBT, when used alongside medication, can help people suffering from severe anxiety disorders maintain their quality of life and gain a more positive outlook on the future.

6.   CBT is used on a wide spectrum of ages.

In cognitive behavioral therapy, the therapist will choose the most appropriate treatment for an individual based on their age and childhood experiences.

This means that CBT can be effectively used with adults, children, and adolescents suffering from severe anxiety disorders.

CBT treats anxiety disorders in children and adolescents because the techniques are consistent with cognitive development (children learn by doing). Therefore, when a child is taught these techniques, it helps them learn how to cope with demanding situations in their everyday lives.

7.   It's beneficial if you feel that you don't want to treat your anxiety symptoms with medication but still want to make some changes in your life.

CBT can be beneficial if you do not want to take medication; however, you still want to make changes to live a happier, healthier, and more fulfilling life.

Because CBT teaches new coping skills, it is a good approach to mental health care for patients suffering from severe anxiety disorders who do not wish to take medications.

8.   It's focused on the here and now instead of dwelling on past events.

The primary focus of CBT is on the patient's current problems and how they can deal with them in their everyday lives.

This means that CBT does not focus on negative memories or events from the past that have contributed to the development of a mental illness.

This helps an individual keep the focus on their life today.

CBT is effective when treating a wide range of mental health disorders because it helps people to view their lives more positively and take things one step at a time.

9.   It takes into consideration the mind-body connection.

Cognitive behavioral therapy uses cognitive techniques that allow people suffering from anxiety disorders to think about and change their thoughts, feelings, and behaviors. This can include changing how they think about themselves, other people, and their surroundings, and how they act on these thoughts and feelings.

This makes cognitive behavioral therapy a good approach to mental health care for patients suffering from anxiety disorders as it focuses on changes in the mind, body, and environment.

10. It helps people to have a more meaningful and productive life.

CBT teaches people how to change their thinking, feeling, and acting to use these skills differently and live a more fulfilling life. Doing this regularly helps people who suffer from severe anxiety disorders gain a better quality of life.

11. It improves relationships, making them stronger.

In cognitive behavioral therapy, the therapist may ask for assistance from family members or friends to help the patient change their behaviors. This can include being more supportive and encouraging and helping them refocus their thoughts and feelings on positive aspects of life.

This is because CBT is focused on improving relationships with others through communication and support. Therefore, it is a good approach to mental health care for patients suffering from severe anxiety disorders as it can improve their relationships with others.

12. It teaches you solution-based techniques that you have learned over time so that they become second nature.

Cognitive behavioral therapy enables you to make changes in your life using problem-solving techniques taught by the therapist.

These techniques should be used in everyday life to help you cope with situations that may trigger feelings of fear or panic at first. However, over time these techniques will become second nature, and you will use them automatically when faced with difficult situations.

Cognitive behavioral therapy is one of the most effective approaches to mental health care for patients suffering from anxiety disorders. With research demonstrating that CBT can be used to treat a range of mental health disorders successfully, it has become one of the most recommended forms of therapy for treating severe anxiety disorders. Research has also shown that people who completed CBT have reduced their anxiety levels after treatment.

Research has shown that CBT can be used to treat patients suffering from severe anxiety disorders who use medications because of varying levels of improvement. Therefore, it is a good approach to mental health care for patients suffering from severe anxiety disorders.

The primary benefit of CBT is the ability to customize and tailor treatment plans for individuals based on their personality, behavior, and cognitive functioning. Cognitive behavioral therapy can be effective for patients who may not respond well to medication.

CBT is effective in treating many different anxiety disorders. This means it is a good approach to mental health care for patients suffering from specific anxiety disorders, as it can effectively treat them. If a patient has more than one type of anxiety disorder, it may be most beneficial to have several therapists working together on their care plan.

Therefore, Cognitive behavioral therapy can help people who suffer from anxiety disorders understand the course of their disorder and find ways to cope with their symptoms, allowing them to lead happier and healthier lives. CBT is a cost-effective therapy for patients suffering from anxiety disorders, with research showing that it does not cost a lot of money and can be easily accessed. This means that cognitive behavioral therapy can significantly affect the quality of life of people suffering from anxiety disorders.

COMMON MISTAKES AND MYTHS ABOUT CBT

Cognitive Behavioral Therapy (CBT) is the most commonly used form of therapy for a wide range of mental health problems. But CBT only works if it is done right; unfortunately, many therapists don't understand how to provide evidence-based, successful CBT. This book post will address some common mistakes and myths in CBT and help you avoid them.

Many believe CBT involves talking about thoughts, using thought records, analyzing negative thoughts, filling out mood charts, etc. This attention to thoughts is particularly important if you suffer from depression, anxiety, or obsession problems. However, if the main problem is things like anger outbursts or substance use, the thoughts are less important, and focusing on changing behavior is more effective. Similarly, the behaviors are most important if you have relationship problems, not your thoughts.

But this doesn't mean that CBT doesn't help you explore and challenge your thoughts on other types of problems. The effectiveness of CBT depends more on how well it addresses behavior than how much time it spends on analyzing thoughts.

There are several mistakes regarding CBT. These include:

1. Being too general or focusing too much on the negative.

This is common in clinical practice. People get referred for a specific problem – for example, a woman who has panic attacks when she rides an escalator at the train station. She comes to you because she wants help with her problem with this one situation.

But then you ignore that and say something like: "The anxiety is caused by your pessimistic expectations of what might go wrong. Let's focus on that".

This general focus seems to make sense, but it can end up ignoring the very problem people thought they were coming to treatment for. This can lead to poorer outcomes.

Secondly, it is easy to get stuck focusing on problems in the past and get stuck in a type of negative rumination which can make things worse. In CBT, we want to focus on what we can do today – and this means that our main emphasis is on planning positive changes for today, tomorrow, and the near future.

This often requires special training for therapists because it means you must interrupt your thinking about the past or worries about the future and concentrate on what's important now.

2. Focusing too much on cognitive issues when behavior change is key.

This is common in clinical practice as well. One of the main differences between CBT and other types of therapy for many problems is that CBT focuses more on behavior rather than thoughts or emotions. After all, thoughts and emotions are a normal part of daily life, but how we behave can affect our thinking, moods, and ability to cope with everyday problems.

For example, when you don't call someone back for a date, you might panic about your lack of confidence.

If you feel more confident, you might call them back and make a date. So there's a clear link between your behavior (not calling them back) and how you feel (anxious).

This doesn't mean we don't learn how to challenge our negative thoughts. But we do it to change our behavior and not because we think it will make us feel better!

3. Focusing on negative emotions or thinking styles.

This is common in clinical practice. It's useful to understand what makes people feel anxious, sad, or depressed because these feelings often become targeted by clients themselves who want to change their feelings with the hope that they will then get rid of the problem. But the problem is that emotions don't have to be something we want to change – they can also be part of a coping mechanism. We might feel anxious because we are worried about something that has happened in the past. But as a coping mechanism, anxiety can help us stay vigilant and cautious or help us deal with or recover from a difficult event.

For example, you might feel anxious when a friend leaves early on a night out. But this could be useful if you want to avoid making the same error! We often overlook the positive aspects of emotions when trying to change them for good.

4. Focusing on thoughts and ruminating about the past or the future.

This often happens in clinical practice, especially if clients don't know what to do with their thoughts or feelings. For example, suppose you are in an argument with someone and get angry and defensive. That can be useful because it helps you feel more ready to handle the situation and develop your arguments so they stick. But if you keep rambling back and forth thinking about what your friend has said, this can make matters worse and make both parties angry without any solution being reached.

5. Focusing on the goal rather than the process of change.

This is a common mistake in mindfulness-based approaches to CBT. Mindfulness is often said to be a way to achieve non-judgmental awareness. But this doesn't mean you can use it to forget why you want to change in the first place. You still need those reasons – they are your goals – and whether or not you achieve them will depend on whether or not you have made changes along the way!

This is why it's important to find out what you want and develop goals based on your values, not just on what seems achievable alone. This also means you can focus on the change process and not just the goal. You might not achieve your goal – but you can still feel good about the fact that you have tried and learned something about yourself or how to achieve what you want in the future.

6. Focusing more on symptom reduction than personal growth

This is common in clinical practice because of its origins in behavior therapy. CBT was originally developed to treat mental health problems as if they were like physical diseases (where treatment should reduce symptoms). But CBT is not just about reducing symptoms; it's about teaching skills that can help you cope with problems and feel more able to respond positively to the obstacles we all face.

For example, we learn that sticking to your goals and not changing them just because of a setback will make you feel more confident as time goes on. But your sense of self can disappear if you just focus on symptom reduction – like trying to avoid feeling anxious or depressed. Feeling bad can be difficult to be strong because the problem will make you want to give up!

There are many other mistakes therapists can make when they fall back on behaviorism rather than embracing some of the key elements of psychotherapy. In clinical practice, it's often difficult to get therapists to see beyond their old habits and techniques. But the most important thing is to remember that we have choices – we can choose where to focus our attention and what skills we will learn.

For example, clinicians often unconsciously assume that clients know the best way to solve problems. When clients come in for CBT – or counseling in general – they tell us they want help with a problem (a symptom). We respond with advice on how we think they should solve the problem or what might be possible future solutions. But clients often end up feeling frustrated that the new problem on the table has been solved without asking them what they want or how they want to solve it.

You can see the relationship between symptoms and goals by looking at your board in mindfulness-based CBT as you walk past it. When you get a symptom, look at your goal and ask yourself: "Is this symptom helping me move closer to my goal?" If it is, then keep focusing on that symptom. But if not, look for something else on your board that might help you achieve your goal.

You can use pen and paper if you don't have a board in your office or home. And you can use any method that helps you move beyond just identifying symptoms and being trapped in a circular problem-solving process. The most important thing is to create something that helps you to focus on the present moment and find out what you want from your board and therapy.

7.   Focusing on the past, present, or future alone

Mindfulness-based therapies are turning a lot of attention to the importance of being here and now. Awareness is helpful for many problems, but it can get in the way if we focus only on the past or just on what's going to happen in the future. To create a mindfulness therapy that works, we have to bring mindfulness into awareness everyday and make it our main focus when doing something unrelated to awareness.

For example, I often find that clients who aren't close to their goals will try too hard when they start the CBT process – focusing on how good they feel about their progress so far. But they can deny that they are not yet where they want to be. They may only think about what they need to do in the future rather than focusing on what's possible.

For these clients, it's much better to focus on the present moment and realize how unlikely everything will go perfectly as planned in therapy – or out in the real world! It's much more useful to find out what you have achieved and understand why you weren't able to succeed yet – as all people fail at some stage.

How to prevent these mistakes regarding CBT:

1.   Focus on awareness and the present moment

Find out what you want in life. This begins with your board and then the process of setting goals. Don't stick to just one goal at a time, but try to think about how you can achieve multiple goals in your life. Don't just focus on what you have achieved so far, but look for things that have gone wrong or that you weren't able to do yet. Use setbacks as learning opportunities rather than seeing them as failures. Think about what you want to achieve in the future and use the goal-setting process to get your focus on that right now.

2.   Cooperate with change, not just symptom reduction

For example, you might choose to start your therapy by focusing on changes in your thinking and behavior (syndrome reduction). But this is only part of the story because there needs to be a balance between personal growth and getting control over your symptoms. If you focus 100% on symptom reduction for too long, this can become an avoidance strategy, which may cause anxiety that will prevent personal growth.

3.   Don't be afraid of setbacks

Setbacks are inevitable, and it's much better to learn to use them as an opportunity for improvement instead of getting rid of every possible setback as soon as possible. When you realize that setbacks are an essential part of the process, you can make the most of them – even if they have been difficult.

4. Avoid blame and shame

People can be afraid of blaming themselves or others when things go wrong, but this often means we blame ourselves more than necessary! When we take a balanced approach, we will be more likely to forgive others (or ourselves) when things don't go exactly as planned in therapy.

5. Avoid the power of self-blame

Many people have been taught to blame themselves for what has gone wrong in their lives. Therapy can be a place to discover your limitations and other people's limitations! But this is only part of the story – instead, we have to look at things from an objective perspective. This is only possible if you accept that no matter how well things go, someone else may still be able to do a better job within their limits than you can!

6. Face your fears and accept your vulnerabilities

For therapy to be beneficial, you have to be able to face up to your fears. CBT is about vulnerability, and you must be willing to use this as a learning process. If you feel uncomfortable with counseling or other therapies, you will probably shy away from them.

7. Be empathetic – not judgmental

This can create conflict if you try to get others to understand how you feel and why you do things. It's much better for everyone involved in CBT to be able to empathize with each other so that we are all working together as a team to understand how things go wrong.

8. Learn from mistakes made by others

As the saying goes, it's always best to learn from someone else's mistakes – even though this can be very difficult! If you make a mistake, learn from it, and don't let it stop you from learning.

If you have been struggling with your therapy and finding it difficult to connect with your therapist, it may be time to take stock. But don't worry – remember that all people struggle when they try to make changes, as CBT can be confusing at times!

But there are some things that you can do to minimize the risk of getting stuck in therapy:

a. Don't just focus on your thoughts and feelings

If you spend a lot of time working on the content of your thoughts (theory or hypothesis) and how you feel about them (emotions), this might lead to problems in therapy. You should also consider what happens next afterthought or feeling. For example, you might work on a thought for a while, and you become aware that a certain situation seems to make you sad. Then you might choose to do something about it or not. Your reaction to the situation will tell your therapist what is needed in therapy then.

b. Don't avoid thinking about personal problems

If we cannot admit that we have personal problems, it may be more difficult for us to make changes in therapy.

c. Face your fears and accept weaknesses

If you cannot face up to your fears, you may never be able to make changes in therapy. Anyone afraid of making changes will not be able to succeed in therapy.

d. Get support from family members or friends

If you cannot get out of a situation that seems stuck with someone close to you, it may be time for further help – and this could mean therapy! Personal growth is often easier with another person involved in the process.

e. Admit that you are not Superman or Superwoman

You may need to hold things together all by yourself, which can be exhausting! When you admit your limitations and ask for help, then you will be able to find the right therapist who can help you.

f. Don't be afraid to get support from a therapist-in-training or trainee psychologist

When finding a suitable therapist, remember that not all therapists are the same. If someone has just started their journey of becoming a therapist, they can still learn along the way! If unsure whether they have the experience and skill required for CBT, ask them about it and say if you think they are not up to scratch. Most therapists-in-training will be glad to hear your feedback and try to get more experience if possible.

g. Don't give up too easily

Quitting can become a habit, and you may find it difficult to stop doing it even when it is not in your best interests! As with most other things in life, perseverance can be challenging but also rewarding. If you feel like giving up, just remind yourself that CBT is only one part of the bigger picture – and in the long term, there are much better things ahead for you!

h. Face your fears instead of trying to avoid them

When you try to avoid something that makes you anxious, then this can cause problems in therapy. You may avoid it because you feel that it is too difficult. But the more difficult tasks are often the ones that can bring us closer to the things we desire in life. When you face your fears, you can start to make progress, which is one of the therapy's most important components.

i. Accept your weaknesses as part of life

We have all been taught that we need to be perfect – but this is often impossible! If something doesn't work out for us in life, we think there must be something wrong with us – when actually, it might be a small obstacle or setback rather than a huge problem!

j. Learn from the mistakes of others

Someone will make a mistake when you try to change things around you. This is a very important aspect of counseling and other therapies – the more mistakes we make in therapy, the better we learn! If you want to continue in therapy, you need to be receptive to other people's experiences – but this may not always be easy!

k. Don't compare yourself with others

If you compare yourself with others or strive for perfection, then this can cause problems. You may feel that you are not good enough or that your problems are worse than other people's. Remember that everyone is different, and some people have different experiences of problems and can face them in different ways.

Therefore, mistakes experienced in CBT must be prevented since they may lead to a possible dropout of therapy. This involves a therapist that can understand their client's problems and needs, we are usually assigned a new therapist, or there might be some other issues that can affect whether we stay in therapy or not.

Some issues that can prevent a client from staying in therapy include:

A therapist is unable to understand what's going on around the individual.

A therapist who cannot offer sufficient support to the client.

A therapist is not going to accept a person's problems as well as their progress in therapy.

A therapist who does not have enough motivation and willingness to help individuals with their problems. A depressed, anxious, or stressed client may feel like there are no possibilities for improvement and may not complete the CBT treatment for longer than intended sessions or completely drop out of the course.

Myths

a.   CBT therapy is just for people with anxiety or depression.

CBT can be used to help a range of mental health problems. It's widely known as the 'gold standard for treating these conditions and other psychological disorders such as OCD and eating disorders.

b.   CBT is used with only specific mental health issues- like OCD and depression

CBT has been used successfully with a multitude of different disorders, including addiction and even ADHD! One common misconception is that CBT involves changing your thoughts to "cure" the problem - but this isn't true. The idea behind cognitive behavioral therapy is that by identifying negative thought patterns which lead to negative emotions (e.g., stress, anxiety, depression) and changing the patterns which cause the negative emotions, you can then change the negative emotions. The idea is that you will have positive emotions once you have positive thoughts.

c.   CBT requires you to spend a lot of time thinking about your problems

On the contrary, clients are encouraged to think as little as possible about their negative emotions or the unwanted thought patterns they experience when doing CBT. When people want to discuss their problems at length - something they often do without knowing - it's usually because they are trying to figure out how they 'should' be feeling in a situation and why things aren't going their way. In CBT, this is not necessary and can even be counterproductive. The focus is on the here-and-now, not what happened in the past or what might happen in the future.

d.   CBT requires you to challenge every single thought or emotion

Again, quite the opposite is true! Cognitive behavioral therapy aims to learn to identify and change only the thoughts causing you problems - those that are negative or unhelpful. You don't want to waste your time challenging each thought you experience as it happens. The idea is to learn to identify your thoughts and then change them so your emotions improve.

"CBT (Cognitive Behavioral Therapy) is a way of learning to be aware of, understand and change the thoughts that cause problems in our lives."

For more information or if you are interested in getting help for issues mentioned above or something else related, read some of my other posts about depression and anxiety treatment.

e. CBT is only used with people who are very depressed or anxious

CBT effectively treats people with severe mental health problems such as depression, anxiety, schizophrenia, and obsessive-compulsive disorder. It can also help people with self-esteem problems, anger, or other issues.

f. CBT involves meeting with a therapist once a week.

CBT usually involves meeting with your therapist once or twice weekly for about 12 weeks, but it can be longer if necessary. If you are doing CBT online, the number of sessions will vary depending on your therapist's advice and how much you need to work on specific issues.

g. CBT involves lots of talking and thinking to "work out" your problems.

CBT is often understood as 'talking therapy' because talking about the past and thinking about what made the situation worse can be very useful when looking at ways to change it or prevent it from happening again. But not everyone needs to talk about their problems, and many people are happy with just seeing their therapist once or twice a week to discuss areas they feel they need help with.

h. CBT involves challenging your thoughts and changing them.

CBT may involve challenging your thoughts if they are unhelpful, but it also involves accepting your thoughts as they are. For example, if you're feeling sad about something which has happened in the past, it will be normal to think about this situation and feel sad for a few days. But what needs to be changed is how long you stay stuck feeling sad, not how often you think about the situation or how intense the sadness feels.

i. CBT doesn't work for everyone

The majority of research shows that CBT is an extremely effective treatment for people with anxiety problems (e.g., panic disorder, phobias, post-traumatic stress disorder), depression (e.g., severe depression, dysthymia, bipolar disorder), and eating disorders (e.g., bulimia nervosa, anorexia nervosa). CBT can also help people who have problems with self-esteem or anger.

j. CBT is expensive

Depending on your area of the world and what type of therapy you opt for, the cost may vary slightly - but it is generally relatively inexpensive. The cost of CBT can also be paid in installments to ensure that people who need help can afford it in a way that suits them best.

These myths must be avoided since they could potentially demotivate or discourage someone who feels they need help. CBT can change people's lives and yours, too, if you're willing to put a little time into it. Moreover, CBT is an excellent way to treat yourself if you feel you have a problem that needs help. If you're unsure whether CBT is right for you, one of the best things you can do is contact your therapist and ask them what they think! They can tell you exactly what they think CBT can do for you and how much it will cost.

Common Errors in CBT

When talking about CBT, it can be easy to get confused and make a few errors in our thinking. These are some of the most common errors that people make and how you can avoid them:

1. Believing that any thoughts or emotions are 'bad' in some way

Many people believe that their thoughts or emotions are somehow 'wrong' or bad for them - even if there is no proof for this being true. This can send negative messages to yourself and lead to more problems due to your beliefs about what is happening in your life.

2. Believing we should be able to 'think positively' no matter what

If we try to avoid negative thoughts or block them out, this can mean that we don't work through problems and fix them in the long run. Some people try to be positive, but this rarely helps them in the long run. Instead of avoiding negative thoughts or emotions, it is better to learn how to accept these as a normal part of being human and then challenge them when they are unhelpful.

3. Trying to think positively without accepting negative thoughts and emotions

If we only accept positive things about ourselves, people, and life in general, then we are unlikely to experience real happiness at any time. Thinking positively is a skill that takes time to build up in the long run. Once we have learned to think positively, we will know that it is okay to have negative thoughts and emotions - but they do not determine who we are. We don't have to let them rule our lives, as this is what unhelpful thoughts can do in the long run.

4. Blocking out negative feelings and thinking about all the 'good' things in life

If we try to avoid our negative thoughts or block them out, some of these emotions can't be worked through and don't get dealt with properly. So if we think about our problems and deal with them, negative thoughts or emotions don't determine our whole life.

5. Blaming ourselves for feeling 'bad' or unable to think positively

It is important to remember that thoughts and emotions are not 'bad' or wrong. For example, if we think negatively about something and react badly. As a result, this is not because we're bad people; we have unhelpful thoughts that need to be changed. If we blame ourselves for not being able to think more positively, it may mean that we don't take responsibility for what happens to us in the long run.

6. Thinking that CBT is a 'one size fits all approach to life

CBT is used for many problems and situations but requires time and effort to work properly; it cannot be done for you. Everyone has their ways of thinking about things, so the way you interpret therapy may not be the same as someone else. But this can also mean that what works for you could be different from someone else's experience.

7. Expecting CBT to be a 'quick fix' approach

CBT is often used as a quick fix in the media and TV. But the reality is that it takes time, effort, and commitment to work through the problems you have. However, the result is that life can become better and more enjoyable when you try to learn how to think differently.

8. Only trying CBT once or twice

Unfortunately, many people give up on therapy too early without giving it enough time and effort to work. Many people go through months of therapy before they start getting better, so you should give CBT plenty of time before making a final decision about whether it helps your problems.

Interventions and Possible Problems in CBT

While CBT is generally a very effective treatment that can help various problems and situations, it still requires you to play an active role in your therapy. Moreover, it may take a while before you start to feel better if you've struggled with depression or anxiety for quite some time. Here are some of the possible interventions you can expect and how CBT can help:

1. Identifying problem thoughts in CBT

The first step in CBT is to learn to identify problem thinking patterns that lead to negative emotions or destructive behaviors. This helps people to understand that they can change their way of thinking and even how they react to certain things in life. If a problem occurs, we don't have to accept it as 'bad' or unchangeable; we just need to work through these problems so they don't run our lives anymore.

2. Challenging problem thoughts in CBT

Learning to challenge these beliefs in therapy is crucial, as full acceptance of negative thoughts only leads to more problems in the long run. The goal is not to ignore or push away negative thoughts but to learn how to examine them and challenge them directly, so they don't determine our experiences. Some people may teach themselves until they fully accept their negative thoughts, and then it can become easier for them to deal with other areas of life.

3. Identifying personal and social triggers in CBT

If you know why you have certain problems, you can then work on things that may trigger your disorder, so the triggers do not cause problems in the long run. For example, if you have panic attacks in public places but only around your boss, you can find ways to manage your stress at work and avoid things that might lead to a panic attack. Learning to identify things that may trigger your disorders is important to avoid them or manage them better.

4. Challenging personal and social beliefs in CBT

Many people believe certain things about themselves which are inaccurate and lead to more problems in the long run - this is known as self-talk. For example, suppose someone believes they're stupid for making mistakes on the job or incapable of relating to others. In that case, this can lead to a downward spiral of negative thoughts and cause even more difficulties in their lives. It becomes easier to manage our experiences if we can challenge these beliefs.

5. Focusing on positive or realistic goals in CBT

Focusing on what you want to achieve in life can help us to overcome problems such as depression and anxiety. For example, if someone has negative thoughts about not being good enough at something, it may lead to a lot of stress and unhappiness that does not resolve after a few weeks of therapy. The goal of CBT is not to completely change the way you view yourself but rather to focus on realistic goals that don't make you feel like a failure - such as improving your performance in certain areas or learning certain skills that are helpful in the long run.

6.   Developing coping skills in CBT

One of the most important aspects of CBT is learning how to manage your emotions and cope with life's challenges when you have serious problems. This is called emotion regulation. For example, someone who is depressed may have unrealistic thoughts about their worth that sometimes make them feel depressed or worthless. They may also have anger directed at others when they think about problems in their lives. By learning skills for regulating emotions and improving coping strategies, we can focus on other parts of life and lead a better existence.

7.   Improving social skills in CBT

Many people with depression, anxiety, or other problems have trouble relating to others or making and keeping friends. This can worsen the problem because it makes them feel like they're in an isolated situation. One of the goals of therapy is to help improve your social skills if you've been struggling with serious problems for a long time. You cannot solve all your problems on your own - so it's important to reach out and connect with others to get the support you need to make life better.

8.   Hiding symptoms in CBT

Many people who struggle with depression and anxiety self-diagnose that they are 'too depressed' or 'too anxious. This often stems from the fact that people may not want to take medicine as it's believed to be potentially dangerous. If someone gets used to using alcohol or drug to deal with their symptoms, they may continue doing so even when they've learned how pointless and harmful it is. One of therapy's goals is to learn what helps you conquer your conditions but also helps you get rid of your self-diagnosis so you can achieve your goals in life.

WHAT IS CBT?

A therapy that looks at how thoughts and feelings play a role in each person's life. It focuses on how thoughts, feelings, and behaviors can be used to overcome difficulties or achieve personal goals.

Cognitive-behavior therapy (CBT) is a practical therapeutic approach used to treat various issues and conditions successfully. Many studies have laid the groundwork for using CBT, identifying treatment efficacy, and helping develop evidence-based practice (EBP). EBP is a research study that tests the effectiveness of treatment protocols on a large group of patients. The goal is to determine if the treatment protocol will successfully treat a given condition or symptom while minimizing adverse effects. As an example, CBT was identified as an effective treatment for depression by numerous scientific studies.

CBT is a behavior change therapy. It was developed in response to the complexity of human behavior and problems. The restructuring of thought and behaviors that occurs during CBT is achieved through the process of applying CBT's results-based approach to PAPs (Problem Assessment and Planning) within a HALT (Helping Allowed Teaching Long Term) mode within an SIT format (Structured Interviewing Technique).

Cognitive-behavioral therapy (CBT) was first described as a new approach in an unpublished paper in 1967 by Aaron T. Beck. He attributed it to the work of Aaron T. Beck, Zev Wanderer, and colleagues and published it in 1969. It has been used to treat various mental disorders, including mood disorders (e.g., depression), anxiety disorders (e.g., generalized anxiety disorder), eating disorders, personality disorders, and substance abuse/addiction. In addition, it is commonly used as an adjunct to alternate treatment approaches, including drug therapy and other talk therapies such as psychodynamic or humanistic therapy.

It is one of the most widely used psychotherapeutic approaches, particularly in the context of cognitive therapy and in the treatment of depression. It is also used as a primary treatment approach in treating anxiety disorders. CBT is growing in popularity among practitioners and has been deemed by many to be both practical and mainstream.

The philosophy behind CBT rests on a belief that psychiatric disorders derive from an interplay between personal history and current life circumstances, combined with a complex set of attitudes about oneself, others, and the world at large. This formulation fits well with the data from genetic research that has found vulnerability factors for developing certain disorders (e.g., substance abuse) in specific brain regions. The goal of CBT is to identify these vulnerabilities and then compensate for them through behavioral modifications.

CBT combines several techniques that have been used to treat mental health disorders. The approach differs from other approaches in that the therapist may focus on what a person did or thought or how they felt, but CBT considers these things by looking at the actual behavior, thoughts, and feelings. CBT focuses on changing behaviors, which can be done by addressing their triggers and helping clients change their patterns of reactions related to those situations. It also centers on helping people deal with their current problems and make changes for the better. CBT also focuses on applying new behaviors in real-world circumstances, which makes it an effective tool for treating clinical depression and anxiety.

Beck first proposed that abnormal behaviors develop through his cognitive triad: (1) negative thoughts leading to negative expectations and assumptions; (2) a negative self-image, leading to failed goals and frustration and (3) a negative cycle of events that made the problem worse. He demonstrated further that this triad develops into a vicious circle, with each element reinforcing the other two. To treat patients with depression, CBT attempts to reverse these processes by changing the way they think about the world and their behavior.

The roots of CBT can be traced to the investigations of George Kelly and others regarding the higher mental processes of humans. However, the theory advanced by Beck and colleagues was first published in 1969 as a monograph entitled: "Behavior Therapy and the Cognitive-Behavioral Approach." This publication brought the work of Aaron T. Beck, Zev Wanderer, Edna Foa, and their colleagues to the attention of a wider audience.

Cognitive-behavioral therapy (CBT) is a child or developmentally new psychotherapy approach based on the cognitive model of human behavior development. Cognitivism states that human beings are not passive organisms but active agents that develop through interacting with their environment. Four primary processes occur in development: (1) the acquisition of knowledge, (2) evaluation of information, (3) patterning, and (4) action. In addition, this approach posits that dysfunctional patterns can be followed or "played out" in various environments, such as families and relationships. Eric Berne developed a taxonomy for understanding the development of behavioral problems based on his observations and experimental studies conducted with children during his research from the 1940s through the 1960s.

CBT was introduced in 1967 by Aaron Beck, who applied to it the methods he had used successfully as a clinician in treating depression. It was later developed to treat anxiety by Albert Ellis, who was trained by Aaron Beck and also influenced Donald Meichenbaum, M.D.

CBT is a cognitive therapy approach grounded in the cognitive paradigm of human behavior. The theory asserts that many problems result from maladaptive or unhelpful cognitions (thinking or beliefs) and behaviors (actions) that develop over time based on one's personal history and life experiences. These thinking and behavioral processes are called schematic representations of the world; they reflect one's expectations, influencing behavior. Individuals can be taught to identify their schemas, recognize when they are triggered, and adapt their schemas to real-life experiences.

According to the theory, schemas develop through learning, conditioning, and personal experience. For example, a person who has battled several bouts of illness or received repeated criticism from a parent may develop the schema: "I am not lovable or worthy." This belief will likely cause the person to behave in ways that elicit further criticism or new illness to fulfill what he perceives as his destiny.

This form of therapy can be thought of as psychoeducation. The focus is on helping a patient to recognize, understand and analyze issues in their life. This information may help the individual develop more adaptive coping skills.

CBT treats various clinical conditions, including mood disorders, personality disorders, eating disorders, and anxiety disorders such as social phobia and obsessive-compulsive disorder (OCD). Its effectiveness has also been demonstrated in several specific situations:

Several pieces of evidence have shown that CBT has effectively treated people with depression in the past few decades. For example, one meta-analysis found that: "Among depressed outpatients, cognitive therapy was significantly more effective than medication management. Although publication bias likely contributes to the apparent superiority of cognitive therapy, this analysis rigorously tested the effects of each treatment strategy and demonstrated its superiority over medication management."

Another meta-analysis found that "Cognitive therapy in addition to standard care was significantly more effective than standard care alone or no therapy." In several randomized controlled trials, CBT is more effective than pharmacological treatment (e.g., SSRIs) for depressed patients. One meta-analysis found that "among depressed outpatients, cognitive therapy was significantly more effective than medication management.

Is there evidence for CBT?

A meta-analysis of studies on the efficacy of CBT for depression by the Agency for Healthcare Research and Quality (AHRQ) concluded that CBT is effective in reducing symptoms of depression but that CBT is not as effective as antidepressant medications in treating depression. This meta-analysis included thirty randomized controlled trials involving over 2,000 patients.

A second large meta-analysis by AHRQ also supported the conclusion that CBT is more effective than no treatment in reducing chronic pain symptoms. This meta-analysis included 15 randomized controlled trials involving 769 patients with chronic pain.

The review concluded that CBT was effective after 6 to 12 weeks of treatment. In addition, it found no significant differences between CBT and treatment in reducing depressive symptoms, pain, or adverse events.

A review by AHRQ of the effectiveness of medications for depression concluded that medication alone is no more effective for treating depression than the combination of therapy and medication. The review assessed a total of eleven randomized controlled trials involving 3,000 patients with depression. The authors concluded that "for most people with major depressive disorder, a combination of therapy and medication is more effective than either intervention alone."

Therefore, evidence for CBT is mixed, and the methodologies employed can lead to different conclusions. Moreover, the concept of CBT is founded upon a developmental model of human behavior. Many studies show that, at least in some instances, CBT has proved less effective than other treatments. In general, a cognitive-behavioral theory is not more effective than psychotherapy.

A 2006 Cochrane systematic review of the role of behavioral interventions in the treatment of depression between 1997 and 2003 concluded: "There was insufficient evidence to allow a firm conclusion as to whether behavioral therapies have any advantages over drug therapy. However, interventions in this area do not seem to be any more effective than drug treatment alone and should be considered a viable, if not preferred, option for treating depression."

The Cochrane review on randomized controlled trials also found that Cognitive Therapy is no more effective than drug therapy in treating mild depression. However, the review also noted that "there is insufficient published evidence [i.e., randomized controlled trials] to allow conclusions on interventions such as cognitive therapy and supportive therapy."

However, given the approach's limitations in gaining scientific consensus, CBT remains one of the most popular methods therapists use. In addition, despite its limitations as an evidence-based treatment model. CBT is a form of effective treatment for several conditions, including social anxiety disorder, depression, marital problems, and post-traumatic stress.

CBT differs from psychodynamic or interpersonal psychotherapy in that the cognitive processes emphasized by CBT tend to be more scientific than those of psychodynamic and interpersonal models. CBT focuses on observable behavior in the here-and-now to determine whether past events may have influenced present thoughts and feelings. CBT is therefore considered more naturalistic than other therapies because it relies less on information from past experiences.

CBT differs from behavior therapy because it focuses on the present rather than the environment or context. In addition, behavior therapy uses reinforcement and punishment as principal tools, whereas CBT does not rely primarily on rewards or rewards for change.

In psychotherapy, patients are typically involved in two-person dialogues, either alone or with a therapist or a group of peers. In general, CBT assumes that humans have an internal voice (the "self"), which is often described as the "inner critic." The role of this inner critic is to evaluate the patient's thoughts and feelings and to tell us whether we are being "good" or "bad," etc.

CBT is known for its focus on core processes believed to underlie many disorders, including depression, anxiety, and obsessive-compulsive disorder. These core processes generally include global evaluations of one's self, others, life, and the belief that events are uncontrollable.

The term "cognitive fusion" in CBT describes how humans relate to their thoughts. When a person is cognitively fused with their thoughts, they engage in thinking at a level at which they experience emotions. When people engage in cognitive fusion, it is common for them to believe that their thoughts reflect reality or that their thought is valid interpretations of reality. However, these thoughts are not necessarily accurate reflections of external reality (as opposed to internal reality), making this person more prone to develop biases and beliefs, leading to more significant negative emotional states such as anxiety and depression. CBT can also be taught to patients in group therapy, which is more effective than individual therapy.

CBT can be used in combination with pharmaceuticals and other therapeutic measures. However, the evidence for CBT's effectiveness as a treatment for depression remains inconclusive. There are several limitations that researchers have identified when assessing the effectiveness of CBT as a psychological treatment, including:

When compared with other therapies, not enough research has been done to determine whether or not CBT is an effective treatment. Also, some studies have suggested that people do well without any additional intervention besides medication, support groups, or self-help organization meetings (like Alcoholics Anonymous).

CBT is often used by people suffering from depression for several reasons. First, CBT often helps sufferers better understand the thoughts that cause their depression and may help sufferers learn skills that increase their ability to resist the negative consequences of these thoughts. For example, CBT may help people with depression cope with social anxiety and interpersonal conflicts and regulate cognitive processes. Second, evidence-based practices are software or a process that combines what is known, what works, and what works better than other practices or interventions.

How are the CBT sessions conducted?

The veteran counselor will begin by asking about the issue the patient faces. The counselor will then ask the patient to describe their thoughts and feelings. The counselor will then ask questions that help the patient identify negative assumptions and evaluate evidence that challenges these ideas. This goal is to help the patient understand their situation better and consider other possible explanations for how they feel or perceive a situation. This helps them develop more productive coping skills, including reducing their anxiety or depression.

The agent is the primary agent of change for the client. The patient identifies and works on the circumstances that create their problems. It is necessary to do a severe analysis of the situation to understand how this affects a particular individual. Every session begins with identifying positive and negative aspects of therapy, skills that need help, and goals that should be achieved by the end of the session. Then, the agent will use specific techniques to communicate with the patient to achieve these goals. These techniques may include expressing approval or disapproval, use of empathetic language, distraction techniques (such as jokes), praise statements, unrealistic statements, change statements (such as "let's start over"), and more. The main goal is communicating so that the patient understands and reacts positively. The techniques are used according to the techniques by which the patient identifies their problem.

The information processing of a human being is the way a person takes in information, decides what that information means, and responds to it. Information processing includes all the steps individuals take to understand their experiences and surroundings.

CBT focuses on four primary processes, such as:

a. Cognitive appraisal

This focuses on how people evaluate their situations, including their thoughts about the world and themselves. People are constantly evaluating situations for things like risk and rewards. As a result, people make predictions about what will happen based on their past experiences with similar experiences. For example, if a storm is nearby, a person may think, "I hope the tree outside my window doesn't fall," or "I hope we don't lose power in this storm." Together, cognition and emotion are called "appraisal processes." In therapy sessions, the counselor will help patients identify their negative thought patterns and evaluate evidence that challenges these negative patterns of thinking.

According to Beck, information processing is biased towards negative experiences in an unhealthy state. As a result, patients tend to ignore positive experiences and magnify the importance of negative ones. In therapy sessions, the counselor will help patients identify their negative thought patterns and evaluate evidence that challenges these negative patterns of thinking.

b. Emotion regulation

Emotion regulation focuses on how people manage and control their emotional responses. Emotions are crucial to an individual's overall psychological well-being. Experiencing intense emotions can sometimes be beneficial (for example, in response to a situation threatening safety). However, when people experience extreme or prolonged emotional states, they can lead to problems like anxiety or depression. Patients learn to identify and challenge negative thought patterns by identifying how these thoughts cause them to act in such a way. For example, if someone is overwhelmed by intense emotion, this person may begin meditating and thinking about their worst possible case scenario.

Interviewing patients allows the psychiatrist or psychologist to determine their mental state at a particular moment. The goal is for the therapist to know where a patient stands emotionally so that they can provide the most appropriate treatment option. In therapy sessions, the psychiatrist will ask questions that help patients identify how they feel in different situations. The psychiatrist will then help the patient identify negative thoughts and evaluate evidence that challenges these negative thinking patterns. In this way, patients learn to manage their emotions more effectively.

c.   Behavioral analysis

The behavioral analysis focuses on how people behave in different situations. For example, someone may react to a stressful situation by feeling depressed or anxious. Still, they may also cope with it by sleeping excessively, overeating, abusing alcohol or drugs, withdrawing from others, becoming aggressive or violent, and so on. The therapist will help the patient identify behavioral patterns in therapy sessions and evaluate evidence that challenges these behaviors. Patients will learn how to replace maladaptive behaviors with adaptive ones through a process called "behavioral analysis.

d.   Cognitive reshaping

Cognitive reshaping focuses on how people think about themselves, others, and their situations. This is typically called self-talk by therapists. People constantly think about themselves and their experiences in terms of "self-schema," or schemas. Schemas are like mental categories that people organize their experiences into (e.g., "I am a smart person who is good at schoolwork"). According to Beck, most individuals have a global schema to evaluate themselves, which often leads to biases in thinking (for example, catastrophizing). Patients will learn to change their negative schemas into more realistic ones, leading to more positive self-talk.

One of the key concepts in cognitive therapy is "automatic thoughts." These are patients' immediate, unconscious responses when they encounter a situation. These automatic thoughts then cause patients to feel and behave in specific ways, which leads them to feel depressed or anxious. The goal of cognitive therapy is for patients to be able to recognize their automatic thoughts and evaluate evidence for patients to correct their thinking and change the way they view situations.

Patients need to take steps to overcome their negative thinking patterns. First, patients must recognize their automatic thoughts and evaluate evidence, allowing them to correct their thinking and change how they view situations.

Recognize negative automatic thoughts: For patients to recognize their automatic thoughts, therapists must help patients identify what a thought is. Once this has been identified, therapists can teach patients how to recognize when they are having these types of thoughts. Most often, a therapist will ask the patient about a recent situation where they experienced anxiety or depression and encourage them to describe their experience. By sharing what happened and how they felt, patients will eventually begin thinking about the situation in a negative way. This is where automatic thoughts are at. If a patient can see that their thought process has gone from one thing to another, it is easier to spot automatic thoughts when they occur.

An example is if someone suddenly becomes upset after someone yells at them on the street. The person will automatically think, "I'm never going to get over my depression because people keep yelling at me," which causes them to feel worthless, hopeless, and depressed. At this point, the patient must evaluate evidence that challenges these automatic thoughts to correct them (see below). Once the patient can identify their automatic thoughts, they must evaluate evidence that challenges them.

Evaluate evidence: To overcome negative automatic thoughts, people must evaluate evidence that contradicts them. Examining this evidence is sometimes called "cognitive restructuring" or "cognition." Essentially, patients will have to examine the same situation from different viewpoints and think about what things may be out of proportion or inaccurate to correct the automatic thought. Taking a new perspective is the goal.

What could go wrong with this therapy?

A few possible problems with this approach are:

1. It takes time for a person to change their thoughts and behaviors. This means that therapy might take more time than the patient is willing to spend. However, this therapy can be beneficial in helping a person work through issues that have been bothering them for years. For example, the therapist could help the patient look at their automatic thoughts, challenge them to be more accurate, and improve negative thinking patterns. After several sessions, the patient should become more accurate in evaluating evidence that challenges their automatic thoughts and, therefore, can change their behavior.

2. Automatic thoughts can be tough to spot. For example, if a person believes for years that they are unlovable and has not been able to develop close relationships, it is hard to know what it will take for the patient to see beyond these automatic thoughts. In this case, the patient may need help from a professional specializing in psychotherapy.

3. It might be hard for patients to identify how they typically think about themselves and their problems. This is especially true if a person does not believe in therapy or if therapy was rejected before. Still, the therapist can ask about something the patient did recently that made them feel better and encourage them to talk about what they thought was wrong with themselves before therapy started.

4. Therapy is supposed to be a trusting relationship where the patient and the therapist feel comfortable expressing themselves. If a patient is afraid they will say something wrong or the therapist will judge them, they may not be able to form a trusting relationship with their therapist. This could lead to negative thoughts and behaviors and even more negative thoughts.

5. The therapist might not be familiar enough with cognitive therapy to be effective. However, cognitive therapy is the most studied and evaluated form of psychotherapy, so therapists should have some training.

6. Cognitive therapy requires patients to be aware of their feelings and think about them simultaneously. If a person is depressed or having a panic attack, this may not be very easy for them to do. It may even make them feel worse by focusing on how they feel instead of trying to change how they think about a situation and what effect those thoughts have on them.

7. Cognitive therapy may not be effective if a person has never been able to work through their problems to overcome their negative thoughts and behaviors. In addition, even throughout therapy, some people may not find themselves more accurate at identifying negative automatic thoughts and evaluating evidence as they learn to change their thinking.

8. Cognitive therapy requires that patients actively work through the sessions, which can be difficult for some people who are having problems with anxiety or depression. In this case, cognitive therapy might not be effective because it does not address the problem that caused a person's troubling behavior in the first place. Instead, the patient needs to find a way to address the root of the problem.

9. Many people might not understand what cognitive therapy is or how it works, which could cause them to reject it immediately. However, a therapist can explain that this therapy helps patients overcome negative thinking patterns that have been preventing them from improving their lives and functioning better in certain situations.

Therefore, cognitive therapy is helpful for patients who are willing to put time into working on changing their thoughts and behavior. This can be difficult for people who have not been able to work through their problems in the past and does not result in immediate changes, but it is beneficial for all people to improve their lives mentally.

The therapeutic relationship forms the foundation of cognitive therapy. What distinguishes the therapist from a mental health professional who sees patients for longer than a year (e.g., psychiatrist, nurse practitioner, clinical psychologist) is that cognitive therapists do not just give advice and direction on how to think about a situation to solve it. Instead, the therapist works with the patient to improve their relationship with themselves and the world beyond to help them overcome negative thinking. To do this, cognitive therapy therapists must be knowledgeable about cognitive therapy and also talk about other psychotherapy methods.

It is essential for a therapist to be well-versed in cognitive therapy and how it differs from other types of psychotherapy. The use of feedback from the patient is one example where it differs from other forms of psychotherapy. In most types of psychotherapy, patients are often given homework assignments such as writing letters home or journaling to give themselves the motivation to continue treatment even after they complete their sessions (e.g., psychoanalysis). Conversely, cognitive therapy focuses on what the patient does to avoid their issues and how to deal with them.

Cognitive therapists also emphasize that it is not enough for a person to overcome a problem with their thinking; they must learn how to think about it in different ways that are not automatic and negative. Therapy is about helping the patient become more accurate at evaluating evidence and how past experiences have affected their current relationships and interactions in life.

The goal of cognitive therapy is not just to solve the patient's problems but to achieve a better quality of life. Thus, cognitive therapists try to demonstrate ways in which they can improve upon their relationships with themselves, other people, and society as a whole.

Cognitive therapy can be beneficial in many ways. For example, one way it can help someone is by helping them overcome depression and anxiety by changing their automatic thoughts to more realistic ones. In addition, with the help of a therapist, a person can learn to develop an accurate self-image.

This kind of therapy could be helpful for people who feel stuck in negative thinking patterns, which leads to depression. A therapist could help the patient understand these negative thoughts and work through them. In addition, the therapy can help patients who feel hopeless about their circumstances, for example, who feel that everyone is out to get them or that they are unlovable.

For example, a person may believe that everyone hates them for what happened in their childhood or because they did not do something right in the past, leading to sadness and low self-esteem. They may feel that everything is their fault and think they are not good enough. With the help of a therapist, however, this person can learn to recognize these automatic thoughts, evaluate evidence that challenges them, and realize how this type of thinking is inaccurate.

Types of CBT

Different types of CBT include:

1. Rational emotive behavior therapy

Rational emotive behavior therapy (REBT) is a type of cognitive behavioral therapy ("CBT") that focuses on changing a person's thoughts and behaviors to overcome depression, anxiety, and other disorders. It was developed in the 1930s by Albert Ellis. This form of CBT emphasizes that people should reason to change their feelings, which are not as accurate as their beliefs (e.g., such as: "I am unlovable" or "I always fail"). People should also try to understand themselves to change their behaviors (e.g., by accepting themselves and others).

2. Interpersonal therapy

Interpersonal therapy ("IPT") was developed by Robert H. Skurnik and Jerome C. Wakefield in the 1960s to treat depression. It focuses on improving relationships with others and enhancing self-esteem through learning more effective communication skills and how to solve problems with others positively.

3. Mindfulness-based cognitive therapy

Mindfulness-based cognitive therapy ("MBT") is an alternative form of cognitive behavioral therapy that emphasizes mindfulness training, relaxation techniques, and other exercises to improve mental health by helping people become more aware of their thoughts and emotions, which help them live happier lives.

4. Solution-focused brief therapy

Solution-focused brief therapy ("SFBT") is a type of cognitive behavioral therapy founded by Dr. David Burns based on cognitive behavioral therapy. This form of CBT does not include the long-term strategies used in other forms of CBT but instead focuses on the past week, two weeks, one month, and three months to improve mental health.

5. Motivational enhancement therapy

Motivational enhancement therapy ("MET") is a type of CBT that focuses on enhancing one's motivation to change problems in one's life. This form of CBT was developed by Dr. David Burns, based on cognitive behavioral therapy, focusing on planning activities to perform positively and finding ways to enhance motivation.

6. Mindfulness-based stress reduction

A mindfulness-based stress reduction is a form of meditation initially developed in 1979 by Jon Kabat-Zinn for medical patients with chronic pain. Still, it has since been adapted for almost any group of people struggling with a mental health problem or emotional disorder.

7. Dialectical behavior therapy

Dialectical behavior therapy ("DBT") is based on a model of mental health developed by Dr. Marsha Linehan in the 1980s. This form of CBT was developed for patients with borderline personality disorder and is currently used to treat others struggling with a mental health problem or emotional disorder.

8. Acceptance and commitment to therapy

Acceptance and commitment therapy ("ACT") is a form of cognitive behavioral therapy developed by Dr. Steven C. Hayes, based on the work of Dr. David Spiegel. CBT aims to improve a person's quality of life and independence through mindfulness exercises, which focus on accepting the present moment, being nonjudgmental, and developing positive relationships with others.

9. Acceptance and commitment to therapy for addictions

Acceptance and commitment therapy for addictions ("ACT-A") is a type of CBT developed by Jon Pincus that focuses on improving motivation to change problems such as depression, addiction, or eating disorders that they face in their lives through establishing an acceptance framework (e.g., accepting the reality of their situation). This form of CBT focuses on how the past cannot be changed and that changing behavior is the only way to improve one's life.

10. Dialectical behavior therapy for borderline personality disorder

Dialectical behavior therapy for borderline personality disorder ("DBT-BPD") is a type of CBT developed by Marsha M. Linehan as a modified version of dialectical behavior therapy ("DBT"). This form of CBT was developed for patients with borderline personality disorder and is currently used for people struggling with mental health problems or emotional disorders. DBT-BPD focuses on helping patients to learn skills to cope with their emotions, control behaviors (e.g., self-harm and suicidal thoughts), improve relationships with others, healthily solve problems, and manage their lives.

11. Visually-based acceptance and commitment therapy

Visually-based acceptance and commitment therapy ("VACT") is similar to "acceptance and commitment therapy" ("ACT") but includes the use of virtual reality exposure to treat anxiety disorders. This form of CBT was developed early in the 21st century by Drs. Matthew J. Friedman, Steven C. Hayes, Anthony Pignone, Sherry A. Stewart, Jon Soderstrom, Matthew McKay, and Arthur Cavanagh help people with anxiety disorders caused by traumatic events (e.g., such as sexual assault).

It is important to note that many people oppose CBT as therapy. They argue that data supports the old approach, or "talk" therapy, as the best solution for mental health problems. For example:

1. Talk therapy has always been the primary form of treatment for depression and other mental disorders
2. The type of CBT used by many psychologists and therapists (such as cognitive behavior therapy and cognitive-behavioral therapy) has shown adverse effects on some types of people (e.g., people with a borderline personality disorder)
3. If you try to force someone to change their thoughts or behavior using CBT, it will probably result in them doing more harm than good (e.g., self-harm or suicide)
4. Using CBT for emotional problems like depression or anxiety can cause more harm than good (e.g., anorexia, bulimia nervosa, etc.)
5. There is little evidence to support the use of CBT in mental health problems
6. other forms of therapy have shown an advantage in treating mental health problems (e.g., yoga, mindfulness exercises, evolutionary psychology, Zen)
7. This type of therapy is very different from what most people are used to when they go to a doctor's office or psychologist's office

Many people oppose this form of therapy, but CBT therapists need to address people's concerns with our approach. Most arguments against this form of therapy focus on how it is not as effective as talk therapy or causes more harm than good. Still, these arguments do not consider what CBT means in a modern context (e.g., many different CBT types have different effects).

CBT- HOW DOES THIS METHOD WORK?

Cognitive behavior therapy (CBT) is a type of psychotherapy that helps people adopt and maintain changes in their thoughts, feelings, beliefs, behaviors, and relationships. It is based on the idea that our thoughts cause our feelings, and then these feelings lead to actions and interpersonal interactions. So to change any of these things, we need to alter how we think about them.

Cognitive behavior therapy is a well-researched, structured, and manualized approach to psychological treatment that is effective in treating many disorders.

CBT focuses on thinking patterns leading to negative or unhealthy emotions and behaviors. It teaches people different ways of thinking about things that help them feel better about themselves and their life. CBT also aims to reduce 'maladaptive' behaviors, such as drug or alcohol use, in favor of healthier coping methods.

For instance, CBT could help you learn how to stop smoking by helping you predict how certain situations trigger your cravings via your thoughts and feelings. The theory behind CBT states that your thoughts about the situation drive your craving to smoke. So, for example, if you're nervous about a presentation you have to give at work, you might think, "Everyone is going to be judging me, and I'm going to fail miserably in front of everyone." These thoughts can trigger anxiety or stress and make you crave a cigarette to feel better. In this way, CBT helps people identify and cope with their dysfunctional thoughts.

Cognitive behavioral therapy teaches basic self-help skills (such as relaxation techniques) individually or within a group setting. These skills are then practiced in between sessions, and over time, people learn to feel better about themselves and their life, which decreases their anxiety, stress, depression and urges to use alcohol or drugs.

Cognitive Behavioural Therapy aims to help patients identify harmful or unhealthy ways of thinking that lead to negative emotions and behaviors. For example, if you constantly tell yourself that you must succeed at everything and anything, you may get very stressed out when you do not. Likewise, if you think everyone must like and approve of everything you do, being criticized may make you feel terrible.

Cognitive Behaviour Therapy helps people develop different ways of thinking about situations to learn to feel better about themselves and their life. No two patients are alike, so the goal is to help people identify how they think, feel and act when feeling down or depressed. For example, if a patient has relationship difficulties, cognitive behavioral therapy aims to help them understand their thoughts and feelings about the relationship. The therapist will help the patient develop different ways of thinking about the partner to decrease negative thoughts and feelings.

How do I get screened for cognitive behavior therapy?

There are several ways to get screened for cognitive behavior therapy. A cognitive behavioral therapist will weigh the patient's motivation, ask them questions about their thoughts and feelings, and determine whether or not they have the capacity to make changes on their own. If they feel they cannot change themselves with proper support, they can be referred to a therapist with more experience in CBT. A self-help book is available for those who feel they can handle it independently.

Ways to get screened for CBT include:

a. By visiting a therapist, who will ask questions regarding what the patient believes about themselves.
b. Through CBT Self Tests.
c. Through assessment tests.
d. Referral by a friend or family member

Cognitive behavioral therapy usually involves four to six sessions per week. However, this may be less if the patient can handle their problems independently or with family and friends' support. In some cases, cognitive behavioral therapy can be a one-on-one treatment, but in other cases, it may need to be done in a group setting. The CBT therapist will also help patients develop skills they can use when feeling stressed or depressed to help them cope with the situation and prevent them from turning to alcohol and drugs for relief.

Medications are not typically used in cognitive behavior therapy because the goal is to stop the thoughts that lead to negative emotions and behaviors. Medication treats problems by altering thoughts, whether anxiety, stress, or depression. Even though medications can alter how you think and behave, they are ineffective in treating depression and anxiety. CBT helps treat these conditions by changing one's thinking patterns rather than altering how people feel or act. So medications are not typically used in cognitive behavioral therapy.

CBT only works effectively when the patient can identify their negative thoughts and feelings and develop strategies to alter these thoughts. Even though CBT is a highly effective treatment, it can be time-consuming and difficult. Some patients do not have the time or desire to work on their problems daily. So the patient needs to understand that therapy may take months or even years before they feel better. Cognitive behavioral therapy requires intense self-help, and many people do not have the motivation or energy to see results quickly. The therapist will work closely with the patient, giving them encouragement and feedback as they progress through therapy. If the patient does not see results or is unwilling to make changes, the therapist may explore other options, including medication or a more intensive form of therapy.

Moreover, evidence-based treatments such as CBT are not the be-all and end-all of treatment. Sometimes the patient's symptoms can be resolved without therapy, or in some instances, and patients will need medication for their anxiety, stress, or depressive symptoms. As with any treatment, cognitive behavioral therapy works best with other therapy and medication.

How long does CBT take?

In most cases, cognitive behavioral therapy can take months to see results, so it is essential to keep up your effort throughout your therapy. It is best to address your thoughts and feelings as soon as you notice them, as this will help prevent you from turning to substances or negative behaviors such as drugs or alcohol in a desperate attempt to feel better. The patient must understand that the therapy can take months or even years to work effectively.

Patients who do not feel like their time is wasted may try to finish the treatment without going into more detail about their thoughts and feelings. However, this may not be possible. Even if you think your therapist is overstepping their bounds with questions such as "Why are you still depressed?" complete honesty is necessary to help the therapist find effective ways to change your thought patterns. It is essential to complete the therapy as best as possible, as it may take months or years to see results.

Cognitive behavioral therapy is based on the idea that you can change your negative thoughts to feel better. If a patient does not see results or is unwilling to make changes in their life, the therapist may explore other options for treatment.

In addition, cognitive behavioral therapy is based on the idea that you can change your negative thoughts to feel better. If a patient does not see results or is unwilling to make changes in their life, the therapist may explore other options for treatment. Therefore, if the patient doesn't believe they need therapy or are unwilling to do what it takes to get better, this type of treatment is ineffective.

This method takes approximately six months to a year. In the case of addiction and substance abuse, the therapy is usually based on a 12-step program. This type of therapy is best if the patient is open to trying it. If they are not open to it, they may do better with cognitive behavioral therapy as it focuses more on changing thinking patterns that are causing addictive behaviors as opposed to your emotional state.

Cognitive behavioral therapy is a crucial component of addiction treatment, as it helps patients better understand their thoughts and how they impact their behavior. CBT teaches patients how to approach negative experiences in a way that does not cause anxiety or depression. This method is best if the patient is open to trying it. If they are not open to it, they may do better with cognitive behavioral therapy as it focuses more on changing thinking patterns causing addictive behaviors instead of your emotional state.

The main goal of cognitive behavioral therapy is to eliminate psychological symptoms and emotional distress that interferes with daily life. This can happen by changing negative thoughts, behaviors, and emotions. In addition, CBT aims to teach patients how to identify their dysfunctional thoughts and develop coping skills through problem-solving. The self-help book "Feeling Good" by David Burns provides detailed instructions on identifying harmful thinking patterns and developing healthy coping skills.

In the case of depression and anxiety, the goal is to help patients learn how to identify their thoughts, emotions, and behaviors that make them feel better. For example, if a patient feels better after doing exercises, reading books, or taking medication or therapy/medication, this demonstrates that CBT worked. The patient needs to understand that changes in behavior may not be immediate but will come with time.

Cognitive behavioral therapy is effective when the patient can identify their negative thoughts and feelings so they can develop skills to alter these thoughts. Unfortunately, cognitive behavioral therapy will not work in several instances because the patient has a psychological disorder. However, many therapists use CBT with other techniques, such as medication or additional therapy, to help patients resolve their problems.

What is a typical session like?

The first cognitive behavioral therapy sessions are essential for the therapist to get to know their patient and the patient to get a feel for how the therapist works. In addition, patients want to feel comfortable talking about their issues and that they can trust their therapists with personal information. For example, if a patient is anxious about going on dates and one of the goals is to go on more dates with different people, then this should be discussed during the first session so that it can be addressed in future sessions.

During the first session, the therapist may ask many questions to help guide the patient. This will give them an idea of whether they need individual therapy or should be referred to a counselor, social worker, psychologist, or another expert in their area.

This helps the patient decide if they want to continue doing cognitive behavioral therapy with the therapist or find a different one. It is usually based on how well they feel after talking with their therapist, how much trust and confidence they have in them, and how helpful they have been so far.

As cognitive behavioral therapy progresses, it may take longer to complete specific exercises because there may be more information to share and ideas about what is going on that might be helpful. Most therapists do not rush their patients and help them work at their own pace.

The therapist and patient may also decide to explore specific topics deeper in future sessions.

The second session may address how the patient feels so far, and the subsequent sessions may help them understand the therapy better. Moreover, the therapist will continue to help the patient identify negative thought patterns and coping skills. This involves looking at the different situations that may have occurred in previous sessions and deciding how the patient can alter their negative thoughts and feelings.

In addition, patients may bring homework to do outside of sessions and discuss it with their therapist during sessions. This helps them understand what they need to work on more when they aren't in therapy.

The therapist will help them identify areas where they are doing well and areas that are hard for them. The therapist will also use various techniques to help the patient work on these problems, including changing their thought patterns or helping them learn new ways to cope with life stressors.

What are the Components of CBT?

CBT components are skills that the patient will learn during cognitive behavioral therapy. Some of the most common components include:

a.   Observation.

Observation is the ability to notice a situation or thought when it happens. This also helps further the therapy by identifying dysfunctional thought patterns and actions. For instance, a patient may say that he or she forgets his keys because they are too focused on other tasks, like applying for another job.

In cognitive behavioral therapy, noticing what is happening and then changing these circumstances to help the patient cope better with life issues helps develop new coping skills that can be used later to deal with similar situations. In addition, thinking helps patients change their behavior and thoughts to feel better emotionally and mentally.

b.   Self-monitoring and reflection (5-second test).

The patient is asked to look at their current situation in this exercise. Then, after noticing the situation, how they think about it (cognitively), and what they feel (emotionally), they are asked to take a 5-second pause before acting on the situation. This helps them make better decisions in future situations by helping them identify their feelings and thoughts before acting on these harmful thought patterns. In addition, this considers that some people have difficulty making quick decisions that negatively impact their lives.

The 5-second test can be performed at any time during a session. Patients can do this exercise any time of the day or night to help them identify unhealthy thought patterns or specific situations or emotions.

The following is an example of how this 5-second test is performed.

1. Notice what is happening (the first two seconds).
2. Think/Identify your thoughts about the situation (the next three seconds).
3. Identify how you feel emotionally (the last two seconds).
4. After the five seconds, identify the situation and think about it for a few more seconds. Still, this time do not overthink or think about it negatively anymore (a few minutes will pass by on average). This helps patients change their perspective of situations, so they have more control over their emotions instead of allowing them to control them.

c. Cognitive restructuring.

In cognitive behavioral therapy, patients learn how to change their thoughts about situations and that these thoughts may not be valid. Cognitive restructuring helps patients change these harmful thought patterns and adjust their reasoning during difficult situations to feel better mentally and psychologically.

For example, A person in a romantic relationship has been caught cheating and is blaming the relationship for this betrayal. The patient may think that if they were not in a relationship, they would not cheat on them, and it is all the fault of the other person for cheating because that person does not treat them well enough.

This is an example of a distorted thinking pattern and one that blames others for the patient's distress. In cognitive behavioral therapy, the patient learns to identify these distortions more clearly and then choose healthy thoughts to replace these to feel better emotionally.

d. Behavioral experiments.

Behavioral experiments help patients change their habits or routines to feel better mentally and psychologically. For instance, a patient may have problems at work because they cannot focus on their job due to being distracted by other things going on in life. So the patient may try this experiment:

1. Notice what is happening.
2. Think about the situation for a few seconds.
3. Identify the behavior that they want to change.
4. Perform the behavioral experiment by making this change in their routine/behavior and evaluate it after a few minutes and hours to see if it can help them feel better emotionally and psychologically later on by helping them identify better coping skills they can use in difficult future situations, so they do not feel so overwhelmed by various factors that are causing their stress and anxiety or depression.

e. Problem-solving and rational thinking (two-column chart).

In cognitive behavioral therapy, patients learn problem-solving methods to feel better mentally and psychologically. In this process, the patient first lists all the problems they are experiencing or have experienced in the past. Next, they choose another column and list ways to solve these problems. This helps patients identify healthy coping skills that can be used later when they are facing similar situations in life.

f. Positive self-talk.

Positive self-talk helps patients use coping skills during stressful situations when negative thinking may otherwise take over and cause them distress or anxiety. For example, in cognitive behavioral therapy, the therapist will help patients unlearn negative thoughts by helping them replace these with positive ones so they can feel better emotionally by changing their thoughts to become more optimistic about life issues.

g.   Rehearsal.

In cognitive behavioral therapy, patients learn to change negative thought patterns and learn new coping skills that they can use to feel better emotionally in the future, which helps them change not only their situation but their uncontrollable behavior.

For example, A patient may become enraged or upset by a friend who constantly makes fun of them in front of others and even disrespects them directly. The patient may think that this person does not like them, and they know that the person only feels tired of being around them, so they will stop putting up with what the other person is doing.

At this point, it is essential to help the patient take a step back and realize that they are the ones who are having trouble with their emotions and not the other person at all. Patients need to learn to separate their behavior from others and be more able to identify why they feel as they do in stressful situations to get better emotionally by changing their thought patterns and specific aspects of their personality.

h.   Relaxation techniques.

Relaxation techniques are used in cognitive behavioral therapy to help patients feel better mentally and psychologically by developing skills they can use to deal with stressful situations more effectively. For instance, a person may be having problems with anxiety or depression because they cannot focus on specific tasks when they need to due to anxiety and depression. The patient identifies this problem and learns different ways to relax his body physically so he can feel better emotionally by focusing on the task at hand instead of feeling as if his mind is racing out of control. This can be done by learning several different relaxation techniques that help them to calm down and feel better emotionally.

i.   Emotional regulation (identifying and replacing negative emotions with positive ones).

Emotional regulation helps patients identify the source of their negative emotions so they can learn how to manage them better when they are having problems with anxiety or depression, and it helps them replace these negative emotions with positive ones. For example, A patient's mother may have died, and he feels depressed because he misses her. He has been having trouble at home because his father scolds him for being inattentive, but he is unaware of why he constantly feels sad. He can identify the source of his depression, but then he must learn how to replace his sadness with positive emotions.

The patient identifies that his father's behavior has caused him emotional pain because he feels like the people in his life do not care about him and treat him as if he is nothing more than an object. You can see why mental health professionals think depression and anxiety are so important. They help people realize that there are things they can change within themselves so they will start to feel better emotionally by admitting their problems and changing their thought patterns.

j.   Understanding your emotions.

In cognitive behavioral therapy, patients learn to identify their feelings about the situation at hand to learn how to change specific thoughts and behaviors (both internal and external) that are causing them mental and emotional pain. For example, A patient may feel sad all the time, and he feels tired of dealing with life issues. However, he has learned that revealing his sadness only causes people around him to feel pity for him, so he hides his sadness by hiding his genuine emotions from others. In addition, he has learned that keeping up with other people's lives helps him avoid focusing on his problems by immersing himself in their lives instead of dealing with what is happening in his own life.

This patient needs to learn how to accept his sad emotions and how to deal with these emotions in a way that does not cause him any pain or stress. In addition, he needs to learn the difference between letting people know that he experiences sadness and being afraid to share his feelings because he has learned that people will not want anything to do with him.

Cognitive behavioral therapy is effective because it helps patients learn skills they can use when faced with stressful situations in their lives so they can get better emotionally by learning ways to cope more effectively with their problems.

What do the Components of CBT do for us?

The psychological components of cognitive behavioral therapy show us how to identify what is causing us stress and unhappiness, and we can learn skills to improve our mental health.

For instance, A patient who has suffered from anxiety or depression for a long time may have trouble experiencing certain feelings or thoughts, so they need to learn how to identify the source of their problems.

A patient may experience distress when his boss yells at him in front of others because he knows that these people will gossip about him later. He must learn to control his behavior when upset with others because he must not act impulsively, which would cause him more stress and unhappiness. In addition, he must learn how to cope with anxiety and depression to feel better emotionally by thinking about his problems differently and changing how he reacts to them.

A person who feels as if no one loves them and believes their life is meaningless may need to learn how to develop positive thoughts and feelings about themselves to feel better mentally. These positive thoughts may be hard to form, but they are crucial to feeling better mentally and emotionally.

A patient may be having problems with anger or other negative emotions because he has learned that being angry is the best way to get his needs met when he feels like he is not necessary at work or in his personal life. Therefore, the patient must learn how to control his behavior to cope with these emotions more effectively.

A person who feels as if no one understands him or cares about him may need to learn how to develop a vision of what his life could be like if only he had better people in it. Doing this will help him develop a better identity for himself through creating goals for his life and a vision for his future.

A patient may have problems because they cannot focus on specific tasks at work or in school when the time comes around, and this causes them to have problems with anxiety and depression. The patient may need to learn to control his behavior better to focus on the task instead of feeling like his mind is racing out of control. He needs to learn to physically relax to feel better emotionally by focusing on the task instead of feeling like his mind is racing out of control.

This kind of patient needs to learn how to develop healthy self-esteem because he believes that changing behavior based on other people's behavior is a good way for them to feel good about themselves. Therefore, he must learn to change this negative behavior by changing his thoughts about himself and how he responds to others.

Cognitive behavioral therapy helps patients learn how to identify their internal emotional problems as well as their external ones, which allows them to develop skills for dealing better with stress, anxiety, and depression. This is one reason why cognitive behavioral therapy is so effective.

The last component of CBT explains an essential factor in helping us feel better. It shows us how to eliminate our mental health problems by identifying their causes so we can feel better mentally and emotionally by changing our thoughts and specific aspects of our personalities to feel better.

Therefore, Cognitive behavioral therapy can be highly effective in helping us control our negative feelings, emotions, and moods when we deal with them in a way that does not cause unnecessary stress. In addition, this treatment helps patients learn about their mental health instead of just treating their symptoms.

This kind of therapy is not invasive or painful like some other treatments. It can benefit anyone who wants to change their behavior to feel better emotionally. In this way, cognitive behavioral therapy is a good choice for anyone who has not succeeded with other treatment forms.

On what basis do I decide whether CBT is suitable for me?

The basis for determining whether cognitive behavioral therapy is suitable for a patient is to determine if the treatment can work with their specific mental health problems.

The therapist uses general questions to help patients discover more about their physical and emotional health. Still, deciding what treatment works best for an individual patient depends on that patient's specific issues.

The psychologist may ask a patient how they or see him or herself physically and in terms of personality, which will help the psychologist provide treatment recommendations. This kind of therapist uses various techniques to determine how best to treat patients with different mental health issues because no two patients are alike.

A therapist will use their clinical experience to determine each patient's best course of action. For instance, in a session, a therapist may ask about which emotions a patient has the most problems dealing with and why.

In another session, a therapist may ask what specific events lead to certain behaviors so that this psychologist can determine why certain behaviors are causing problems.

In yet another session, a psychologist may ask how to deal with depression because it is hard for the patient to think positively when he feels down on himself, and nothing seems right in his life. The psychologist can provide practical solutions by teaching him how to change his negative thoughts into more positive ones so he will be happier when dealing with difficult situations in the future.

This will help a therapist determine the treatment plan best for the patient. A patient can also ask questions about other forms of treatment and how they work to see if cognitive behavioral therapy is suitable for them.

For instance, an individual who does not like taking medications might feel more comfortable with a different form of treatment. In addition, their doctor may have some information about CBT available to help the patient decide whether it is likely to be more effective than other forms of treatment in dealing with his specific mental health problems.

Other patients might never ask about this treatment, but their doctors might recommend it because it is designed to help people with various mental health issues. However, no two patients are like the next, so one patient may not be able to benefit from this kind of therapy if they do not keep track of their emotions, and a therapist cannot heal other people's problems for them.

Therefore, the doctor can only give a general recommendation as to whether CBT will work best for a specific patient by asking questions and discussing the patient's past experiences in dealing with their mental health issues to find out which issues are their most significant need immediate attention.

What about cognitive rehabilitation for those with brain injury?

Cognitive rehabilitation is the principle of helping patients with brain injury learn how to handle and adapt to their new lifestyles after injury. In addition, this kind of therapy helps a patient learn about his actions and the actions of others for his good.

This therapy demonstrates that people who have experienced brain injury have specific mental health issues. Still, in this case, their mental health problems are caused by their changes in lifestyle after their injuries. For instance, an individual may deal with certain aspects of brain damage through positive thinking.

Similarly to this form of therapy, cognitive behavioral therapy can also be used to deal with many forms of mental health problems.

Cognitive behavioral therapy can help individuals from a wide range of backgrounds to learn how to change the activities in their lives so they do not feel negative about themselves and thus become happier.

For instance, if an individual is dealing with anxiety or depression, they can learn that other people have perspectives different from their own and thus will feel better by understanding why others are thinking differently than him.

On the other hand, understanding this kind of therapy can help an individual deal with social situations more successfully because he will know what he does not have control over as opposed to what he does have control over.

To help an individual with brain injury learn this form of therapy, the therapist can teach him to control his behaviors, so he does not have to worry about his brain injuries and thus become happier. Furthermore, this kind of therapy can benefit patients with various mental health problems.

For instance, to treat depression, cognitive behavior therapy will help the patient deal with negative thoughts and emotions to feel more positive about himself. Patients who have experienced shootings and other forms of violence may also benefit from cognitive rehabilitation because they can learn how to handle the situations they are dealing with.

How does CBT relate to other approaches to anxiety and depression?

Cognitive behavioral therapy is a form of psychotherapy that treats depression, anxiety, and other mental health issues. Cognitive behavior therapy is based on the premise that thoughts, emotions, and behaviors are all connected.

For example, suppose a person is depressed because they recently experienced a breakup with her boyfriend. As a result, she had to take a new job at her company to help pay for the loss she suffered with their relationship. In that case, the therapist will help her learn how to deal with these problems by changing how she feels about them.

The therapist will first assess the patient's feelings to determine precisely what is causing their negative emotions by asking open-ended questions about what makes him feel sad or angry.

The patient will then learn how to take control of his emotions by practicing specific exercises, such as cognitive restructuring, which is the modification of negative thoughts to make them more positive to change how a person feels about himself.

For example, suppose a patient feels depressed after a breakup with his boyfriend and feels his life has no direction or purpose. In that case, the therapist may help him learn how to deal with this by reminding him that he has made mistakes along the way despite his successes.

The patient will repeat these positive and realistic statements until these thoughts become habitual within his mind and he can feel better about himself.

As another example, if a person has an anxiety attack after experiencing criticism from a coworker, the therapist will help him feel more confident by trying to change his thoughts to make him feel like he can deal with the critique.

Similarly, cognitive behavioral therapists will also learn how to motivate their patients by providing them with resources that help them learn how to deal with their mental health issues and the tools they need to overcome those issues.

The therapist's goal is generally to teach patients how they can control their emotions and behavior to overcome obstacles in their lives. For example, cognitive behavioral therapy treats various mental health issues, including anxiety, depression, eating disorders, and other forms of aggressive behavior. This kind of therapy is particularly effective when used to treat addictions because the patient is given a safe environment in which he can learn how to control his actions.

Cognitive behavior therapy has also been effective in treating PTSD because it helps patients deal with trauma by allowing them to understand that they have had some control over the events that have occurred in their lives, so they do not need to worry about these events and become stress about dealing with those issues. Furthermore, it has been proven that CBT is more cost-effective than many traditional therapeutic approaches.

PRINCIPLES AND CHARACTERISTICS OF CBT

Cognitive behavior therapy (CBT) is an evidence-based psychological treatment that aims to help people who have problems with anxiety, depression, addiction, and other mental health problems. It focuses on how patterns of thoughts and behaviors affect emotions and moods. CBT also has a strong emphasis on the development of practical coping skills to reduce the impact of these maladaptive thoughts and behaviors.

CBT is a 'talk therapy in various settings, including doctors' surgeries, hospital outpatient departments, counseling, and community health services, and can be delivered by several professional practitioners.

This therapy has several principles and characteristics that differentiate it from other psychotherapies. Moreover, this therapy reaches people who need to use their initiative to make changes in their lives necessary for recovery, rather than doing things 'on the list. CBT involves the active participation of patients in their treatment and is focused on facilitating self-management of symptoms and recovery.

CBT integrates, improves, and focuses on the patient's present functioning (across all domains) and does not focus on past events or future forecasts. In addition, it strongly emphasizes being outcome-based (aiming for positive outcomes) instead of behavior-based (targeting negative behavior). This is because it believes that change happens only when patients desire it.

Principles of CBT

These CBT principles have been the subject of many empirical studies in recent decades. The contributions of the principles to therapeutic outcomes have been found to vary across disorders, patients, therapist styles, and different types of therapy. However, there has been agreement that these principles are essential ingredients in a CBT model.

The effectiveness of CBT relates to an active collaboration between therapist and client. The goal is not simply to provide advice or insight but to help patients work through their problems by facing their fears. This is accomplished by developing personal coping strategies through exercises that enhance personal control and responsibility over one's life.

CBT-based interventions are structured, goal-oriented, and collaboratively developed by the patient and the therapist. CBT can be delivered in various modalities—individually, face to face, via computer, telephone, or videoconferences.

CBT has clinical applications for patients with chronic or severe mental disorders, including major depression, anxiety disorders, eating disorders, substance abuse disorders, and personality disorders.

The principles of CBT (with some differences) are used to treat non-psychiatric problems such as weight loss and relationship difficulties. In recent years CBT has been applied to a wide range of physical illnesses such as diabetes mellitus, chronic pain, cancer recovery, heart disease, and irritable bowel syndrome. There is also increasing evidence that it can play a role in treating chronic diseases (such as asthma).

The Cognitive model emphasizes an understanding of how an individual's thoughts affect one's emotions and behavior. It views thoughts as a chain reaction relating to feelings, resulting in different actions. In general terms, negative thoughts lead to negative feelings, which lead to negative actions and outcomes.

Psychotherapy is a unique intervention because the therapist (together with the patient) directly engages in cognitive and behavioral activities that focus on changing maladaptive patterns of thinking and be-having. This process often occurs within a particular therapy setting that emphasizes personal attention, active listening, and the use of behavioral techniques for change.

Instead of simply talking to patients about their problems, CBT therapists will often request specific be-haviors, which are considered homework or even ask patients to experiment with new coping skills. For example, many CBT therapists ask their patients to try using relaxation techniques such as deep breathing before an upcoming stressful situation or even in the middle of the day just before a challenging task at work.

The principles of CBT include:

1. Self-management of symptoms – CBT focuses on personal changes of behavior that help control and reduce the impact of emotional reactions in situations that can trigger anxiety or depression. The goal is to achieve a level of comfort, relaxation, hope, and optimism during challenging situations that would not otherwise be present.
2. Client-directed therapy—Therapy sessions are developed in collaboration with the client based on the patient's individual needs and issues rather than according to a preconceived plan. This technique focuses on how a particular session can benefit both parties. They will also focus on making the best use of their time together by developing strategies to keep clients engaged and interested throughout counseling sessions.
3. Collaborative and work-focused relationship – CBT therapists believe that change is most effective when clients feel comfortable and willing to experiment with new ideas or ways of doing things. The therapist's goal is to have patients actively participate in their treatment to create a "cooperative therapeutic alliance." The therapist will often work with clients to develop specific goals and agree on techniques for working towards those goals.
4. Self-discovery – CBT helps individuals recognize patterns of thinking and behavior that trigger feel-ings of anxiety or depression while also exploring factors that may contribute to these conditions, such as childhood experiences, personality traits, social support systems, and other environmental variables. As a result, CBT clients can develop more realistic and practical coping skills by better un-derstanding these behaviors.
5. Mindfulness – The principle of mindfulness is often used as a component technique for reducing anxiety or stress. It involves focusing on one's perceptions, emotions, thoughts, and behaviors in a non-judgmental way that helps individuals become more aware of their current state of being. With-in this technique, it is often helpful to observe various patterns in one's life and then notice what thoughts are associated with them and how they alter feelings or behaviors.
6. Striving for success – CBT teaches clients how to overcome their emotional difficulties. They are encouraged to explore their options and use specific skills and techniques to cope with anxiety or depression. These strategies can include:

1) Relaxation techniques such as breathing or meditation

2) Plain, everyday activities that can be used simultaneously with one's usual activities, such as giving up watching television instead of going home early

3) Imagination exercises, such as focusing on positive thoughts during difficult situations or using an optimistic self-talk

7. Reciprocal reinforcement – CBT therapists often request that clients actively attempt new coping skills rather than simply listening to the therapist and accepting one's diagnosis and treatments. The therapist will explain how coping techniques work and will often provide immediate feedback on whether or not clients are responding appropriately. CBT therapists will also request that clients make a conscious effort to acknowledge and reward themselves for their successes at specific tasks, such as being able to remain calm during a stressful situation.

8. Problem-focused coping – CBT is known for dealing with specific problems or issues in one's life, such as difficulty sleeping, relationship difficulties, chronic pain, self-esteem issues, and work-related stress.

9. Relaxation techniques – There are many relaxation methods in CBT, including meditation, guided imagery, and progressive muscle relaxation. These tools are often used during stress to help reduce anxiety while developing other coping skills.

Common cognitive distortions include:

a. All-or-nothing thinking – This type of thinking tends to exaggerate the reality of a situation by viewing things in absolutes. The individual will think that something is either good or bad rather than have the ability to appreciate both the positives and negatives of a particular situation.

b. Overgeneralizing – This type of thinking occurs when individuals view adverse events as indicative of a more significant problem without recognizing other factors that may not be related to the targeted event. For example, a person may start to believe that they are completely incompetent, even though there is evidence that some regions of their life are not affected by these poor skills.

c. Mental filter – This type of thinking leads individuals to focus on and amplify only certain aspects of a negative situation without considering the fullness of the context. For example, a person may focus on the one task or aspect that they performed poorly during the day but ignore all other positive events or completed tasks.

d. Disqualifying the Positive - This occurs when individuals accept positive experiences as accurate (or valid) but qualify them with negative thoughts and feelings to remove their validity. For instance, if a person feels they are a valued family member, they may still find a way to disqualify this positive experience by believing their parents only wish for them to keep them company.

e. Jumping to Conclusions – This occurs when individuals make assumptions about other people, situations, and events without concrete facts. For example, an individual may believe that a friend's lack of response to an email is due to anger before trying to check in with their friend.

f. Magnification and Minimization – These distortions involve exaggerating the severity of negative events or minimizing the value of positive experiences. For example, a person may expect to fail at a task and dwell on how they will be embarrassed if they do so, thus magnifying the negative experience. Alternatively, people may find ways to minimize their positive experiences by assuming that others are not impressed by the same accomplishment or event.

g. Personalization – This type of cognitive distortion occurs when individuals believe that things that happen are directly linked to them or their behavior when there is no evidence to back up these claims.

h. Labeling – This occurs when individuals place a negative label on themselves without considering that other people may not view them the same way. For example, a person may believe that their personality is so unique and different from others that they will be considered rude even if they do not mean to be.

i. Catastrophizing – This distortion involves assuming catastrophic outcomes when a situation is perceived as more complicated than it is by including extreme possibilities based on one's fears and expectations.

10. Problem-solving

a. Cognitive restructuring – This technique involves individuals recalling and challenging distorted thoughts to help them adopt a more realistic perspective. For example, if an individual believes that everyone will be upset if they admit to having anxiety and anxiety symptoms, cognitive restructuring can focus on the fact that other people may not share this assumption. But even if they do, the individual can still benefit from taking action while open to new possibilities. For example, an individual may believe their coworkers will discover their disability and fire them for being on medication for anxiety or depression. However, cognitive restructuring can focus on the fact that this is an unlikely scenario and that one must still accept that coworkers may be frustrated instead.

b. Cognitive coping – This coping focuses on placing oneself in a better position to handle negative events by finding ways to make these situations less stressful. For instance, if a person believes that other people will think they are lazy, cognitive coping can help the individual focus on being more productive and putting forth effort throughout the day so as not to be confused with a person who is not willing to work as hard.

c. Changing perspectives – When individuals feel trapped and unable to control their lives, they may become paralyzed by overwhelming feelings of anxiety and depression. Changing perspectives allows people to feel in control and take positive steps towards their goals by challenging negative thoughts and assumptions about themselves. For instance, individuals who have problems with their health may adopt different perspectives around their negative thoughts about being unable or unwilling to take care of themselves. Individuals can be more proactive in navigating difficult situations by changing their focus from caring for themselves to caring for their family or helping others.

d. Active role – To find ways to break negative cycles and cope with distressing situations, individuals must take an active role in their recovery. For example, by focusing on how one can approach challenging situations instead of engaging in problem-solving based on how one can cope with negative outcomes, individuals can focus on more positive and effective methods. e. Positive self-talk – This type of coping focuses on believing in a positive outcome and repeating positive thoughts to keep one's spirits up.

11. Interpersonal effectiveness

a. Social support – This type of coping involves having others in one's life that can provide emotional support and help more effectively manage thoughts, feelings, and behaviors that may become problematic. For example, suppose an individual is not feeling well but does not know how to reach out for emotional support. In that case, other people in their life may be able to provide helpful resources or personal connections without trying to fix them or make them feel better.

b. Problem-solving – This refers to how one can approach distressing situations that may otherwise become overwhelming. For example, suppose individuals are having trouble socializing with others. In that case, problem-solving can help them identify and tackle the issues that may influence their behavior in these settings and provide better solutions for communicating with others more healthily.

c. Communication – This type of coping relates to how one communicates with others and helps them better understand challenging situations in their lives and themselves. When individuals can communicate effectively with other people, they may feel less isolated and more supported when they face difficulties.

CBT was initially developed by psychiatrist Aaron Beck in the 1960s through the 1970s through his pioneering studies on depression and anxiety disorders. He also developed cognitive therapy, which deals primarily with thoughts, helping people change the way they think to overcome negative self-beliefs such as negative cognitions and dysfunctional beliefs.

Some CBT approaches use a "Cognitive Therapy" technique that alters one's thinking patterns. On the other hand, other approaches use "Behavioural Therapy" as a guiding principle of treatment.

CBT practitioners typically work within a different setting than medical doctors, who are trained to diagnose and treat mental disorders solely by medications. CBT therapists believe that people can deal with their feelings and problems by taking an active approach to suffering through different strategies that can be learned within the therapy sessions.

These principles are essential since:

a. CBT is considered more effective than other psychotherapies, with most patients receiving positive results as long as they are willing to work and be active in the therapy process.
b. CBT is available in various formats and types, including individual sessions, group therapy, self-help books, computer programs, and Internet applications.
c. CBT mainly focuses on patients' participation to help them take an active role in their treatment.
d. CBT can be used with medications and other treatment modalities, such as traditional psychotherapy or behavioral techniques.
e. CBT does not require patients to address their early experiences, which is a common framework for other types of therapy.
f. CBT is cost-effective since psychiatric hospital stays and physician visits are unnecessary for this type of treatment.
g. Recent studies have suggested that some forms of CBT may positively affect patients with schizophrenia or obsessive-compulsive disorder (OCD).
h. CBT therapy is typically shorter than other types of psychotherapy, such as psychoanalysis, since it often takes less time to achieve results than more traditional treatments.
i. CBT is more effective at treating anxiety disorders than other types of psychotherapy.
j. CBT is often used to help patients deal with various life issues, including depression and panic disorder, eating disorders, alcohol abuse, and substance abuse.

CBT is sometimes used with medications to treat severe mental illnesses such as bipolar disorder or severe depression. In some cases, it replaced medication altogether.

CBT can also be used to improve skills in dealing with anxiety/ stress reactions, child/ adolescent counseling, couple's therapy, and family therapy. CBT has been proven effective in treating most types of mental health disorders.

CBT Characteristics

CBT has several characteristics. These are also essential since:

a. CBT is considered an effective form of psychotherapy, with most patients who undergo this type of treatment showing noticeable improvements.

b.　CBT is a short-term therapy that takes about 12–15 weekly, depending on the patient's specific needs and goals.
c.　CBT has been proven effective in treating anxiety disorders, depression, and other mental illnesses.
d.　The right combination of CBT principles, psychology, and social work techniques can effectively treat any mental health disorder.
e.　In most cases, patients don't require medications or hospitalization while they undergo this type of therapy to help them overcome their issues and improve their well-being over time.
f.　CBT is cost-effective since the therapist helps patients identify their problems and implement solutions to manage their symptoms within a short period.
g.　CBT is based on scientific evidence and practice, making it a more reliable approach to help people overcome different issues.
h.　CBT works well with other forms of treatment, such as medication or dietary changes, because this approach may combine different techniques to provide better patient outcomes.
i.　Generally, CBT can be implemented in various settings and formats, such as individual therapy sessions, group sessions, phone sessions, or online counseling (e-therapy).

Therefore, some of the characteristics of CBT are explained below:

1.　It is time-limited than other therapies

CBT is a time-limited therapy. Therefore, patients need to identify the reasons why they need clinical treatment and the goals they want to achieve. Thus, CBT therapists and patients work together to develop appropriate psychotherapeutic treatment strategies to apply certain CBT techniques within a specific period.

2.　It focuses on changing current ways of dealing with problems and incorporates other types of therapies

CBT makes patients aware of their options for dealing with or solving issues in their lives by changing how they respond to specific situations.

CBT does not always work alone. Some patients may have to combine CBT concepts with other forms of psychotherapy, such as interpersonal therapy, family therapy, or dialectical behavior therapy (DBT).

3.　It is based on scientific evidence and realistic practice

Most CBT techniques have been proven effective in clinical trials and research studies. On the other hand, CBT practitioners are well-educated professionals trained to help patients overcome their mental health issues through different therapeutic interventions based on scientific evidence.

4.　It is cost-effective

Since most CBT therapies can be implemented within a short period, this type of treatment tends to be more cost-effective than some traditional approaches.

5.　It is based on cooperation and collaboration between patients and their therapists

Patients are expected to be active in the therapy process by taking an active role in the treatment. Therefore, patients should have good communication skills that help them express their feelings, thoughts, experiences, or other issues they want to change over time. In some cases, it may be helpful for patients to keep a journal or record their thoughts and feelings on different situations that affect their mental health status during the CBT treatment period.

6.　It can be used in various settings

CBT can be applied in different settings, such as individual, group, face-to-face, or phone sessions. It can also be used to treat patients with various mental health disorders alone or in combination with other therapies.

7.   It helps patients identify and deal with their emotions and other psychological factors

CBT helps patients identify the negative thoughts or beliefs that affect their coping mechanisms and make managing their symptoms difficult. For instance, some people may feel upset because they tend to feel guilty when they make a mistake at work or home. Other individuals may become anxious when faced with specific situations because they create negative interpretations (i.e., "I failed this time, and it will happen again").

8.   It helps patients develop more effective ways to handle stressful situations

During the CBT treatment process, patients learn how to control their thoughts, behaviors, and emotions to manage stress levels better. Some of these skills are useful for managing specific mental health disorders after completing their sessions.

9.   It is a short-term therapy

Most CBT programs last for about 19 to 21 weeks. However, there are some cases where people may benefit from more extended treatment periods (such as one or two years). The length of CBT programs depends on the patient's specific needs and goals.

10.   It is a combination approach

CBT involves different types of therapeutic techniques that can make it more effective than the use of single techniques on their own. For instance, CBT practitioners will help patients explore relevant emotional issues, such as suicidal thoughts and feelings, and address other emotional sources based on their assessments and observations over time.

11.   It can be used to treat several mental health disorders

CBT has been proven effective for various mental health disorders such as depression, anxiety, panic disorder, eating disorders, post-traumatic stress disorder (PTSD), social anxiety, and addictions such as alcohol addiction and substance abuse. CBT is a few psychotherapies considered a first-line treatment option for patients with major depressive disorder (MDD).

12.   It is used together with other evidence-based treatments

Although CBT is highly effective, it may be combined with other therapies to improve patient outcomes. For instance, patients struggling with anxiety may benefit from using CBT combined with exposure-based interventions, such as imaginal desensitization and relaxation (IDR). Some patients may also benefit from using DBT, a cognitive behavior therapy performed online and face-to-face. These therapies can be combined with medication to increase treatment effectiveness and reduce the risk of other side effects.

13.   It helps patients deal with their unwanted thoughts and emotions

CBT can also help patients develop ways to deal with their unwanted thoughts and feelings. The therapist will help them explore why they tend to experience particular negative or unpleasant feelings in specific situations, such as episodes of intense depression, anxiety, or anger over time.

14.   It can be applied to a wide range of different populations

Some CBT programs are gender-specific such as the Heidelberg Cope Program for men, which focuses on issues unique to men, such as alcohol dependency and relationship concerns, while others (such as DBT) are designed for women.

15. It can reduce the risk of relapse

CBT has been proven effective in preventing people from relapsing into depressive or anxiety disorders. Based on the research presented in several CBT studies, reduced symptoms and improved overall functioning are associated with an increased chance of treatment dropout among patients who do not adhere to their treatment protocols.

16. It is more effective than some other therapies

CBT is generally considered one of the most effective non-pharmacological treatments available today. It also has fewer risks than medication and other standard therapies used for treating major mental health issues over time.

Adjunctive Interventions

Education

There is evidence that CBT can be effectively delivered to groups of patients in educational environments to spread the skill set and make them available to more people. Several E-learning platforms provide online CBT, making this delivery method more accessible and affordable. These online resources provide a cost-effective way of disseminating CBT skills worldwide.

Self-help Books

CBT self-help books are used as an adjunct to other forms of therapy or by individuals wishing to address particular issues for themselves without being seen by a therapist. These books allow the reader to work through the material at their own pace and have the added benefit of being relatively inexpensive. Books can be purchased online or at local bookstores.

CBT in Schools

CBT is being used increasingly in schools to teach children how to deal with various issues, such as anger management, social skills, and emotional intelligence. It is becoming a standard part of the curriculum in schools nationwide. The use of CBT and other methods is increasing, and many teachers are now trained specifically to deliver this treatment when it's required.

Inpatient Rehabilitation Programs

CBT in acute care rehab programs for patients suffering from depression or anxiety disorders has been proven effective for reducing symptoms and improving functioning and quality of life. In addition, this approach is inexpensive and effectively reduces recidivism rates by allowing patients to address their issues while under close supervision.

Online CBT Programs

CBT is now being delivered using a variety of online platforms. These programs blend face-to-face therapy, video conferencing, and internet exposure techniques. Sometimes, the therapist will be local and available for a phone or Skype session whenever required. The patient can work through the material at their own pace, and the online program will automatically score them after each step so they can see where they are in the process at any time. This type of approach has the advantage of being relatively inexpensive and allows access to the therapist at any time.

CBT in Public Settings

CBT is now offered in public settings such as daycare centers, rehabilitation centers, prisons, and community mental health clinics. CBT works best when delivered to large groups of patients at once. This was first done by the Beck Institute in California and has now been expanded to many other countries worldwide. This method has also been proven effective in reducing recidivism by allowing patients to work through their issues under close supervision.

Parent-Child Relationship Therapy

A form of a family program initially developed by John Gottman, this therapy focuses on improving communication between parents and their children. It seeks to help parents understand their child's emotional needs, set clear boundaries regarding this behavior, improve communication skills and establish an emotional connection at home. The program also seeks to teach children fundamental skills for communicating effectively and appropriately, such as giving feedback, apologizing for mistakes, and accepting criticism.

A recent study has shown that the program can be used in the online environment to treat children with social anxiety issues. The program is designed for parents and children and uses a series of exercises to strengthen family relationships.

Cognitive behavioral therapy is based on a theory of maladaptive learning. It suggests that maladaptive behavior patterns are no more than faulty associations automatically learned by individuals as they cope with their day-to-day life experiences as they age. CBT aims to identify these patterns and provide strategies to change them into adaptive, healthy, productive behaviors and thoughts.

Many different therapies have used elements of CBT, but they are often not included in the therapeutic manual. Some examples of therapies that include cognitive behavioral therapy are rational emotive behavioral therapy, rational behavior therapy, cognitive integration, acceptance and commitment therapy, dialectic behavior therapy, and more. Cognitive Behavior Therapy differs from other types of psychotherapy because it focuses on the present behavior rather than the client's past experiences.

Cognitive Behavioral Therapy has been used to treat children as young as five. It was thought to be well suited for them because it was straightforward and practical. This treatment aims to change specific thought patterns and create healthier relationships among family members or peers.

There are several groups of cognitive distortions that CBT focuses on changing. They include:

CBT attempts to rewire the person's negative thinking style by providing them with strategies to identify and re-evaluate their negative biases and assumptions. Therefore, CBT aims to have a client or patient accept things and then make informed decisions rather than fall back on the inaccurate information they had previously.

Behavioral activation is often used to treat depression, anxiety, and phobias such as agoraphobia by encouraging clients and patients with these issues to engage in behaviors related to avoidance.

CBT Theory

Many therapists use CBT for conditions other than depression, anxiety, and phobias. CBT is a helpful treatment for many psychological disorders, but its specificity makes it most appropriate for treating depression and anxiety. This is because most forms of CBT are based on the theory of cognitive therapy and subsequent assumptions about depression and anxiety.

Similarly, to Beck's model, most modern CBT theories are based on the assumption that depression and anxiety result from negative thoughts about the self or others; what we think about ourselves or others can, in turn, lead to unhealthy thoughts and behaviors. For example, the belief that one is not good enough to get a job causes a person to think and act in ways that prevent them from getting the job. This culminates in feelings of depression and anxiety. The opposite applies if the person believes they are good enough for the job: a healthy set of thoughts and behaviors results in positive outcomes, preventing feelings of depression and anxiety.

CBT emphasizes how these thoughts lead to unhealthy behaviors. Still, it also allows therapists to examine dysfunctional emotions, which are negative emotions resulting from a thought process. This assumption allows CBT theories to distinguish between different types of depression and anxiety disorders and individuals with both types of disorders simultaneously.

CBT is a set of cognitive behavioral strategies that attempts to change dysfunctional thoughts and behaviors. To do this, therapists must use positive interventions and strategies (such as focusing on the present) while also being able to challenge dysfunctional thoughts and emotions.

Therapists believe that depression and anxiety result from negative thoughts about the self or others, which can lead people to act in unhealthy ways. Therapists are there to help patients identify these negative thoughts, evaluate them accurately, clarify the truthfulness of their beliefs, and replace them with healthy alternatives. These adaptive thoughts can then guide decisions about treatment options, decreasing feelings of depression or anxiety.

CBT is based on the cognitive model of emotional distress. This model consists of several interconnected components: the target (or client or patient), the event (sometimes called "stimulus"), the thoughts that follow, the feelings, and finally, behavior. The diagram below depicts this relationship.

CBT Practice

Many different therapies have used elements of CBT, but they are often not included in the therapeutic manual. Some examples of therapies that include cognitive behavioral therapy are rational emotive behavioral therapy, rational behavior therapy, cognitive integration, acceptance and commitment therapy, dialectic behavior therapy, and more. Cognitive Behavior Therapy differs from other types of psychotherapy because it focuses on the present behavior rather than the client's past experiences.

Basic assumptions or beliefs that comprise a large part of CBT theories make diagnoses more specific to certain disorders. This is important for therapists to consider when deciding which model to use in their case. In addition, CBT requires therapists to be able to make distinctions between several different types of depression and anxiety disorders.

Depression is a mental disorder in which people experience low mood (depressed), an inability to experience pleasure or both. Some people with depression may also have feelings of guilt, worthlessness, hopelessness, and suicidal thoughts. Common symptoms include anhedonia (lack of interest in enjoyable activities), problems with concentration and sleep, poor appetite, fatigue, or weight loss.

Constant sadness or hopelessness are associated with anxiety disorders. This includes an intense fear of anxiety ("Fear," panic attack), leading to an avoidance of anxiety-provoking situations ("Flight" response) and results in excessive worry ("Rumination" response).

CBT INTERVENTIONS

Cognitive Behavior Therapy is a type of psychotherapy developed to help people with various mental health disorders. It uses cognitive processes, such as thoughts and behaviors, to help change the way one's brain functions. This therapy has been proven effective for treating people suffering from anxiety, depression, insomnia, and panic disorders. In this book, we'll discuss how CBT interventions work to treat these conditions.

CBT interventions are often used for treating patients with mental health conditions such as anxiety disorders and depression by helping them become more aware of their negative and potentially destructive thoughts, which lead them towards emotions like fear or sadness. These interventions aim to replace these negative thought patterns with positive and constructive beliefs.

One of the most common CBT interventions is Cognitive Reframing, which involves examining their thoughts, feelings and negative behavior patterns to acknowledge them and then change them if necessary.

In some cases, Cognitive Behaviour Therapy may be used in conjunction with medications for treating mental health conditions such as depression as a stand-alone treatment or with traditional psychotherapy. However, it's essential that any woman who is pregnant, nursing, or thinking about becoming pregnant speak to her doctor before taking any medication.

Cognitive behavior therapy aims to help people with mental health conditions to recognize their negative thinking patterns and to see how those patterns directly influence their behavior and emotional state. For example, a person suffering from panic attacks might acknowledge that they tend to view even small physical sensations as dangerous; by practicing relaxation techniques, they may be able to re-train themselves from this negative thinking pattern. The goal, in general terms, is for people undergoing cognitive behavior therapy to learn more constructive ways of thinking about things and behaving. CBT interventions are most effective at treating patients with mental health conditions when the treatment is comprehensive.

What are Cognitive Behavioral interventions?

Cognitive behavioral interventions are a treatment system that focuses on helping people with mental health disorders change their behaviors and emotions by changing their internal thoughts. In CBT, we try to make the changes that would benefit your mental state, even if they don't seem evident at the time.

We used several methods, including prompts, self-help exercises, behavioral experiments, and thought records. These are all ways we can help you look more carefully at where your thoughts and behaviors are coming from so you can address them more effectively in the future.

Hopefully, with some guidance, you will be able to learn what to focus on and change to make your life better. Depending on your response, we may use several different CBT interventions or treatments for the same condition.

CBT interventions are used for many different purposes. The primary ones are self-help, promoting a more positive outlook, and helping with emotional well-being and behavior modification.

Cognitive behavioral therapy effectively treats anxiety disorders such as social anxiety, panic attacks, OCD, phobias, and post-traumatic stress disorder. It is also commonly used to treat depression, particularly in women during pregnancy and postpartum. However, it should be noted that CBT interventions do not work for everyone with these disorders. Still, it can be tremendously helpful for people without immediate access to therapy or medication.

CBT interventions include:

1. Thought records

A thought record is a tool designed to help you recognize your negative thinking patterns so that you can change them. You will be asked to record how you are feeling and what you are thinking about. This may seem like a simple task, but it can be difficult when we don't see our negative thoughts as problems or believe that those thoughts are ok. Thoughts should ideally not be treated like beliefs or facts but instead looked at and assessed for false, misleading, or distorted information.

With some practice, making a thought record may feel awkward at first, but after gaining some experience, it can become somewhat natural and enjoyable. Thought records may also be used to help you focus on the positive aspects of your life by recognizing and recording what you're feeling and thinking about. Thought records can be used for a variety of situations and purposes, such as:

a) How you feel about yourself or your life

b) Your relationship with others

c) Your religious, spiritual, or personal beliefs

d) What kinds of things make you feel the way you do?

2. The negative assumptions worksheet

In this worksheet, we will ask you to write down as many negative assumptions or expectations as you have about yourself and your life. These are things that you believe to be facts about yourself or others, even though they might not be accurate.

When doing the negative assumptions worksheet, most people have more difficulty with the positive listing of expectations, which is just as important. Therefore, when first completing this worksheet, it is a good idea to take your time, write down what you come up with, and don't be discouraged if it takes a few efforts before you feel like you've covered all of them. Moreover, once you've completed the worksheet, it is essential not to skip over any lines - instead, keep filling out the sheet.

3. Thought records manipulation

A thought record manipulation is designed to help you identify negative or generally unhelpful thoughts and patterns. For example, you may have some negative beliefs about yourself or others even though they are not true, and when these beliefs are set in stone, they can be challenging to change. For this kind of intervention to be effective in helping you alter your negative thinking patterns, you must recognize and acknowledge them.

For this reason, you are asked to think about a specific problem and write down your thoughts and feelings about it. The thought record manipulation helps you look at this information and put it into perspective to develop a more productive way of thinking.

4.   The ABC worksheet

The ABC worksheet is designed to help you identify what happens when you have certain emotions or moods. When we experience an emotion or feeling, we tend to attribute the emotion to something in particular. When we feel angry, for example, it may be because someone said something rude or because of some other outside stimulus; similarly, when we feel anxious or stressed out, it is often attributed to some environmental factor.

The ABC worksheet helps you to identify what makes you angry, anxious, or sad and why. These facts can be used to help you alter your moods or reactions in a healthy way so that they will not affect your everyday life in the way they do now.

5.   The relaxation response and breathing meditation

By learning to control your breathing, you can relax and calm down, even if you are having a difficult time doing so at the moment. The relaxation response is a state of deep relaxation achieved by short periods of controlled breathing.

Breathing more effectively can help us decrease physical and mental stress levels. Various breathing exercises help improve sleep, reduce pain, and ease feelings of anxiousness. These techniques include diaphragmatic breathing and tummo (Tibetan yoga breath).

6.   Metacognitive therapy

Metacognitive therapy (MCT) is a form of CBT concerned with how people think about their thinking. It is a popular treatment used primarily for anxiety disorders, but it can also be used for other conditions. For example, a person suffering from an anxiety disorder tends to worry excessively about what they believe could go wrong in their life. Even though some people may be more naturally prone to having these thoughts than others, a person can develop them through life experiences.

MCT helps people with anxiety disorders to understand how their current behaviors and fears prevent them from leading healthy, productive lives. As a result, it can help people reduce the intensity of their anxiety, learn how to relax, and handle stress in more productive ways. MCT also helps the person recognize that they are not alone in thinking these thoughts, that they are common and other people have them too; this realization often helps individuals feel less isolated and therefore less depressed or anxious.

7.   Cognitive behavioral therapy

Cognitive behavioral therapy (CBT) is a treatment that is effective in treating many psychological conditions. CBT aims to provide people with a way of thinking about the problems in their lives that will help them progress towards their goals, no matter how large, small or irrelevant they may seem.

In CBT, people are encouraged to recognize and acknowledge disturbing thoughts and beliefs to learn how to imagine different scenarios and how they might affect their lives. This helps people identify situations in which they might otherwise be anxious or stressed so that they are more likely to cope with them by trying new coping strategies instead of taking on unwanted behavior.

8. Mindfulness and acceptance

Mindfulness and acceptance are two common approaches to CBT that are also used to treat several psychological disorders. The purpose of mindfulness is to help people become more aware of how they react to their thoughts and feelings and stop identifying these reactions as being outside their control. For example, if you feel anxious about speaking in front of an audience, this anxiety may result from an issue with your self-confidence or performance, but you might see this feeling as your fault. The idea is that the more you become aware of these reactions, the less they will influence your behavior.

With acceptance, people are taught to accept their thoughts and feelings instead of trying to change them. This approach can be helpful for people with anxiety disorders who are bothered by a constant flow of intrusive thoughts. The idea is that the more you practice accepting these thoughts, the less they will bother you.

9. Cognitive therapies

Cognitive therapy seeks to help individuals change their thought processes to form more rational and realistic beliefs about their lives and the future. This typically involves learning how to use your memory well to recognize distorted or mistaken information you may have been receiving.

The goal of cognitive therapy is to help people learn how to focus their attention on events that are important to them and those that are not. For example, a person with an anxiety disorder might focus on the thoughts and feelings they associate with worrying about something happening in their lives, when there is nothing of importance to worry about. Unfortunately, this distraction from more essential hassles prevents people from focusing on more positive aspects of their lives.

Cognitive therapy can also help people make more effective judgments about the future by helping them become aware of how they think about events in their past and present.

10. Psychodynamic therapy

Psychodynamic therapy focuses on improving a person's sense of well-being by teaching them how to make the most of their inner resources and strengths instead of focusing on their weaknesses. This approach is often used for people who feel anxious about things that are out of their immediate control, such as people who are afraid of contracting HIV or other infectious diseases or a person who feels uncomfortable going out to meet new people because they do not know how to behave in social situations.

This treatment teaches people that specific thoughts and feelings are irrational and harmful, but they tend to experience them anyway. In addition, this approach helps change how these thoughts come to be or create new ways of reassuring themselves that they are not as stressed or upset as they are experiencing.

11. Rational emotive therapy

Rational emotive therapy (RET) focuses on helping people with frightening thoughts and feelings by helping them challenge their negative beliefs about the situations that cause them to fear. This approach has been used successfully with various anxiety disorders, such as phobias, panic attacks and PTSD, because it helps people understand that their irrational fears do not have to be true for them to feel anxious and stressed.

RET aims to help people become more self-aware and recognize the irrational thoughts they have that cause their anxiety in the first place. This approach is beneficial for people who tend to be extra cautious about controlling the situations that make them worried or anxious.

12. Experiential therapy

Experiential therapy, also called exposure therapy, helps people learn how to tolerate the things they fear without succumbing to them. This treatment is beneficial for people with phobias who fear certain situations or objects, such as a person who is afraid of dogs or a spider; it can also be used for those afraid of heights, enclosed spaces, or flying.

This type of therapy focuses on exposing people to the type of situations they fear as often as they feel they can handle them. For example, if a person is afraid of dogs and is struggling to walk by one, they may be required to walk by a dog on their way to work slowly. If this causes anxiety, they could be taught to walk through the dog in question and keep walking.

13. Acceptance and commitment to therapy

Acceptance and commitment therapy (ACT) takes a more direct approach to examining how people react when confronted with troubling thoughts that normally trigger their anxiety. This therapy is particularly useful for those who feel overwhelmed by guilt or shame but struggle to actively express these emotions to others.

ACT encourages people with anxiety disorders and phobias to think about situations that give rise to the feelings of guilt or shame they are experiencing. This approach helps them work through the thoughts that cause their anxiety and change how they express these emotions.

14. Dialectics

Dialectics is a branch of learning theory that teaches people how to learn better by actively engaging in dialogue with others. This approach identifies ways in which people can challenge their ideas by first becoming aware of why they feel the way they do about certain subjects.

Dialectics helps people recognize and become aware of the various emotional and cognitive processes that cause them to be stressed when faced with certain situations or events. By recognizing these thoughts, people can identify situations that cause them stress and then decide whether or not they are worth worrying about.

15. Transcendental meditation

Transcendental meditation (TM) is a unique form of treatment that uses a series of words known as mantras while sitting in a comfortable position to help you achieve complete mental stillness. This program works by using positive affirmations or thoughts that can be said to oneself to improve your state of mind and remind you of a beneficial feeling or situation.

Though there are some similarities between transcendental meditation and other therapy programs, such as Cognitive Behavioral Therapy and Cognitive Therapy, it has a unique philosophical basis that centers on self-regulation. TM teaches people how to regulate their thoughts and feelings to become more aware of how they think about certain situations.

How do these CBT interventions work?

CBT interventions work by helping people gain insight into the thoughts, feelings, and behaviors that are causing them anxiety or stress.

Reality therapy can help people gain insight into how they react to social situations by teaching them to become aware of their thought patterns and how they make judgments about the future.

Dialectics works by helping people examine the thoughts that cause their anxiety and stress rather than relying on listening to their irrational beliefs.

Acceptance and commitment therapy helps people learn how to regulate their emotions by identifying situations in which they feel anxious. For example, a person could be taught to focus on one thing at a time instead of trying to accomplish multiple tasks simultaneously during stressful times.

Transcendental meditation helps people become aware of the negative thoughts that cause them anxiety by helping them gain a sense of stillness in their minds, allowing them to identify this negative thinking more easily.

Overcoming anxiety and stress is a challenge that requires the help of a trained mental health professional. Some people with anxiety disorders may be able to overcome them alone by using anxiety self-help strategies and therapy, such as CBT. However, more people benefit from the help of a therapist trained in CBT interventions and other anxiety-related treatments. This can include Cognitive Behavioral Therapy (CBT) and other forms of psychotherapy for anxiety disorders, such as psychodynamic therapy and client-centered therapy.

These interventions have been proven effective in treating anxiety disorders and can help people overcome their fears, worries, and feelings of panic. Moreover, there are many other ways people can learn to manage their anxiety and stress, including professional anxiety treatment, acupuncture treatments, exercise, and medication.

Even though hundreds of different types of anxiety disorders can affect people in specific ways, the good news is that many different types of interventions are available to help overcome these fears. Learn more about how you can get help for your anxiety or stress-related condition by speaking with a mental health professional today.

CBT is a therapeutic approach that employs skills to manage to worry, stress, and other symptoms associated with psychological disorders. CBT is effective in the treatment of a variety of psychological conditions, including panic disorder, generalized anxiety disorder (GAD), social anxiety disorder, obsessive-compulsive disorder (OCD), post-traumatic stress disorder (PTSD), depression, personality disorders, and eating disorders.

Some CBT interventions are generally preferred over others because they have been proven more effective in treating certain disorders and episodes of anxiety than other similar approaches. However, the overall effectiveness of CBT, as well as whether a particular intervention is more or less effective than others, depends on a variety of factors, including the severity and duration of emotional disorder symptoms experienced by the patient, their experiences, and personal history with emotional disorders, cognitive abilities, personality traits and previous treatments they have received.

CBT interventions involve different strategies designed to assist people experiencing mental health problems such as stress or anxiety by working with them to overcome their feelings of distress or reduce their reliance on irrational beliefs that may be causing symptoms.

CBT interventions also involve techniques designed to change people's thoughts, feelings, and behavior. For instance, some interventions focus on helping people understand how their feelings and thoughts are causing symptoms such as anxiety, depression, or irritability. Other interventions help people to identify and make positive changes in their thoughts, beliefs, and behaviors that may prevent them from experiencing mental health problems in the first place.

CBT does not only involve behavioral changes such as changing your diet. It includes several other strategies to change your thoughts to feel less anxious and stressed. CBT encourages people to think positively about themselves rather than focusing on negative experiences in their life. Changing how you think about yourself is changing how you feel, which can help improve almost all symptoms of psychological disorders.

CBT interventions are not for everyone. They can be very challenging and require dedication and commitment from the person receiving CBT interventions to overcome their feelings of distress, anxiety, and irrational beliefs. In addition, some people do not enjoy being made to change the way they think and behave because they would instead continue in their old way of thinking or behaving, which may have been causing them problems in the past.

CBT is based on the idea that it is possible to change how we think about ourselves and our environment by changing our behavior and helping us take positive steps towards improving our life situations.

Trained psychologists can use CBT interventions with people experiencing mental health problems, especially those experiencing anxiety and stress. These psychologists can also employ behavioral therapy techniques that are not part of traditional CBT interventions but are similar, such as cognitive restructuring.

Cognitive restructuring involves a person changing their beliefs about themselves or the world by challenging their irrational beliefs or challenging their negative self-talk. For example, a person suffering from depression may challenge the negative thinking they have associated with feeling depressed to improve their mood.

Cognitive restructuring is often used with other CBT interventions to make them more effective. This can include changes in a person's behavior learned by practicing different skills during CBT sessions.

CBT interventions can be tailored to the needs of a particular person and are designed to help you understand your feelings and thoughts and how these are causing your psychological difficulties.

Some people may benefit from receiving CBT interventions over a more extended period than others, depending on the severity and duration of their symptoms and their ability to cope with their anxiety or stress. Other people can benefit from receiving just one CBT intervention and then being referred to a psychologist for further counseling to address their psychological needs.

CBT is a very practical approach for treating many mental health problems because it focuses on helping you understand your feelings and thoughts and how these feelings and thoughts are causing your irrational beliefs. In addition, by understanding how these feelings, thoughts, and beliefs are all connected, you can begin to work on changing them so you feel less anxious or stressed in the future.

Post-traumatic stress disorder (PTSD) is a type of anxiety disorder that can develop following the experience or witnessing of a terrifying event. The type of event that triggers PTSD can vary and may be directly experienced, witnessed, or even learned about.

The symptoms of PTSD are wide-ranging and include emotional distress, mood changes, increased or decreased arousal, and changes in sleeping patterns or a combination of these symptoms. These symptoms can also vary from person to person, depending on the trauma they have been exposed to.

Those people experiencing PTSD feel emotionally distressed and re-experience their traumatic event over time as if it were happening all over again. Often people with PTSD experience "flashbacks" where they feel as if they are experiencing their traumatic event all over again, as well as nightmares where they dream about aspects of their traumatic event.

Essentially, PTSD is a psychological reaction to an experience that has been difficult or even traumatic to cope with. This means it can develop as a response to any event, such as witnessing, taking part in, or experiencing physical violence, abuse, terrorist attacks, or natural disasters. Often anxiety disorders develop after trauma individuals receive little support and hope from others regarding their experiences, which can lead to PTSD.

PTSD is often associated with other mental health problems, such as depression and anxiety. Cognitive Behavioral Therapy (CBT) is an effective treatment for people with PTSD by helping them learn how to change their thoughts about themselves and their traumatic experiences to find more effective coping methods.

Cognitive Behavioral Therapy can help people with phobias because it helps them to:

Learn how to understand better the thoughts and feelings that cause their fears and phobias.

Identify maladaptive thought patterns which make the fear worse. For example, a person afraid of dogs may believe that all dogs are dangerous, even though they have not come into contact with any hurtful dogs in the past.

Learn how to better deal with their fear by facing the object of their fear and reducing their triggers, such as eating disorders.

So, cognitive behavioral therapy is a type of psychotherapy that can help you understand where irrational beliefs or thought patterns are causing your stress and anxiety to teach you new ways of coping with them.

To be most effective, CBT interventions need to be tailored to the individual's experiences and personality. This means that these interventions are likely to be conducted by a trained mental health professional who will ask questions about your thoughts, feelings, and behaviors to help you understand where your negative thinking patterns are coming from.

What are CBT interventions used for?

CBT interventions are used for a wide range of psychological problems. These include:

Cognitive behavioral therapy is used to help people understand the relationship between their thoughts and feelings, how their thoughts and feelings are related to their behaviors, and how they can change these cognitions to feel more relaxed and cope better with their emotions.

Developing a greater understanding of your thoughts, emotions, and behaviors is often the first step in positively changing them. The CBT interventions will then help you learn new ways of coping with anxiety or stress by focusing on specific skills that need improving or other areas where changes may be beneficial.

Learning these new coping methods will help you become more confident in managing your emotions rather than relying on other people for support. CBT interventions encourage you to take control of your own emotions rather than leaving them under the control of other people.

This approach may be particularly helpful for people experiencing stress, anxiety, or depression if they wish to feel more in control over their emotions and reactions. However, if you regularly feel anxious, stressed, or depressed, it is best to discuss your concerns with a trained professional who can carefully consider the specifics of your case and provide you with the appropriate CBT interventions.

CBT can also be helpful for people experiencing depression, anxiety, or stress if they are unable to cope with their emotions, either due to a lack of understanding about their thoughts and feelings or because their thoughts and emotions are causing them excessive levels of grief.

Many different types of CBT interventions are available depending on the specific issues that need to be addressed. For example, there are various interventions for anxiety disorders, such as panic disorder, generalized anxiety disorder, specific phobias (such as fear of dogs), and social anxiety disorder.

Therapy for generalized anxiety disorder (GAD), a chronic and excessive worry about everyday problems and life in general, is intended to help you understand how your thoughts cause you to feel anxious and act in ways that worsen your problems. In addition, these interventions will help you learn new coping methods so that you can better manage your emotions without allowing your worrying to create more problems.

There are also different interventions for specific phobias, such as fear of heights or public speaking. These interventions teach you how to change your thought patterns so that you see the object of your phobia as a regular everyday occurrence rather than something which causes excessive fear and anxiety.

Psychotherapy interventions for social anxiety disorder are intended to help you feel more comfortable in social situations. These interventions often include exercises where you practice your skills in a safe environment, such as with a trained therapist, so that you become more confident using them alone.

Psychotherapy interventions can also be tailored to people experiencing stress, anxiety, or depression and wishing to develop new ways of managing their emotions and feelings. This can be particularly helpful for people experiencing difficulty when it comes to expressing their emotions, such as bottling them up rather than sharing them with trusted friends or family members.

Psychotherapy interventions can help you learn ways of expressing your emotions and thoughts to manage intense or overwhelming feelings better.

CBT interventions can help you deal with your problems, even if they aren't related to feelings of anxiety or stress. Once you understand how your negative thoughts and feelings are causing you trouble, CBT interventions can help you develop better ways of coping with feeling more relaxed and confident in managing your emotions and reactions.

CBT interventions can help you better understand your thoughts and emotions and become more confident in managing them. This is often the first step in learning how to cope with your problems and prevent them from worsening, which can make you less stressed, anxious, or depressed in the future.

Disadvantages of CBT interventions

Despite the many benefits CBT interventions can provide, they have some limitations. These include:

a. CBT interventions are often only as effective as the skills you learn. Without these skills, CBT interventions may not achieve their full potential

b. Some people may not benefit from CBT interventions in certain circumstances or because they do not fit their situation or personality. For example, some people may already have a strong support network in place, so there is less need for them to develop their coping strategies. Others may be too attached to traditional psychotherapy and resist learning new ways of thinking about their problems. In these cases, it is best to consult with a trained professional who can provide an alternative approach suited to your needs

c. CBT interventions may not be effective for people with severe mental health problems or substance use issues. For these cases, it may be best first to consult a trained professional who can determine if inpatient treatment is necessary or if there are other ways of helping you address your issues

d. Some people may be uncomfortable with the idea of psychotherapy and believe that their problems don't need "fixing" or would instead learn new coping mechanisms on their terms. Since CBT is mainly about learning to cope with your own emotions, it may not be a practical approach for these people.

CBT interventions are a middle ground between traditional psychotherapy and more practical approaches like cognitive behavioral therapy. In the past, therapists were only trained to provide long-term psychotherapy interventions that help patients explore their thought patterns and identify areas where they may be causing problems. This was often beneficial for those experiencing severe mental health issues which needed long-term therapeutic support and guidance to learn the skills necessary to cope with their problems. However, this approach may not be appropriate for people who want to learn new coping strategies or manage their problems.

CBT interventions are also a valuable complement to psychotherapy interventions, especially for people with milder anxiety disorders struggling to manage their symptoms even with the traditional techniques that therapists have been trained in. In addition, CBT interventions can help you learn better ways of dealing with your emotions and thoughts in different situations to develop more effective techniques when facing similar future situations.

CBT interventions are also helpful in helping you manage your other problems related to mood and mental health rather than just anxiety or depression. Many different types of CBT interventions exist, each with its benefits. This means a CBT intervention is available to help you deal with any problem you are experiencing.

The most accurate way to determine the best type of CBT intervention is by consulting a trained professional who can carefully consider your specific situation and provide the appropriate interventions to help you feel better and manage your emotions effectively in the future.

BASIC CBT FRAMEWORK

Cognitive behavior therapy is a form of psychotherapy that aims to change thoughts and behaviors by addressing their underlying cognitive processes. It has been applied to many disorders, but treating anxiety and depressive disorders is the most well-known.

It is based on the theory that thoughts are triggered in response to events/situations, including bodily sensations, memories, or questions. These thoughts often (but not always) lead to feelings such as anxiety or depression.

For instance, when one is alone in a room, one may think, "what if someone comes in." This thought may make them feel anxious. They may think: "I must be experiencing a heart attack" (because they feel so anxious). This thought makes them feel more anxious.

However, if they think: "It's okay to be anxious sometimes." They may then feel better. It is important to note that these thoughts are automatically triggered by the situation and are not consciously chosen by the person. However, people can learn that their thoughts follow a certain pattern and eventually challenge their automatic negative thoughts with alternative/positive thoughts.

In cognitive-behavior therapy (CBT), patients are taught to challenge their automatic negative thoughts with alternative/positive thoughts, to address their anxiety and depression. By changing how they think about themselves and how they interpret their experiences, the patient can change their emotional response. As the patients' anxiety begins to decrease, they can also use this new barrier to manage physical symptoms of anxiety (such as trembling or sweating).

Four principles underlie the cognitive-behavioral model. They include (1) automatic thoughts, (2) dysfunctional attitudes, (3) core beliefs, and (4) self-esteem.

The first principle is automatic thoughts. These thoughts occur in reaction to an event/situation before we even have time to think about them. They are sometimes called "hot" thoughts because they are elicited by something in the environment. For example, one may feel a sensation and then experience a negative thought (e.g., hot flashes). Automatic negative thoughts tend to be highly exaggerated or unrealistic.

The second principle is dysfunctional attitudes. These negative beliefs result from one's automatic thoughts and responses. Negative attitudes (e.g., "I am worthless") can lead to self-destructive behavior, such as alcohol or drug abuse or severe depression in the patient. Self-esteem is a term used to describe a person's positive views about themselves, their abilities, and their beliefs about the world.

The third principle is core beliefs. They are statements that persist over time despite contrary evidence because they have been formed with strong emotion by using logic when forming them initially (e.g., "I am helpless" and "I will never be happy"). These core beliefs tend to be negative and can make people feel fearful, anxious, and worried about certain situations.

The fourth principle is self-esteem. It is a person's overall evaluation of their worth, including their actions and attitudes; it is often used synonymously with the term "self-worth." Self-esteem affects how people interact with others, cope with problems, and handle criticism. It can change in reaction to positive or negative events in one's life (e.g., being praised or criticized). Self-esteem is an important concept when dealing with depression because research has shown that when self-esteem goes down, depression increases.

Cognitive-behavioral therapies can treat various disorders, including somatic anxiety – anxiety rooted in the feeling of physical symptoms triggered by an event/situation. For instance, a person may experience the sensation of cold, then feel anxious about the sensation that occurs. Another example would be getting stressed when seeing a spider in their room at night. The patient must learn to recognize these somatic sensations and challenge their automatic negative thoughts with alternative/positive thoughts (e.g., "It's okay to get cold sometimes.").

Consequently, there are different phases of the CBT framework, such as:

Phase one: assessment

This phase includes a detailed clinical evaluation to determine the type of disorder the patient suffers from. The evaluation includes questions about the patient's symptoms, social and occupational functioning, history of mental disorders, and personality. In addition, the patient's negative automatic thoughts are identified, and the consequences of these thoughts are assessed. The patient is also asked to complete a questionnaire regarding their negative beliefs such as "I am helpless," "I will never be happy," etc. Cognitive-behavioral therapy generally includes many sessions with the patient and the therapist.

Assessment first looks at the patient's symptoms and underlying beliefs. The therapist then asks the patient to complete self-report measures of their negative thoughts, feelings, and behaviors (such as the Beck Depression Inventory). These measures give the therapist important information regarding how much thought problems contribute to a patient's referral symptoms. Moreover, the patient learns what is causing the symptoms and why. As the patient's negative automatic thoughts and feelings decrease, they learn that they can cope with situations better.

Consequently, recovery in CBT involves the establishment of new beliefs, behaviors, and value systems that are more congruent with who the person wants to be. This will also lead to increased self-esteem and decreased feelings of helplessness.

This phase is essential since it allows the patient to understand the triggers and consequences of their maladaptive beliefs. It is also important because it gives patients time to recognize their maladaptive thoughts and practice coping with these situations. In addition, these beliefs are now so patients can apply them in the future.

Moreover, assessment is important since it gives the patient a chance to think about how they see themselves and how others view them. This helps the patient change negative perceptions about themselves, develop more effective coping strategies for dealing with their emotions, and learn to accept that other people have different opinions than theirs. The assessment also includes a medical history and clinical interview for physical causes of symptoms. Therefore, there is a need for accurate, thorough, and consistent assessment before proceeding to the next phase.

Phase two: re-conceptualization

The second phase involves the re-conceptualization processes. This is the stage where patients learn about their negative thoughts and how distorted they are. Patients also develop alternative, positive thoughts and other ways to cope with their stressors/situations to help decrease negative symptoms. Re-conceptualization includes:

a.   Identifying the negative thoughts:

This phase is important because it allows patients to identify their automatic thoughts and underlying meanings.

b.   Identifying the negative emotions:

This process is important because it allows patients to recognize how these distorted thoughts can lead to maladaptive behaviors, such as depression. It also allows the patient to develop coping strategies for dealing with their stressors/situations. For example, if a patient feels hopeless and helpless in a situation, they can talk with someone about it or try to find another solution for this problem. In addition, self-monitoring is another tool patients can use to recognize their automatic thoughts and develop a plan of action based on those thoughts.

c.   Identifying the consequences of negative thoughts:

This is important for patients to see how their distorted beliefs can contribute to their symptoms and feelings of hopelessness, helplessness, and worthlessness. Patients learn to be successful by accepting that they can change negative thought patterns and learn to use alternative positive behaviors. They also begin to see that other people have different opinions, which will help them accept other people's opinions without feeling threatened or rejected.

d.   Identifying alternative, positive thoughts:

This is important because it allows patients to develop alternative ways of thinking about themselves and more healthy and realistic situations. As a result, patients come up with alternative beliefs regarding themselves and their patients, which leads to a self-esteem increase that helps them deal with situations more healthily. Furthermore, patients learn more effective ways of coping with their negative feelings and stressors.

e.   Developing alternative behaviors and coping strategies:

CBT can be beneficial because it helps patients develop alternative and positive behaviors that are more congruent with their characteristics, values, and needs for attention. In addition, the patient learns how to better manage their emotions by developing new coping methods (such as actively seeking out sick leave or talking to someone). The goal is for the patient to learn that they can change or cope with situations without needing medication. This phase is important for identifying the patient's negative thoughts, beliefs, and consequences of their maladaptive thinking. It is also important because it allows patients to view other options as ways to cope with situations. In addition, this phase allows the patient to learn that they can change and cope with situations independently without medication. This helps them develop self-esteem so they can deal with situations more positively.

Re-conceptualization involves the identification of maladaptive thoughts, emotions, and consequences. For example, if the patient believes they are not good enough or unlovable, they may feel and act differently in the future. These maladaptive beliefs can contribute to symptoms such as depression and suicide attempts. In addition, this phase involves identifying alternative ideas that are more congruent with the patient's positive characteristics. These positive ideas help diminish maladaptive thoughts and increase self-esteem. By recognizing the negative effects of these distorted beliefs, patients better understand their emotions and behaviors to change their ways of coping with stressors/situations. In addition, patients learn more effective ways to cope with their emotions and dissociation thoughts.

In general, re-conceptualization is when patients learn to change the meaning of their thoughts by recognizing the negative consequences of their distorted beliefs. It involves identifying the beliefs and negative emotions that lead to maladaptive behaviors such as depression and mood swings. The goal is to develop new ideas congruent with their positive characteristics. In addition, this phase involves identifying alternative ways a patient can cope with stressors/situations on their own without overusing medication. It also involves learning more effective coping strategies for dealing with stressors/situations. Finally, this phase involves the patient accepting the idea that they can successfully change their behaviors, thoughts, and emotions by not over-relying on medication. It is important to identify when patients over-rely on medication because this can lead to negative consequences by inhibiting their natural ability to cope with stressful situations.

Re-conceptualization helps patients develop positive traits to become more optimistic, stable, and coherent. Generally, re-conceptualization is important for developing positive characteristics that will help increase coping skills, reduce maladaptive thoughts/behaviors and alleviate symptoms of mental illness. In addition, it is important because it helps patients realize how they can successfully change their maladaptive thinking and behaviors. Finally, this phase involves re-conceptualizing thoughts, behaviors, and emotions to deal with situations more healthily without medication, which helps patients develop self-esteem.

Therefore, this phase is important because it allows patients to learn alternative beliefs, behaviors, and coping skills to help them overcome and manage their symptoms. It also increases self-esteem, which helps the patient cope with negative feelings and stressors/situations healthier. This phase is important for eliminating distorted thoughts, accepting other people's opinions, and learning how to cope with emotions healthily.

Although this phase is important because it helps patients realize alternative ways of thinking and behaving, one may argue that it is also unrealistic. Many people believe that medication should always be given to patients, no matter how much they believe it does not provide any real help. This may be true because a patient may become dependent on the use of stimulant medication and other psychiatric drugs to provide relief from symptoms and behaviors. In addition to this, many people believe that the patients will not benefit from CBT because it can lead to anxiety and stress for the patient. Therefore, psychotherapists, psychiatrists, family members, and friends must educate themselves about alternative treatments for patients with mental illness before choosing between two treatment options. Moreover, patients must be educated about the benefits of both treatments to make informed decisions when choosing treatment options. The process of CBT can be time-consuming, but many believe it is beneficial to learn new ways of thinking and to behave to become more stable, coherent, and healthy.

Phase three: skills acquisition

This phase generally involves the patient learning alternative ways to cope with stressful situations. This can be accomplished by learning new ways of thinking concerning the patient's symptoms (to learn healthier alternative definitions and behaviors). This allows for more mature and effective ways of coping with stressful situations. However, this may be difficult if a person feels that their maladaptive thoughts are realistic or accurate. This can be accomplished by identifying alternative ways they can cope with stressful situations, including practicing healthy behaviors such as seeking treatment at their local mental health clinic. In addition, this phase involves the patient learning new skills to help them maintain a stable lifestyle by reducing maladaptive behaviors such as excessive drinking or medication intake. For example, a patient may learn to find new ways of coping with stressful situations and emotions that decrease the risk of relapse of symptoms. An example of this would be if a patient drinks too much alcohol; they could understand that they have developed a negative thought such as "I drink too much, I'm worthless as a person, I am an alcoholic" or another maladaptive thought and ask someone for help (ex: their therapist or psychiatrist).

In addition, patients can work on developing alternative ways to cope with the symptom by learning new skills to decrease maladaptive thoughts, emotions, and behaviors, such as recognizing that these thoughts are not factual and in tune with reality. Moreover, patients can work on developing coping skills by learning new alternative ways that they can think and behave to reduce stress and negative emotions. However, this may be difficult because some patients have redefined their maladaptive thoughts as realistic, believing that their negative thoughts are accurate. In addition, some patients may have unrealistic thought patterns that cannot be changed. For example, some people may believe they are superior or inferior to others based on their race or social class, which cannot be changed. In general, this phase involves the patient accepting new ways of thinking and behaving to help them become more stable and reduce symptoms of mental illness to lead a more coherent lifestyle.

In addition, this phase is important because it teaches the patient to cope with stressors and symptoms of mental illness by learning new skills. It is important to note that patients are not taught how to cope with stressors while in the hospital or taking medication. Therefore, this phase helps develop coping skills to help prevent relapse and undesirable consequences of mental illness. Although the process is time-consuming, many patients believe it is beneficial because it helps them develop useful skills that will help them manage their symptoms more effectively without medication. Moreover, some may argue that teaching patients how to cope with mental illness is unnecessary because patients can learn how to cope with stressors independently, and psychiatric drugs will help them cope with the stressors and symptoms of mental illness.

In addition, this phase may be important in helping the patient develop a relationship with the therapist or psychiatrist they seek treatment from. This is because they are working together to overcome the symptoms of their mental illness. This phase may also be beneficial because it allows patients to express themselves more effectively and helps them deal with their emotions healthily. These new coping skills can help organize behaviors and thoughts that will allow patients to lead healthier lifestyles, leading them toward recovery. To help the patient reach this stage, the therapist or psychiatrist must know about alternative mental illness treatments.

However, this phase is difficult because there may be a lack of communication between patients and their therapist or psychiatrist due to different cultures and values. This can be overcome if the therapist is well-versed in alternative treatments for mental illness, such as CBT, and understands that alternative treatment does not necessarily mean that a patient will become dependent on medication. Some argue that care should always be provided to patients with mental illness regardless of their treatment (such as medication). Others argue that care should not always be provided because it contributes to dependency, stigma, and lack of recovery.

This phase involves the patient learning alternative ways to cope with stressful situations and symptoms of mental illness through different methods such as cognitive restructuring and new behaviors. The patient can communicate more effectively with their therapist or psychiatrist through these new techniques.

Moreover, these skills help patients reorganize their thoughts and behaviors, which helps them recover from symptoms of mental illness. However, this phase may be difficult for some patients because some cultural values and beliefs may not be compatible. This can be overcome by being well-versed in alternative treatment methods (such as CBT) and how they can benefit the patient's recovery process.

In addition, this phase requires a patient to believe that mental illness is biological and treatable. However, some argue that this belief may be inaccurate because mental illness may not be biological. However, these patients understand that symptoms of mental illness are caused by their thoughts and behaviors, and they do not have any other explanation for why they have symptoms of mental illness. Moreover, these patients understand that if they continue to drink alcohol, they will develop another mental illness, such as alcoholism. However, this phase is difficult for these patients because they often believe that their symptoms are always caused by their lifestyle and their current environment. This can be overcome by educating patients on the importance of healthy lifestyle choices and encouraging them to increase control over their thoughts and behaviors.

This involves prescribing medication to help control symptoms of mental illness. In general, people tend to receive psychotropic medication for their symptoms of mental illness to be controlled. In addition, patients need to receive psychotropic medications to treat future relapse or undesirable side effects to get better results from treatment and reach a positive outcome.

Phase four: skills consolidation and application

This phase involves the patient becoming more independent because they have learned effective coping skills to manage their symptoms of mental illness without medication. Medicine can still be prescribed to help reduce symptoms; however, patients often believe medication is unnecessary because they have learned healthy methods to cope effectively.

This phase is difficult for some patients because if they are not complying with the prescription, it may be viewed as a failure on their part as a patient. However, this phase benefits patients because it helps them become more independent and healthier. For example, the patient may learn how to avoid or reduce stressors or situations that trigger anxiety and other symptoms of mental illness. Patients may also learn new behaviors (e.g., physical activity) that can help reduce symptoms of mental illness.

Furthermore, this phase is important because it helps the patient realize that their symptoms of mental illness are real and that they need to take control of them. Patients usually believe it is best to avoid symptoms rather than manage them. For example, patients may use alcohol to suppress stress instead of communicating with others if they find the situation stressful or confront the person causing the stressful situation. Moreover, these coping skills can help organize behaviors and thoughts, allowing patients to lead healthier lifestyles and prevent relapse more effectively than medication.

Therefore, this phase is beneficial for patients because it helps them develop the necessary skills to prevent relapse and the undesirable consequences of relapse more effectively than medication does.

Skills consolidation is important because this stage is where patients develop the necessary skills to prevent relapse and undesirable consequences related to relapse more effectively. For example, the patient learns new ways of coping with symptoms, such as using relaxation exercises instead of drinking alcohol. In addition, the patient learns to use stress management techniques, such as meditation, breathing exercises, and physical activity. These skills help the patient relieve symptoms triggered by stressful situations and reduce the overall negative impact of stressors on the body. As a result, patients feel more in control of their mental illness because they have learned to manage symptoms without medication rather than just suppressing them.

In addition, this phase requires patients to comply with their treatment plan and continue taking medication for a specified period. Many believe patients should take their medication as prescribed instead of "gambling" with their mental health. The patient needs to have a strong desire to get better because they must follow the prescribed exercise plan, which may include taking medication for some time. Nonetheless, this phase requires the patient to comply with medication to get better results from treatment and reach a positive outcome instead of focusing on symptoms of mental illness or relapse. Furthermore, medications should be taken as prescribed because they play an integral role in successful recovery by controlling symptoms and preventing relapse.

This phase is difficult for patients because it requires them to understand that the medication works slowly. However, this phase can be overcome by educating patients on the benefits of medication, how their body processes medications, and why it takes time to see results from treatment.

This is important because patients need to learn what causes relapse and how to prevent it. Patients who use alcohol or drugs in this stage are more likely to relapse than those who do not.

Therefore, this phase helps prevent relapse because people are on medications for a specified period instead of "gambling" with their mental health and experiencing undesirable relapse-related consequences. Furthermore, it improves compliance with treatment and increases the quality of life while managing symptoms of mental illness.

A medical home expands the medical system where all aspects of care are considered to ensure that the patient receives quality, safe and coordinated care. Inclusion of mental health professionals in the medical home is possible as long as they work within a multidisciplinary team with physicians, nurses, and other health professionals who provide highly effective care.

The usual starting point for a person with a medical illness is the office visit, where the patient meets with a physician who examines them and determines if their condition needs to be addressed. If not, the patient might be referred back to their primary care physician or direct primary care physician, depending upon which doctor visits first.

Skills application is important because it allows patients to apply skills learned in earlier phases to do better without symptoms of mental illness. Furthermore, this phase helps people learn how to manage symptoms without medication or with less medication.

This phase is difficult for patients because they may not remember how to use their coping skills when applying them to daily activities or situations. However, this can be overcome by using relaxation techniques and practicing new coping skills in stressful situations. Furthermore, a patient can use the support of their family and friends to help them apply their learned coping skills to stressful situations in their daily life, thereby preventing relapse more effectively than medication does.

This phase is important because it helps patients maintain progress through continued self-care, monitoring, and skills. This ensures that the patient will not relapse for a long period. In addition, this phase gives patients the chance to learn to manage symptoms of mental illness more effectively than medication does.

This is a difficult phase for patients because they must stick with their treatment plan and avoid situations and circumstances that could cause relapse or the undesirable consequences related to relapse.

Therefore, that phase is important because it helps improve compliance with treatment by enhancing motivation and dedication to get better without symptoms of mental illness or with fewer symptoms or medication than before treatment started.

This is the most important phase because it helps patients avoid relapse and the undesirable consequences related to relapse and improves compliance with treatment. In addition, this phase enables patients to stick with their treatment plan, including abstaining from alcohol or drugs.

This is important because it helps maintain the gains achieved in earlier phases and leaves patients more in control of their mental illness. Therefore, it helps people learn how to manage symptoms without medication or with less medication.

In addition, drug holidays can be taken to help control symptoms of mental illness and prevent relapse. Furthermore, this final phase allows people to learn how to feel better by managing symptoms with fewer medications than before treatment began.

Phase five: generalization and maintenance

Treatment is not complete until the skills a patient has learned and practiced in earlier phases are applied to future situations. Therefore, when a patient leaves an inpatient or outpatient facility, their treatment provider needs to assist them with generalization to ensure that they do better at home rather than worse.

This phase is more important because it enables patients to apply their coping skills and learn how to cope with symptoms without medication or with less medication. Therefore, it helps people do better without symptoms of mental illness or with fewer symptoms or medication than before treatment started.

This phase may be difficult for people who are not as motivated to do better, but it is necessary for their mental illness. Furthermore, it helps people learn how to feel better by managing symptoms with fewer medications than before treatment started.

This is a difficult phase for patients because they need to learn how to deal with their lives at home and the stressors associated with everyday life. In addition, patients with difficulty adjusting or accepting life changes usually find it difficult to cope with their mental illness and relapse.

Therefore, this phase encourages patients to adjust or accept change while focusing on maintaining progress without symptoms of mental illness. This helps them do well without symptoms of mental illness or with fewer symptoms or medication than before treatment started.

This is important because it helps prevent relapse or the undesirable consequences related to relapse. Furthermore, this phase allows patients to maintain progress through continued self-care and monitoring symptoms.

This is a difficult phase for patients who do not want to comply with treatment and maintenance. If a patient refuses treatment, they must receive a strong message from their doctor that they need to comply with their treatment plan if they are going to feel better and prevent relapse.

This is an important phase because it helps maintain the gains achieved in earlier phases and leaves patients more in control of their mental illness. Therefore, it helps people learn how to manage symptoms without medication or with less medication.

This is a difficult phase for patients who have difficulty adjusting to or accepting life changes. Unfortunately, patients with difficulty adjusting or accepting change usually find it difficult to cope with their mental illness and are likely to relapse.

Generalization and maintenance are important because they help patients maintain progress through continued self-care, monitoring, and skills. This ensures that the patient will not relapse for a long period. In addition, this phase helps people feel better by managing symptoms with fewer medications than before treatment started. This is important because it helps people learn how to manage symptoms without medication or with less medication. Therefore, this phase helps people do well without symptoms of mental illness or with fewer symptoms or medication than before treatment started.

In addition to helping patients learn how to apply their coping skills and feel better by managing symptoms with fewer medications than before treatment started, this phase allows people to use the support of family and friends to help them cope more effectively with stressful situations in their daily life.

Generalization involves the patient learning to apply their coping skills and feeling better without medication or with fewer side effects than before treatment. This is important because it helps people learn how to feel better by managing symptoms without medication. This helps people do well without symptoms of mental illness or with fewer symptoms or medication than before treatment started. In addition, generalization helps patients use the support of family and friends to help them cope more effectively with stressful situations in their daily life. Moreover, it helps people do well without symptoms of mental illness or with fewer symptoms or medication than before treatment started.

Maintenance involves the patient learning how to feel better by managing symptoms without medication or with less medication than before treatment started. This helps people do well without symptoms of mental illness or with fewer symptoms or medication than before treatment started. This is important because it helps people do well without symptoms of mental illness or with fewer symptoms or medication than before treatment started.

The benefits of this phase degrade as the disease progresses and the patient's abilities decrease. The patient may not be motivated to continue the maintenance phase, but the benefits remain. In addition, these benefits need to be monitored during routine visits in an outpatient department (at home) because they can change at any time and may get worse.

This phase is more important because it allows people to do better without symptoms of mental illness or with fewer symptoms or medication than before treatment started. It helps patients use family and friends' support at home. In addition, it helps people cope more effectively with stressful situations in their daily life at home. In addition, a person may want to go back and do more after feeling better. However, continuing the maintenance phase is a good idea because it helps patients use their skills and feel better without and with less medication than before treatment started.

Psychotherapy is any therapeutic interaction between a trained professional (e.g., psychologist, psychiatrist) and a client or patient, focusing on issues concerning mental health. In particular, psychotherapy refers to "a goal-oriented, intentional relationship between a mental health professional and someone experiencing significant intrapsychic and emotional problems."

"Emotions can be maintained if they are repeatedly evoked by events that trigger them, and the emotions that are triggered are usually those which have been most recently experienced. Therefore, one must change one's experiences to change one's emotional reactions."

This is important because it helps people learn how to feel better by managing their symptoms without medication or with less medication. For example, a depressed patient who feels something bad will happen when they get angry and avoids feeling angry is likely to continue feeling depressed for a long time.

Phase six: post-treatment assessment

The last phase is the post-treatment assessment. In terms of research and practice, in this mental health process area, "post" means after the treatment has gone on for a while: "the period following a course of clinical intervention (e.g., psychotherapy) or a course of social support or psychosocial interventions over time."

In this process area, the post-treatment assessment is any event or activity that concerns how people are doing after psychotherapy for patients with mental disorders or depression. The post-treatment assessment is also known as "termination," which means "to stop or end something" or "the act of making an end to."

In this phase, any changes are monitored to ensure that the patient is making progress. If necessary, the treatment should be changed or adjusted to fit the patient.

Components of post-treatment assessment may include:

a. The patient's mental illness diagnosis, symptoms, and severity.
b. The patient's response to treatment and psychotherapy and mood before the onset of relapse.
c. The patient's readiness to begin psychotherapy or treatment with medications to effectively manage their mental illness to help prevent relapse or recurrence.
d. The patient's support systems and ability to cope with stressors outside therapy for relapse and recurrence prevention.
e. The patient's adherence, or compliance, with therapy and treatment to prevent relapse or recurrence.
f. The patient's level of functioning is measured by their ability to maintain employment, complete education, manage their relationships and social interactions effectively, etc.
g. The patient's response to the psychotherapy and treatment that they received to prevent relapse or recurrence of their mental illness with less staff involvement in therapy and more independence for the patient in daily life activities such as employment training, school attendance, peer relationships, and interactions with others (e.g., family members), managing finances on an ongoing basis.
h. The patient's response to the psychosocial interventions and support systems they received to prevent relapse or recurrence of their mental illness.
i. The patient's ability to effectively manage their emotions as revealed by their responses in psychotherapy, social support, and family relationships.
j. The patient's insight about the causes and persistence of emotional problems for relapse prevention; this usually requires psycho-education about the causes of mental illness and strategies for managing emotional problems in daily life.

Post-treatment assessment involves checking the progress of the therapy and psychosocial interventions. The patient's progress can be checked by monitoring symptoms, medication levels, and psychotherapy skills. The results of the treatment and psychotherapy are also checked. If the patient does not agree with the change in treatment and progress, they should be invited to discuss it with their health care provider. Post-treatment assessment helps determine whether the patient has responded well to therapy and psychotherapy and whether the treatment is working.

The results of post-treatment assessment influence how therapy should continue. If therapy is effective, it should be continued until the patient can adjust without medication or with lower medication dosage. The clinician must decide whether a person who can survive without mental illness medications needs regular therapy or more social support, such as family and peer support.

In the end, post-treatment assessment helps people learn how to live better with their mental or emotional problems. Moreover, the treatment and psychotherapy results are used to make more informed decisions regarding future treatment.

Therefore, the post-treatment assessment phase of mental health is an ongoing process that varies from one individual to another, depending on their needs and circumstances. In addition, the post-treatment assessment phase is a process that must be repeated repeatedly to keep the person with mental or emotional problems from relapsing.

A common question about post-treatment assessment is whether patients should continue taking psychotropic medications or if they can stop taking them on their own. The answer depends on a few factors:

a. Patients with severe mental disorders, such as schizophrenia and bipolar disorder, are more likely than others to need to stay on psychotropic medications for life.
b. Patients who take medication inconsistently or forget to take them should be reminded of their need to do so and helped in every way they can to remember and adhere to the treatment plan.
c. Psychotherapy goes hand in hand with the use of medication because psychotherapy addresses emotional issues and social supports (e.g., family or peer support) that affect how patients cope emotionally, socially, and behaviorally. Psychotherapy helps patients to develop new thoughts and patterns of behavior that have a positive effect on their mental and emotional status.
d. Patients with a mental disorder (e.g., depression) that has been successfully treated with psychotherapy may not need psychotropic medications. But these patients are still at risk for relapse unless they continue to practice the skills learned in therapy and develop strong social support for themselves.

The results of the post-treatment assessment phase will depend on the clinician's conclusions about a person's symptoms, severity, and level of functioning before beginning therapy or treatment with medication.

Mental illness is a serious issue affecting millions worldwide. It is important to understand that there are different types of mental illness, and treatment varies depending on the form. Treatment depends on the type of symptoms the patient is experiencing; therefore, different treatment methods may work better for some patients than others. Treatment options include psychotherapy, medication (such as benzodiazepines), electroconvulsive therapy (ECT), group therapy, and other alternatives such as diet and exercise. According to Kahn et al. (2010), patients should choose from these options based on their preferences and be open to discussing all aspects of their lives with healthcare providers at any time during treatment.

Over the last few years, researchers have used neuroimaging to find out how CBT works for people with mental illnesses. There has been a focus on the hippocampus (which is important for long-term memories). This area becomes activated during CBT as well as when people are retrieving memories from long-term memory. It has been found that hippocampal volume decreases when people have depression compared to healthy controls.

Cognitive therapy has been used for several problems that are affected by emotion. For example, depression has responded well to cognitive behavior therapy (CBT) for patients with agoraphobia in tests on children and adults. In addition, the International Journal of Eating Disorders has published research showing that cognitive therapy can effectively treat bulimia.

Although cognitive behavior therapy is effective against depression and bulimia, it has not been as successful for patients suffering from eating disorders. However, treatment usually focuses on disordered eating behavior, which may lead to decreased symptoms of other emotional problems such as depression.

Therefore, the CBT framework should be expanded to include positive emotions, coping and emotion regulation problems, and social relations. This would make it more effective in dealing with eating disorders such as bulimia nervosa.

In the past decade, cognitive exposure therapy has been used to help depressed adults and children. Cognitive exposure therapy is a therapeutic method where people are exposed via imagination to situations related to the onset of their disorder or mood disturbance. For example, people who fear flying will be exposed repeatedly to images of flying on the Internet or in films until they no longer fear flying. In addition, people with agoraphobia will have many opportunities via graded exposure exercises to be out in public and learn ways to deal with their anxiety.

HOW TO IDENTIFY EMOTIONAL TRIGGERS

Cognitive behavioral therapy is about retraining the way your brain responds to events, ideas, and "triggers." For example, if you have been struggling with anxiety, you might want to recognize the times when your anxiety spikes in intensity. When do you feel it? What are you doing? Who are you with? What specific thought pops into your mind at that moment?

Beyond these anxiety triggers, it can be helpful to start identifying "idiosyncratic" triggers—those things or activities that work as a cue for a strong emotional response. For instance, you may be anxious in certain social settings but not others. You may face similar situations repeatedly, and each time react differently. If so, you could try to identify a particular pattern: "When I attend a play at an arts festival, I normally experience some anxiety. Today, though? It was fine."

Each trigger can be considered a weakness to the patient's ability to maintain control of their emotions. The goal is for the patient to change these weaknesses so that specific external cues no longer trigger the feelings. This process is known as "autonomic regulation."

Autonomic regulation can be accomplished by identifying the cue (the "trigger"), determining the emotion that is associated with it (i.e., anxiety), thinking of negative emotion, then practicing this new response to the trigger until it becomes habitual. Examples of emotions opposed to anxiety are calmness, relaxation, and happiness. For example, Agitated patient – Calm response: "I am feeling anxious, but I'm going to choose a calm response. Maybe I'll go sit down, relax my shoulders and breathe deeply."

Determining the key emotion involves paying attention to the patient's face and tone of voice. If the patient appears anxious or upset, the therapist might ask questions or do other things to draw out the emotions: "What happened that made you get anxious? What is it like when you get anxious?" The therapist might determine what type of anxiety is experienced: Is it fear? Is it worry? "When you are worried about something, your body tightens up, and your muscles tense up. When you feel fear, your body prepares to run or fight."

The therapist will then help the patient identify an emotion opposite the trigger. This may be a distraction tactic. For example, A person who is anxious while driving might choose calmness as the negative emotion. The person might say, "I'm going to count backward from 100," or "I'm going to try and relax my shoulders and take deep breaths."

Once the patient has identified a calm response to the trigger, they can learn to employ it using practice strategies. For example, the therapist might ask the patient to think of a stressful situation likely to provoke the trigger. The patient imagines themselves in this situation but instead thinks of the soothing response. The therapist then asks the patient to rate their anxiety on a scale of 0-10 (0 being no anxiety and 10 being extreme terror). New triggers can be chosen if it's too difficult to imagine something stressful.

Empirical studies suggest that people with post-traumatic stress disorder (PTSD) do not get relief from their symptoms by imagining pleasant memories as much as other patients do.

Instead, they often get relief by imagining the trauma that caused their symptoms. In this case, it is suggested that the trauma is too prominent in their minds and needs to be reduced.

To do this, the patient should imagine triggers and practice the positive cue until it becomes a habit. Rewarding yourself for doing so can be helpful, as it can be difficult to change habitual behavior. For example, it may help to think of a reward associated with a positive response: "If I feel angry when my boss yells at me, I'll take a few deep breaths and remind myself how much I like my job.

Why emotional triggers occur

Many researchers believe that people suffer from anxiety because they don't master (or forget) how to regulate the automatic responses of their bodies and mind.

It can be helpful to think of your body as a car. Your brain is like the car's computer: It processes information about your environment and makes decisions, including when to remove your foot from the gas pedal and step on the brake. The brain decides when you have had enough food, when you are too hot or cold, and when to relax or contract your muscles. It regulates your breathing, your heart rate, and hormone production.

The computer (your brain) must work properly. But if you are stuck in "high gear" without the ability to switch to "low" or "park," stress can build up. Therapy aims to understand what causes your anxiety and ways to change reactions so you can respond more appropriately.

Emotional triggers occur when we react too strongly to a situation that we perceive as threatening. We are experiencing such a threat because of our experience with similar situations. Our brain has stored information about this situation, which was experienced in the past, and makes us feel so strongly about it that we feel terrible. For instance, an abusive father might leave his child at the store, causing her to feel terror. The child's fear is then stored in the brain, and she may react similarly if she sees or hears something related to the actual situation, which triggers memories of the abuse.

People experience many negative emotions, such as anger, sadness, and anxiety. Emotions are processed automatically, outside of our conscious control. Think of an automatic reaction to an emotional trigger like a voice recording. When you hear your voice recorder go off in the morning, you might say, "Oh no!" You may do this without thinking about it or even being aware of what you are doing—your body reacts automatically.

Many people who have experienced trauma find themselves reacting to certain situations similarly over and over again. For example, if you were stuck in a car accident when you were 16, you might find that certain sounds or feelings cause you to flash back and feel the same way as you did when it happened. If that happens, try to bring yourself back to the present moment, reminding yourself where and when. This can be difficult, but you must learn to keep yourself here.

Many people who have experienced traumatic experiences are confused about their reactions and behaviors. For example, they may be afraid of a certain situation yet feel an urge to run toward it or act scared even when there is no danger. The confusion makes it hard for them to see what they are feeling or what they need to do next.

Often, we automatically go to extremes when we are feeling angry, fearful, or upset. In a car accident example, if you are scared and the door is opened suddenly by someone standing behind you, your automatic response might be to jump and scream. However, if you have experienced a traumatic event, this reaction may not be appropriate for current situations. Many people with anxiety problems find they have a hard time knowing what their reactions mean. For example, if someone tells you it is cold outside, you see them wearing a coat and know it is not cold outside for them. But because of your past experiences, you feel upset and cold (your brain is telling you something is wrong). Many people with anxiety problems think, "this person must be a threat to me," when the truth is that it is the cold weather itself. This is another way your brain and body react automatically without knowing the context of the situation.

Many people who have experienced trauma find it hard to control their reactions to emotional triggers. As a result, people often respond when they are triggered, even if they know that the response is not appropriate or helpful in any way. This can cause frustration and confusion because you do not understand why you reacted so strongly or felt so much anxiety.

It is important to learn how to control how you react and feel to reduce your anxiety with help from a professional therapist or instructor. Once you understand what triggers your anxiety, you will be able to respond differently each time it happens. This will help you gain control of your body and mind.

Therefore, emotional triggers occur when we react too strongly to a situation that we perceive as threatening. Moreover, people often respond when they are triggered, even if they know that the response is not appropriate or helpful in any way. This can cause frustration and confusion because you do not understand why you reacted so strongly or felt so much anxiety.

There are other reasons as well, as I have described above, which you can see in the above passage. It is important to learn how to control how you react and feel to reduce your anxiety with help from a professional therapist or instructor. Once you understand what triggers your anxiety, you will be able to respond differently each time it happens. This will help you gain control of your body and mind.

Therefore, you can reduce your anxiety. The above passage tells you where the cause of anxiety comes from and gives some practical ways by which you can deal with it. However, anxiety can also be reduced in other ways. So it does not depend upon any one way, but many ways too – that is, by reducing your anxiety with many different methods- by medicines and so on.

The causes of anxiety are different. What causes anxiety for one person may not cause it for another person. The causes of anxiety in different cases differ from those of the same case according to differences and similarities among the cases experienced by persons suffering from illness or being healthy.

Stressful events: Traumatic experiences can cause emotional triggers to develop and become conditions that are difficult to overcome. Usually, the reaction is more severe and intense than the first reaction.

Psychological/emotional/mental triggers: The stress and anxiety caused by these events can cause emotional triggers to form, causing a condition that is difficult to overcome.

Psychological/emotional/mental health issues: People suffering from psychological or mental issues often develop emotional triggers. Combining both situations can be very hard to deal with, whether the trauma occurred before or after these issues.

Psychological/emotional/mental problems usually appear in one's teenage years, while a trauma can happen at any time of life. Emotional triggers can cause one to experience anxiety and depression, which can be hard to control.

Psychological/emotional/mental issues are likely to cause an individual to become very self-critical. Trauma usually causes one to blame him or herself, which contributes to low self-esteem and can be hard to overcome.

Psychological/emotional/mental problems tend to make one feel isolated from others, and this feeling of loneliness is a trigger for trauma survivors. Therefore, it is important for individuals struggling with psychological or mental issues and trauma survivors alike to seek guidance from a trained professional to overcome emotional triggers.

Traumatic experiences usually result in emotional triggers that are not as severe but can still create anxiety. These episodes of mild anxiety often occur when the person is triggered by a specific event or situation instead of responding to a random occurrence. Learning to detect these mild cases helps you manage your anxiety better.

Repetitive thoughts: Repeated thoughts may occur because the trauma was intense and allowed the memory to be stored in the brain more easily. Though once learned, the thought will continue to resurface unexpectedly unless it is dealt with on a conscious level.

Most people with anxiety are affected by their past experiences and their anxiety. Adapting to these triggers and mastering the situations or situations that cause them to happen can be difficult, even if you have control over your current situation. Therefore, knowing what causes anxiety is important to deal with it effectively.

Breathing exercises are an excellent way to deal with anxiety because they help you center yourself, reduce muscular tension, and relieve stress. Breathing exercises are a great way to reduce anxiety because they can help you center yourself, reduce muscular tension, and relieve stress. Moreover, they help you to be more in control of your reactions to stressful situations.

Psychological treatment is also an effective way to deal with anxiety, as it helps you learn how to react and respond appropriately in different situations. For example, the therapist might ask about your past experiences, which may release some buried feelings that can cause anxiety.

Psychotherapy can also be very helpful in dealing with anxiety and emotional triggers because it allows the person to work through their issues psychologically. The therapist will help the person learn about themselves and how they react in certain situations, allowing them to see why they may feel anxious or depressed when triggered by something from their past.

Deep breathing is a technique to calm the body and mind and regain calmness and focus. This natural relaxation method engages all major muscle groups while calming the mind and creating a sense of self-control. Unfortunately, many people turn to deep breathing techniques as natural stress relievers without knowing the proper way to do it or how beneficial they can be in anxiety disorders. One of the most effective forms of deep breathing involves slow abdominal breathing.

How to identify emotional triggers

Emotional triggers are complex, and it is easy to misinterpret them. Here are some tips that can help you identify and manage the emotional triggers:

1. Write down your thoughts and feelings.

Thoughts and feelings are important parts of emotional triggers. Write them down in a journal, which will help you evaluate yourself and reduce the stress of the emotions. Moreover, it will help you identify the triggers and learn how to deal with them.

2. Stay away from unnecessary stressors.

To effectively deal with emotional triggers, stay away from unnecessary stressors. For example, if you know that a certain situation is usually a trigger for you, avoid being in that situation by all means. Even if it is unavoidable, try to relax before entering the situation, so the emotional trigger does not worsen the situation or affect you as much because of your reaction to it.

3. Take time for yourself and ensure you enjoy life by doing what you love.

Stressful situations or people often trigger emotional triggers. To deal with them, take time for yourself and do what you love to help you enjoy life and relieve stress. Even if you cannot take time for yourself because of work or school, try to make sure you are doing something that brings enjoyment to your life by something that makes you happy and relaxed at the same time.

4. Improve your relationships with people who can help ease your emotional triggers.

You can learn how to deal with emotional triggers by improving the relationships with people who can help ease them, such as a friend or family member willing to listen to how you feel and put things in perspective. Talking to friends and family can help reduce anxiety and provide an outlet to share what is happening. Moreover, it allows them to see who you truly are instead of who you pretend to be.

5. Identify the cause

Individuals need to identify why they feel upset about something by evaluating the issue thoroughly. This can help the individual realize the importance of an event or situation and understand why they feel anxious or depressed when triggered by it. It is also important for individuals to learn how to react optimally in situations that might trigger an emotional trigger to avoid being physically and mentally affected.

6. Stay in control of your emotions

There are many ways to reduce anxiety, such as deep breathing and meditation. These can help you reduce stress by allowing you to stay in control of your emotions so that an emotional trigger does not affect you as strongly. Furthermore, these methods can help you identify your feelings and deal with them effectively so that the emotional trigger will not affect you negatively.

7. Learn to say no and be assertive

You need to learn how to say no when you cannot finish something so that you will not feel overwhelmed by stress in your everyday life. Moreover, you need to learn how to be assertive and stand up for yourself in the face of anxiety triggers. You should also learn to ask for help, when necessary, from someone who can provide you with the help you need. Always remember not to be defensive when dealing with someone else's opinion on the situation because it can hurt your feelings and make you more upset because of the emotional trigger, which can result in a physical response as well as an emotional response that can affect your day-to-day activity negatively.

8. Learn to relax

Relaxation is an important strategy to reduce stress and manage emotional triggers. There are many relaxation methods, such as deep breathing, meditation, and yoga. In addition, relaxation is also helpful in reducing any physical pain that may be experienced as a result of being triggered by an emotional issue.

9. Connect with nature

You should also connect with nature and enjoy the beautiful scenery to reduce stress and tension that can lead to trigger because of anxiety. Nature can help you relax, de-stress, relieve tension, and reduce anxiety by putting you in a good state of mind. Moreover, connecting with nature is a healthy way to enjoy the wonders of our world, which can sometimes feel overlooked by hectic schedules and stressful jobs or school life.

10. Do not avoid a trigger

You should not avoid a trigger when it is unavoidable, such as in social situations that can be uncomfortable. When triggered by something, you may feel overwhelmed by anxiety and depression, but do not avoid the situation after thinking it through. If you have to go somewhere anyway, try to be prepared with things that can help reduce anxiety before entering the situation. For example, you can wear a meditator's hat or take deep breaths before entering an environment or event that causes anxiety.

11. Relax before entering the situation or event

It is important to relax before entering an uncomfortable situation because it can help reduce anxiety. You can take deep breaths, use a meditator's hat, and listen to soothing music to help you relax before you enter an uncomfortable social situation.

12. Try not to worry about what will happen

You should try not to worry about what could happen in that stressful event or situation because worrying can bring negative thoughts and emotions. When triggered by anxiety, individuals often focus on what might happen instead of how to deal with the problem. Worrying about the issue will only worsen the trigger because of increased stress and tension.

One of the best ways to control anger is by identifying your triggers so that you know how to deal with them effectively. Unfortunately, work and school are places where many triggers tend to occur, such as competing with co-workers or students for a big project that has a large sum of money attached to it; not getting what you want at work; experiencing personal disagreements with co-workers and managers; or being teased by co-workers and peers for things such as race, religion, gender identity, or sexual orientation.

Before you can identify your response to a trigger, you must first identify the triggers you may experience. You can learn about possible triggers by talking to people who have experienced similar things and have learned how to deal with them effectively. For example, when you feel upset about a situation, consider what feelings it could bring you, such as anger or depression. In addition, find out whether any triggers happen before or after that event or situation when it causes stress and tension in individuals, such as reading negative news reports on the internet or watching news reports about national disasters affecting people worldwide.

Therefore, identifying your triggers is essential since it lets you know possible situations that can affect you emotionally, mentally, and physically. You can then take time to prepare yourself before entering a situation or event that triggers your emotions. Moreover, learning how to cope with emotional triggers will make you more capable of dealing with various issues in your everyday life by avoiding anxiety or depression. First, you need to know whether the trigger is simple or severe; once you know this, you can decide on an appropriate strategy that suits your needs.

Lastly, emotional triggers are not something to feel ashamed about because they are a normal response under certain circumstances. Always remember that each person has their emotional triggers, so it becomes easier for people to understand why they have different reactions and feelings when facing similar situations.

Take a break from the situation if you feel stressed about a large project or competition. It is important to take time to relax and reduce stress. Also, prepare yourself before entering the situation so that you don't have to worry about emotions caused by certain situations.

Use relaxation techniques such as meditation, deep breathing, and listening to soothing music before entering stressful situations if necessary because it can help reduce anxiety.

It would be beneficial for individuals dealing with stress and anxiety to try all possible ways of managing their stress or anxiety even if they do not work in a stressful environment or do not have access to a psychologist or mental health professional at this moment in their lives.

How to identify your body's response

To identify your body's response to social situations, you can read about various experiences people have had in their lives about their feelings and emotions when they are put in the same scenario. This will provide useful information on how individuals deal with stressful situations when asked to perform or complete a certain task.

For example, when dealing with a stressful job, you may read stories of how people deal with relationships at work and how they cope with their performance pressure by reading positive and negative feedback from others. Remember that responses to a task or situation can differ from one individual to another.

You can also talk to other individuals who have experienced similar situations to help you identify whether you are experiencing your body's response or an emotional trigger. Talking about your experience will let you learn more about the social environment where it takes place for individuals to grow and become more confident as they gain valuable experiences that could improve their skills.

Therefore, these tips can help you identify your body's response:

1. Observe your body and emotions

Observing your body's response can be useful when you are stressed while working. To do this, observe whether you feel anxiety or not while going through the task or situation. Take note of how you feel after completing the task, such as relaxing and having a good time with your friends and family.

2. Identify triggers

When confronted with stress in a social setting, it is important to identify your triggers so that you can take steps to prevent such situations from causing negative emotions. Try reading books online about individuals who deal with similar situations in their daily lives about what works for them and what does not when they have problems at work or school.

3. Do note-taking

Take note of your emotions or feelings when in a stressful situation at work. These can include anxiety, depression, and anger. You should also determine whether you felt any response before and after the stressful time at work.

4. Go through your actions while dealing with stress

Because actions trigger emotions, it is important to conduct a self-analysis by going through your actions or behaviors while handling the stress at work or school. Ask yourself questions such as "What do I do when I experience stress?" and "Why do I get stressed?" By understanding why you feel frustrated with certain situations, you can identify what triggers you consistently experience before and after stressful situations.

5. Identify possible solutions

When you understand your body's response, you can identify possible solutions for dealing with stressful situations. You can either look for ways to reduce anxiety or try to avoid stressful situations altogether. If the situation is too serious and persistent, you may need to seek a psychologist or psychiatrist specializing in dealing with emotions like depression and anxiety.

6. Remove distractions

Removing distractions will be a good idea if you are in a stressful situation at work. This will keep your mind focused on the task at hand, allowing you to reduce anxiety and stress and focus on the task without being distracted. You can do this by working alone or turning off all internet devices.

7. Focus on one step at a time

When dealing with stress or anxiety in social situations, it is important to focus on one thing only while doing so. For example, if you are studying for an exam, focus only on the text you are reading and not the other things happening around you, as distractions can keep your mind from focusing.

8. Control your breathing rate

When you feel anxious, stressed, or panic in a social setting such as work, try to control your breathing rate. This will help keep your thoughts clear while calming yourself down to keep stressful emotions away. Deep breaths can do wonders in helping with stress and anxiety attacks during stressful situations at work and school.

9. Stay positive

It is important to stay positive during stressful times. During such situations at work, think about what you can do to improve it instead of dwelling on the problems. If you are trying your best, do not think about failures or what other people say about you because these can only cause negative emotions.

10. Be in control

If you feel stressed out at work, try focusing on what you can do to improve it. For example, if your boss demands a project within a week while other co-workers fail to finish their tasks, it would be a good idea to set goals and think about completing them in time without sacrificing quality and accuracy. You can gain positive results from your efforts at work and school by being in control during stressful situations.

11. Establish a routine

It is important to establish a routine when dealing with stress and anxiety. It can help you reduce anxiety and stress when you do the same things before going to work and during stressful times at school or work. If you continue the same routine every time, it will be easier to deal with stress as unwanted thoughts will not often occur, which can bring negative emotions.

12. De-stress

If you are stressed out at work or school, try doing something that may take your mind off. This can include listening to music, watching funny videos, and doing something you enjoy, as these can distract your mind from the stress.

A great way to manage stress is by using self-help books and listening to relaxation music. These can help you stay relaxed, calm, and focused throughout stressful situations, giving you more time and opportunity to do the tasks.

Another helpful way of reducing stress is taking a walk or exercising before entering a stressful situation. These activities help lower stress levels, leaving you with a better mind for work or school.

Lastly, cultivate positive thoughts when dealing with stressful situations because these reactions can benefit your body in numerous ways. Some benefits include improved mental health, coping with feelings of worry and depression, and reduced feelings of anxiety.

How to identify your thoughts

Identifying your thoughts involves acknowledging your feelings first, then thinking about why you're feeling the way you do.

It is important to identify your thoughts if you want to deal with stress effectively. The following are five questions that will help you think about how you feel:

a. What made me feel this way?
b. What else could I be doing?
c. Am I getting all my needs met in life?
d. How does my family view me?
e. What am I good at?

After you have identified your thoughts, write them down. Then, put these aside and come back to them later. You may realize that they are unnecessary thoughts or fears.

These tips can help you identify your thoughts:

1. Recognize your emotions

Instead of ignoring your feelings, you should recognize them. Writing down how you feel and identifying the triggers is a good way to deal with stress.

2. Experiment to see what works best for you

There are many stress management techniques, and one will work best for each person. Therefore, you should try different techniques to find what works best.

3. Tell someone how they make you feel

Share your thoughts and feelings with someone close to help them understand how they may affect you. This step might seem simple, but it's the key to understanding yourself better.

4. Identify your triggers

Triggers are things that cause you to feel stressed and anxious. Think about where you feel negative emotions and write them down to identify your triggers. Triggers may include bad thoughts when you see certain people, smell scents, hear loud noises, or even at certain times of the day.

5. Observe your reactions

After identifying the three steps to identifying thoughts and feelings, try to observe what happens in your head in stressful situations at work or school. Note how these situations make you feel by writing down what happened during stressful times at work and school so that you can overcome stress easier later on.

6. Evaluate

After you have identified your thoughts, write them down and evaluate them a few days later. Try to see if they are helpful or not by analyzing how they make you feel and how you respond to them.

7. Never apologize for your feelings

There is never a need to apologize for your feelings because it is normal to have negative and positive thoughts about certain situations in life. Your emotions will keep changing for good and bad, so do not feel guilty about thinking the way you do because other people understand that it is only natural to think this way, even though it seems irrational sometimes.

8. Realize your feelings are not facts

Feelings can lead to thoughts that aren't true, so it is important to separate emotions from the factual reality of situations. Thoughts about how other people think about you can be invalid, so you should never feel guilty for being who you want to be and doing what will make you happy.

9. Accept your feelings

Accept your thoughts and feelings as a part of who you are because it may seem difficult at times, but it is necessary if you want to manage stress more effectively.

10. Take care of yourself

Dealing with stress is very personal, and you must take time to understand yourself better. While trying to identify your thoughts and feelings, it is important to focus on your physical well-being by drinking lots of water, eating right, exercising, getting enough sleep, and having fun.

Identifying thoughts can be challenging for everyone, so be patient throughout the process. Moreover, be persistent and keep up the good work, as stress management will pay off in the end.

Anxiety is a part of everyday life, whether you're feeling anxious due to something that happened in your life or regularly feeling anxious about worry. Anxious feelings can be controlled through proper self-care, a healthy lifestyle, and other coping strategies.

Once you have taken stock of your negative thoughts, managing them is important. Here are ten tips that will help you manage them:

a. Practice positive thinking.
b. Be in the moment.
c. Learn how to quiet your mind.
d. Have faith in yourself and your abilities.
e. Get a good night's rest.
f. Try not always be perfect; it's okay to fail sometimes too!
g. Don't blame yourself for things that aren't your fault (i.e.: blame others for their faults or not being perfect)
h. Don't be so quick to trust others.
i. Practice breathing techniques for stress.
j. Get out and live your life, don't spend all your time worrying about the computer and with friends or family!

Using self-talk is a way to talk yourself into believing positive statements about life in general and coping with stressful situations. Start by choosing one negative thought and writing it down in a notebook or journal, being sure to write it down in detail rather than just analytically saying it aloud. Once you have written the negative thought, turn the thought into an opposite positive statement that will help you cope with stress better.

WHY CBT WORKS FOR ANXIETY

The premise of cognitive behavior therapy is that thoughts, rather than external events, cause you to react with anxiety. If it seems like everyone has anxiety these days, it could be because they are thinking a lot more about their worries and the possible consequences of these worries. It is not obvious on the surface, but this type of worry can lead to feelings of helplessness and overwhelm that contribute to health problems like high blood pressure and heart disease.

While CBT may work for some people in addressing chronic worry, many people struggle with mental health conditions such as stress-related disorders or bipolar disorder, where thoughts cannot be ignored because they are overwhelming or unrealistic as obsessive-compulsive disorder (OCD). This is where mindfulness training can help.

Mindfulness training and CBT complement each other in a mutually beneficial way. Mindfulness is the ability to pay attention to the present moment without being distracted by past or future events. Sound familiar? That's just like one of the components of CBT: distraction techniques that allow you to focus on your breathing to ground you in the present moment.

CBT may also help boost your ability to use mindfulness techniques effectively and vice versa. Increasing your mindfulness skills may enhance your ability to think through better options for solving problems and removing compulsions rather than retreating into a dissociative state.

Mindfulness training can aid in improving your mental well-being using cognitive behavior therapy. At first glance, CBT may seem like a rational process that allows you to assess situations and then make decisions from there clearly. However, while it does involve this thinking, CBT is more of a process than a magic bullet solution. As such, it can be better compared with mindfulness therapy than many other forms of treatment for anxiety and depression.

Mindfulness training, on the other hand, can be applied mindfully while working to eliminate unhealthy habits or compulsions that you may have. Even if mindfulness seems like a passive activity and not something that you can focus on while doing something else, it can help take your mind off of overwhelming thoughts or the natural tendency of one's mind to judge others based on their appearance and background rather than focusing on what's important. You'll find that through practice, mindfulness will eventually become a habit.

By extending the helpfulness of mindfulness to a situation where you can experiment with CBT, your mindfulness skills can strengthen your ability to think through things better. This is why many people with anxiety and depression report greater success in thinking through their problems while incorporating mindfulness techniques into their daily lives.

Mindfulness meditation and mindfulness techniques can help you better cope with your anxiety symptoms because it brings your attention back to the present moment rather than allowing your mind to wander and become distracted by unimportant things.

While treating the underlying cause of your anxiety is important, focusing on mindfulness can help you remove the "disguises" that prevent you from thinking clearly about the world. For example, if a person is trapped in a negative thought pattern, mindfulness can help them recognize this pattern so they can deal with it appropriately. In addition, they may recognize that these thoughts are associated with anxiety disorders or depression rather than something that is factually true.

What does CBT do for anxiety?

Cognitive behavior therapy does more than teach you to distract yourself from negative thoughts effectively. It also teaches you to recognize your "triggers" to form a plan of action when these triggers are set off. This allows you to remove the overall anxiety from an event or experience and prevents triggering strong negative emotions.

CBT allows the recognition that you may have been using avoidance as a coping mechanism for some time and teaches new coping mechanisms in place of avoidance. For example, if talking about death may cause a person to feel anxious, CBT can teach them new ways to cope with their anxiety without avoiding the subject altogether and how they can best talk about things when necessary. CBT aims to help you reflect on your thoughts, feelings, and behaviors and learn how they contribute to the problem.

While it is not often used in mental health care centers today, CBT has been a mainstream therapy since the 1960s. In addition, Charles Darwin and other cognitive psychologists have also contributed greatly to cognitive behavior therapy.

Cognitive behavior therapy can treat anxiety disorders by helping people recognize that positive thinking doesn't necessarily mean you will feel happy or calm. It can help people think more clearly about specific thoughts and identify when those thoughts or behaviors are bringing them down in the long run. CBT is a great tool to help people address their negative thoughts and actively replace those thoughts with ones that feel more helpful.

CBT works for anxiety by assessing the negative thoughts that cause stress and anxiety and then teaching new ways to cope with these thoughts. CBT guides you in the process of exploring your emotions and recognizing when you get stuck in a negative thought pattern.

CBT is appropriate for people suffering from debilitating anxiety disorders and teaches them new coping mechanisms to live healthy life while coping with their disorder. People who have learned effective methods of coping with their anxiety can also better recognize when they're slipping back into old patterns and easily regain control over their thoughts.

CBT will teach you to recognize your triggers and how your negative thoughts contribute to the problem simply by identifying them. It's an important tool for anyone who suffers from anxiety disorders because it impacts your thoughts and behaviors when they're unhelpful.

CBT is a good way to treat anxiety because it allows you to focus on what's happening now without letting your mind wander. In addition, by helping you recognize the triggers of negative thoughts, CBT can help you address these issues directly.

CBT can also teach you to recognize when your negative thoughts are taking you down a negative spiral that can keep you stuck in an unwanted pattern. CBT helps people focus on the positive by giving them new ways to look at their anxiety and their experience of it.

Cognitive behavior therapy is often effective because it addresses the inner work of your brain and teaches new ways of coping with negative thoughts and emotions. It also focuses on specific issues that cause anxiety and teaches people how to approach these situations differently.

People who suffer from anxiety disorders or depression often have an unhealthy relationship with their thoughts. The main focus of CBT is to show people how to respond to their thoughts instead of letting the thoughts control them. This is why CBT is a good tool for anxiety and depression.

Cognitive behavior therapy uses a method known as exposure therapy to help people process their emotions, thoughts, and experiences so they can heal. Exposure works because by addressing the underlying problem directly, you also address the symptoms of that problem. For example, if you're afraid of dogs because your parents were bitten by one when you were young, exposure therapy can help you face your fear head-on in a safe environment and learn how to cope effectively.

CBT allows you to remove the symptoms of your anxiety by eliminating the behaviors that may be causing it. It also allows for a deeper look at the root cause of the problem so you can address it accordingly.

Cognitive behavior therapy can often help us understand why our thoughts are so negative and how we can make them more positive. In addition, it teaches you to recognize when your thoughts are causing anxiety.

It may be helpful to speak with a professional regarding cognitive behavior therapy if you think it could be a good fit for your anxiety problems and concerns.

One thing that CBT does is teach you to identify when a thought feels irrational so that you can learn to respond with more positive thoughts and actions. Cognitive behavior therapy can also help you slow down your thoughts, and better handle them.

CBT is a great way to help people identify how their negative thoughts, behaviors, and emotions contribute to the problem. In addition, it teaches people new coping methods that are more effective than avoiding what may cause anxiety.

Cognitive behavioral therapy is best known for treating the underlying problems behind stress and anxiety disorders through recognizing your thoughts and feelings and changing your actions in response to your feelings. Moreover, cognitive behavioral therapy also enables you to address emotions healthily so that they don't control your thoughts and behavior.

Cognitive behavioral therapy targets the underlying issues that cause anxiety to help people learn new coping methods.

CBT can also be used to treat depression and other mental health disorders through each condition is best treated individually. Cognitive behavioral therapy focuses on the client's thoughts, feelings, and behaviors and teaches them how to make better decisions to help them feel better about themselves and their lives. Cognitive behavioral therapy can take time, like any other medical treatment. Therefore, sessions are scheduled on an as-needed basis, although there may be follow-up sessions after the initial ones if necessary.

How can I use CBT to control my anxiety?

Behavioral therapists are trained to identify your emotions and behaviors contributing to your anxiety and take them in a healthy direction. They will address these issues one at a time, which allows you to regain control of your anxiety.

CBT helps people recognize thoughts, feelings, and behaviors that may be causing their anxiety. CBT is an effective treatment for anxiety disorders like generalized anxiety disorder (GAD), post-traumatic stress disorder (PTSD), social anxiety disorder, panic attacks, and obsessive-compulsive disorder (OCD).

Cognitive behavioral therapy can be helpful if you're suffering from any mental health condition because it addresses the underlying cause of your problems.

Cognitive behavioral therapy also targets thoughts and emotions that can contribute to anxiety. It teaches you how to recognize your anxiety symptoms and pressures you healthily.

CBT is a good treatment for anxiety disorders that focuses on the relationship between thoughts, feelings, and behaviors so that you can develop new habits and behaviors to help manage your symptoms effectively.

Cognitive behavior therapy uses relaxation techniques, breathing exercises, positive self-talk, and other methods of managing stress. Behavioral modification is one of the most common ways cognitive behavioral therapy treats anxiety. It targets the root of your problems by changing your behavior instead of trying to change your thoughts alone.

Therefore, these tips can guide on how to use CBT to control anxiety:

1. Mindfulness: Learning to be present and in the moment is an effective way of managing anxiety. Mindfulness helps people see their anxiety for what it is - a passing emotion that may not mean what they think it means.
2. Focused attention: Focusing your attention on one thing can help make you feel centered and less anxious. You should focus on everyday things like your breathing, your feet hitting the ground, or something other than anxious feelings or emotions.
3. Relaxation techniques: Relaxation techniques can help you regain control of your anxiety symptoms and behavior by helping you manage stress physically and mentally.
4. Distraction: Distraction can be very helpful in managing anxiety. Distracting yourself by listening to music, reading a book, taking a walk, calling a friend, or meditating are all ways of helping you calm down and gain a better perspective.
5. Try hard to be positive: Positive self-talk is key in managing anxiety because it helps you change negative thought patterns into positive ones and change your behavior accordingly. Moreover, positive self-talk helps you see your anxiety as a passing feeling that you can learn how to manage.
6. Look at what makes you anxious: When you realize the things that cause you to stress, it's easier to handle them and think more positively. Make a list of everything that causes you anxiety. As you respond to these things more positively, your anxiety symptoms will decrease because your negative thoughts will stop controlling your behavior.
7. Take care of yourself: Managing your symptoms and learning new coping methods takes time, work, discipline, and patience, so be sure to treat yourself well. Don't beat yourself up if the process takes longer than expected. Remember, you're trying to change your life, so it's okay if it doesn't happen immediately. Be proud of your accomplishments, and know that you're learning to manage your anxiety by taking small daily steps.
8. Talk: Talking doesn't just mean visiting a professional counselor or therapist weekly. Talking can also

include talking with family, friends, coworkers, etc., and sharing what's going on with you healthily (not complaining or criticizing). You may want to try journaling alone or with someone interested in helping support and encourage you along the way.

9. Practice: Practicing and learning new coping techniques is just as important as the others on this list. Knowing what works for you and what doesn't takes time and practice. Don't give up! Take notice if you feel stressed, anxious, or become obsessed with something that you think is causing your anxiety.

10. Look after yourself: When you're feeling overwhelmed with stress, it's easy to forget about your needs as a person. Make sure to get enough sleep, eat well, exercise regularly, go out for frequent walks or runs outside, or take a hot bath once in a while! Get some fresh air by breathing in the wind, or do some yoga or meditation.

11. Seek help as needed: It's important to seek professional counseling if you feel you need it. Working with a therapist can let you talk about feelings and emotions you may have previously avoided.

12. Have fun: Life is too short not to get outside your comfort zone and have fun! Go out with friends, volunteer, socialize in public, or try something new, like learning how to play an instrument or dance. The most important thing is that you take care of yourself and enjoy yourself so that you stay healthy and happy!

13. Be yourself: Being comfortable in your skin is key to success. Don't compare yourself with others; remember that it's okay not to have answers or solutions immediately. The point is to keep moving forward even when you don't know where you're going.

14. Take action: Don't just think about things - take action! Start by making a list of what you would like to change in your life, and then seek the help of friends, family, or professionals as needed. Getting started on changes will significantly affect how you feel and how much control you feel over your anxiety symptoms!

15. Get out of the house: If you spend most of your time alone at home, it's important to be around other people and socialize! The more you get out and do new things, the less anxious you will feel because your mind won't feel like it's constantly stuck in a rut.

16. Practice: Don't stop practicing these tips once you feel better because continuing to practice will help build up your self-confidence and make change easier with time.

17. Learn from mistakes: If something doesn't work or you make a mistake, learn from it and move on. Remember that mistakes happen but learning from them matters most in the end.

Many methods allow CBT techniques for treating anxiety disorders effectively in clients with a higher level of thought processing and concentration, for example, giving homework that the client completes before subsequent sessions or asking them to carry out tasks between sessions e.g.

The impact of fear and panic

The impact of fear is an automatic pattern of responding to danger, which is perceived as a threat to the person's well-being and influenced by the content of a fearful thought. Panic attacks trigger panic sensations in vulnerable individuals who live with anxiety disorders. This triggers the person's reaction and alertness. Fear can be induced by certain stimuli in situations that are threatening to people (danger cues), such as stairways, elevators, bridges, and driving under bridges. The response to threatening situations depends on how effective the person believes they are at coping with those situations (self-efficacy beliefs). The challenge for CBT is creating or enhancing motivation for change.

The cognitive model of panic disorder is well established in clinical and research literature. According to that model, panic attacks manifest a dysfunctional response learned by sufferers to cope with the anxiety naturally associated with certain situations (for instance, being in a situation from which it would be difficult or embarrassing to escape). Situations that result in this feedback are called "goals." People with panic disorder are conditioned to respond incorrectly when they find themselves in threatening situations because they fear that intense anxiety and physical symptoms will be experienced if they don't get away quickly. The panic attack consists of the feared sensation plus a strong fear response, whose only function is to prevent the person's actual exposure to feared public situations.

Cognitive behavioral therapy helps to counter the effects of panic by teaching patients that their responses to situations are not catastrophic and do not need to be avoided. People are taught to ask when they panic, "What is the worst that could happen?" Since nothing catastrophic happens in most situations that trigger anxiety in people living with panic disorder, it often follows that the answer is nothing at all or something that can be readily endured. For example, flight initiation may be accompanied by shortness of breath and an increased heart rate. The sufferer may believe these sensations indicate a serious illness, only exacerbated by catastrophizing about their symptoms (e.g., "I feel like I'm going to die!"). However, the anxiety and other unpleasant sensations accompanying panic attacks are usually not life-threatening. Inventing a catastrophic event does little to help the sufferer in real life. This can be overcome by keeping a re-evaluation of all of one's prior experiences in mind (the so-called "reality testing"). The goal is merely to recognize that panic attacks do not lead to catastrophes and that panic is a response to a feared situation, which is often not at all dangerous. Note that this use of thought testing does not mean one should be fatalistic about their health. If they had a heart attack, they should seek help. Even though the sensations of a panic attack are unpleasant and terrifying, what is feared is not dangerous.

The cognitive-behavioral model proposes that people with panic disorder misinterpret harmless body sensations as signs of imminent death or catastrophic illness. This leads to an immediate increase in anxiety (a panic attack) which makes the person hypervigilant to bodily sensations and provokes them to administer emergency response behaviors such as fleeing or avoiding situations where anxiety symptoms are predicted to occur. These symptoms are believed to be maintained by the mistaken belief that they prevent the adverse event and keep it at bay. This hypervigilance maintains and exacerbates the problem, in which people are not exposed to situations where they can learn that their anxiety symptoms are not harmful. Relative to this model, cognitive-behavioral therapy aims to reduce misinterpretations of harmless bodily sensations and decrease maladaptive emergency response behaviors.

The fight-or-flight response during a panic attack is similar to that during a traumatic event in which an individual perceives themselves to be threatened with mortal danger. The American Psychiatric Association, the National Institute of Mental Health, and the American Academy of Pediatrics have identified numerous therapies for panic attacks. A type of therapy called cognitive behavioral therapy (CBT) is particularly effective.

Cognitive behavioral therapy (CBT) is a short-term counseling treatment that helps people change their thoughts and behavior by teaching them to view their world more positively to help them deal with difficult situations more constructively. In addition, CBT resets the reaction pattern of chronic anxiety, allowing the body to respond normally to stressors without resorting to fight-or-flight responses or maladaptive avoidance.

CBT for panic attacks is a short-term counseling treatment that helps change irrational thoughts, overcome fears and phobias, accept oneself and one's surroundings, and learn how to modulate responses to stress. CBT has been found to help many adults deal with their fear of bodily symptoms and unfamiliar situations in everyday life. CBT aims to help the person gain control over their emotions by helping them recognize their irrational thoughts as irrational thoughts rather than facts. CBT exposes the person to the belief that they can control their feelings and have a positive view of themselves regardless of situations. It is also hoped to allow the person to realize they have a high responsibility for changing difficult situations.

Propranolol is effective in treating panic disorder when administered immediately following a panic attack. Although its effects do not last forever, they are long-lasting enough to give panicked individuals time to defend themselves and flee the situation where the panic took place. In some cases, patients may not experience immediate relief from symptoms at first but usually experience them within the day or two following the dosage of propranolol. Another study involving propranolol administered before exposure therapy (as opposed to immediately after) did not reduce symptoms as effectively. This may have been due to the timing and dosage used. These findings suggest that propranolol should be taken at the first sign of symptoms.

Propranolol may work by decreasing the activity of the amygdala or helping the subject control their sweating or both. It is thought that propranolol helps patients control their symptoms due to its ability to be metabolized into a beta blocker, which tightens blood vessels and reduces physical responses to emotional stimuli. Studies involving propranolol have shown it to be effective in treating panic attacks immediately following them (as stated earlier) and throughout treatment.

The cause of anxiety

The cause of anxiety attacks is a combination of genetic and environmental factors. The disorder is thought to have a genetic component, meaning that biological and environmental factors may contribute to the development of the disorder. But an anxiety attack can also be triggered by a traumatic event, such as receiving news of a divorce or losing a loved one.

Panic attacks are common among those who have been diagnosed with panic disorder. According to the Anxiety and Depression Association of America (ADAA), about two-thirds of people with panic disorder develop irrational fears (phobias) during their life. The ADAA describes phobias as unrealistic or exaggerated responses to situations involving intense fear or discomfort. These fears can cause people to avoid the situations that trigger their panic attacks.

Psychological factors can also play a role in developing panic attacks and other anxiety disorders. For example, studies have found that when compared with those who had not been diagnosed with an anxiety disorder, individuals who had responded to feeling needed security by seeking help from psychologists or psychiatrists were at greater risk of later experiencing anxiety or tension-related attack. This suggests that helping someone feel secure can trigger a panic attack.

Research has shown changes in the brain, particularly in the amygdala, during states of anxiety and fear. For example, studies have shown increased amygdala activity when people are threatened. These changes in brain activity are believed to result from long-term (beginning as early as infancy) exposure to stressful events and environments, which may include traumatic experiences.

The result is that many patients experience anxiety without any identifiable cause or trigger. You can only hope that your symptom is triggered by a specific event, such as a car accident or public transit incident – usually, a stressful one that leaves you shaken up by the symptoms of your panic attack.

Anxiety is a normal response to danger and stress, but unlike fear and other emotions associated with danger, anxiety attacks are often unexpected and unprovoked. In contrast, to fear, the hallmark characteristic of anxiety is having feelings of apprehension or dread about an upcoming event or situation that is perceived to be no threat. Anxiety attacks usually occur "out of the blue" because they are not associated with a specific situation around which nerves can be calmed down.

The only treatment proven effective for panic disorder is cognitive behavioral therapy (CBT), a specialized type of psychotherapy. CBT teaches you different ways of thinking, behaving, and reacting to the symptoms of panic disorder. CBT aims to help you recognize and change the negative thoughts, emotional responses, and behavior patterns that affect your ability to function.

CBT has been shown to help improve various symptoms associated with panic and other anxiety disorders. CBT has also been shown to help lessen the frequency of panic attacks when combined with pharmacotherapy. In addition, CBT has been shown to help improve outcomes when combined with a treatment such as exposure therapy.

Adolescents and children can benefit from short-term psychodynamic psychotherapy, but only if there are no clear signs of dangerousness, such as attempts at suicide or self-harm.

When panic attacks occur infrequently or are isolated events, a therapist may suggest that the person with panic disorder focuses on coping strategies such as relaxation training, cognitive restructuring, and exposure therapy. Relaxation training involves beginning a hierarchy of graded exposure to situations that might cause panic, starting with situations that are likely to cause less anxiety and progressing towards more challenging situations.

Cognitive restructuring helps the person challenge irrational beliefs about the self and the world by developing more realistic ways of thinking. A specific technique is called "thought stopping." Despite not being supported by empirical evidence, cognitive restructuring is still used in treatment today. For example, it is considered equally effective as behavioral therapy when treating an isolated panic attack.

Exposure therapy involves exposing the person with panic disorder to situations or environments that cause anxiety in a controlled manner while being accompanied by trained therapists. This can involve exposure to different situations intended to trigger anxiety and facing the individual's fears about such situations. Exposure to these situations without supportive people can cause more extreme panic symptoms.

Psychoeducation is recommended to prevent panic attacks in children and adolescents (10–18 years). There is evidence that adolescents who are actively informed about their condition and what they can do about it may be less likely to have a period of intense fear and distress when they first begin to experience symptoms. Parents, guardians, and teachers are good resources for information. In addition, anxiety can be managed effectively in children and adolescents by establishing ongoing relationships with the child and family that have a positive and reassuring effect. This is done by actively ensuring that the place, time, and circumstances are as comfortable as possible. In addition, care should be taken to ensure that environmental conditions are adequate to minimize exposure to hazards such as smoke or second-hand effects of drugs, alcohol, or volatile chemicals.

Panic disorder can occur with other psychiatric disorders. It frequently occurs with depressive disorders, particularly major depressive disorder (MDD), which mild depression-related setbacks may trigger. It is also common during manic episodes of bipolar disorder. In addition, it has been diagnosed comorbidly with a generalized anxiety disorder (GAD), where the patients may constantly worry about the future and have difficulties in routine activities.

Anxiety disorders are associated with major functional impairments. The likelihood of panic disorder and agoraphobia is estimated at 10% to 23%. The risk is higher among women than men. Agoraphobia without panic disorder produces an increased risk of being unable to leave home alone due to fear of experiencing panic symptoms. Panic disorder can be effectively treated with various interventions, including psychological therapies and medication, which can relieve symptoms and help prevent future episodes.

Benefits of CBT for the long-term anxiety

There is limited evidence to support the use of CBT as a first-line treatment for anxiety disorders in adults. However, CBT can be an effective component of treatment in adults and adolescents with anxiety disorders.

One meta-analysis concluded that CBT is more effective for reducing anxiety than other treatments, including pharmacotherapy, recommended for treating GAD. In addition, treatment duration was significantly longer with CBT than with medication alone in the short term. Three randomized controlled trials compared treatment as usual (TAU) to a combination of TAU and CBT (CTST) for anxiety disorders. Two studies indicated that CTST improved anxiety symptoms more than TAU. Although the third study reported no difference between the groups, this may have been due to problems with the randomization process.

Some people have only a single attack and then never have another one, while others have many attacks in a short period. Some people have recurrent attacks that come on suddenly and last only a few minutes, but others experience anxiety that lasts for weeks or months before they go away.

Agoraphobia can develop suddenly in children or teenagers due to situations that usually do not cause panic. The condition usually lasts at least six months but is often recurrent and can continue into adulthood.

Panic disorder and agoraphobia are a basis for developing panic attacks in conditions such as social anxiety disorder, obsessive-compulsive disorder (OCD), post-traumatic stress disorder (PTSD), and phobias. When this occurs, the main symptom is recurrent panic attacks that may involve all of the symptoms previously described in this book or some combination thereof. These attacks are temporary and can end in a few minutes or last months. Psychiatrists describe this as a temporary condition that causes significant impairment in functioning due to the intensity of the symptoms. When the individual is experiencing distress during an attack, the diagnosis of panic disorder is made.

Therefore, these are some of the benefits of CBT as a treatment method for long-term anxiety:

a. It is considered a highly effective treatment for anxiety disorders.
b. CBT is effective in the long-term treatment of anxiety disorders.
c. It has a lower dropout rate than other treatments such as pharmacotherapy (e.g., antidepressants and benzodiazepines).
d. It allows the patient to learn coping skills that can be applied even after the treatment ends. Reports indicate that these skills can be transferred to other types of anxiety disorders, including post-traumatic stress disorder (PTSD).
e. It has also been shown to be an effective component of a combined treatment involving pharmacotherapy, often prescribed to treat anxiety disorders.
f. It has been reported to be an effective treatment in adults, children, and adolescents.
g. In addition, CBT is considered a treatment of choice for many anxiety disorders.
h. CBT has also been effective in treating depression and generalized anxiety disorder (GAD).
i. It leads to restoring the functioning of patients affected by panic attacks, leading them back to the activities they were able to do before having panic attacks.
j. Due to its effectiveness, high client compliance rate (the patient must follow all sessions closely and attend all appointments), and low dropout rate compared with other treatments, it is often considered a first-line treatment option when no other treatments are available, or they fail.

TREATMENTS

Cognitive Behavior Therapy for Depression is psychotherapy that looks at how the patterns of thoughts and beliefs are related to depression. This includes thinking too much about the negative events in our lives or not thinking enough about positive events. A key element of cognitive behavior therapy is identifying distortions in our view of ourselves, others, and our world so we can change things.

The National Institute of Clinical Excellence (NICE) in the UK has recommended that CBT be used for mild to moderate depression and prevention (to keep the number of people who become depressed low).

Cognitive Behavior Therapy should be thought of as a skill to be learned. It is a set of skills that you can use to solve your problems. So while it will have time limits in a clinical setting, it will have no time limits if you learn how to use it on your own.

Social anxiety and CBT

CBT treats social anxiety through a process of education and awareness of the nature of anxiety and its symptoms. Individuals are encouraged to become more aware of their anxiety symptoms, identify the thoughts and situations that trigger them, and learn how to maintain control.

Researchers have found that CBT effectively reduces social phobia, while other studies show that it is comparable to pharmacological treatment concerning effectiveness.

CBT is an effective treatment for people with a diagnosis of schizophrenia. It helps patients interpret their experiences in more realistic terms, identify distorted thoughts that lead to emotional distress, and develop coping strategies to deal with distressing feelings or situations.

Social anxiety and CBT are helpful in the treatment of borderline personality disorder (BPD). Through these skills, CBT helps patients develop a sense of self, feel more in control over their emotions, lead more fulfilling lives, and improve relationships with others.

CBT also treats eating disorders like anorexia nervosa and bulimia nervosa. By helping patients recognize their unhealthy thoughts and develop healthier behaviors, CBT can help patients overcome their eating disorders.

Moreover, social anxiety is a key feature of a generalized anxiety disorder (GAD) and post-traumatic stress disorder (PTSD). CBT is effective in reducing social anxiety. In addition, patients who were treated with CBT experienced a significant reduction in avoidance symptoms.

The process of using CBT for social anxiety involves:

a. Self-monitoring of social anxiety: Patients are encouraged to become more aware of their symptoms of social anxiety and monitor their responses to specific situations such as public speaking, eating in public, etc.

b. Cognitive restructuring: This involves identifying distorted thoughts that lead to the patient's negative feelings and developing more realistic ways of thinking about the situations.

c. Behavioral experiments: Patients are encouraged to test their unrealistic thoughts through a series of behavioral experiments in this step.

d. Reducing safety behaviors: The fourth step involves reducing safety behaviors, such as distracting oneself from an imagined negative evaluation by focusing on something else or leaving an uncomfortable situation.

e. Exposure to feared situations: Within a controlled setting, patients are encouraged to experience their feared social situations without using safety behaviors and exclusively through a long-term goal-oriented perspective ("arrivederci").

Social anxiety and cognitive behavior therapy are effective in reducing depression. The underlying assumption is that depressed individuals experience negative events in their lives as more intense than healthy individuals do. For this reason, CBT tries to teach people how they think about these events and change their thoughts so they are less intense. This process involves CBT skills like rehearsal, role play, and imaginal exposure (putting ourselves into a situation where we predict how we would feel). This can also be used to prevent depression by reducing the intensity of negative events.

For example, some people think: "Nobody likes me," and they are afraid that no one would like them. Cognitive behavior therapy would try to change this thought into a healthy one. Therefore, the treatment starts by considering why it is important to make the person you treat to feel like others like them. The focus is to ensure they understand what it means to be liked.

CBT can alter how people view themselves by focusing on the benefits of social relationships, such as feeling loved or valued.

Techniques that are being taught must be ones that can fit in with all situations. Therefore, if a person has had some personal experience of using CBT techniques and it is not working, they need to be taught new techniques and retested. If problems still occur, referring them to their GP for medical assessment is best.

CBT and Negative Core Beliefs (NCBs)

CBT is used to treat individuals who have had traumatic experiences in their lives, such as cancer patients, soldiers, and victims of sexual abuse. CBT is useful because it can help patients develop healthier behaviors to relieve the distress caused by their traumatic experiences. In the case of cancer patients, one of the coping mechanisms that help reduce anxiety involves NCBs. NCBs are beliefs about oneself (such as I am worthless) or beliefs about the future (such as I will never get better). People use NCBs to make sense of stressful situations, but in some cases, they can also increase feelings of helplessness and hopelessness and become harmful. There are two ways in which CBT helps treat individuals with NCBs, and the first is that it reduces their sense of helplessness. A study shows that after eight sessions of CBT, participants experienced less hopelessness and helplessness than those who did not receive CBT.

The second way CBT addresses NCBs is by helping the individual reconstruct the meaning of their experiences. When individuals go through a traumatic or potentially traumatic experience, they can cope with it using two different methods: via constructive (meaning-making) or destructive (meaning-maintaining) processes. The latter involves a person having negative thoughts about themselves or their environment and then trying to find a way to maintain these negative thoughts. The constructive way of coping with a traumatic experience is by having positive thoughts about the environment or themselves. CBT is useful because it helps individuals to reconstruct their experiences and constructively recover from trauma.

The benefits of CBT have been demonstrated for people suffering from mood disorders such as major depression, bipolar disorder, and dysthymia. The most noticeable effect of CBT is an improvement in mood, but generally, functioning and quality of life are often improved. This is partly due to the direct effects of CBT on mood and functioning, but also indirect effects such as increased motivation, more activity, and more positive social interactions.

For individuals with bipolar disorder, the most established and evidence-based way of preventing a depressive episode is to reduce or eliminate drinking alcohol or using drugs. Because both substances have a depressive effect, reducing intake often helps to prevent depression. Unfortunately, some individuals with bipolar disorder are unable and unwilling to reduce their substance use.

The main aim of CBT for substance misuse is to reduce the frequency and amount of substance use and any associated problems such as health issues, unemployment, or relationship problems. Therefore, the first step in treatment involves identifying goals related to reducing usage or stopping altogether. A therapist will then help the person identify how their thoughts about using substances might maintain their problem. They can then work on reducing the frequency of substance use and sabotaging their thoughts.

CBT is useful in treating adolescents with depression because it is a short-term therapy that gives young people the skills to deal with their depression in the future. Most teenagers that suffer from major depression will recover within a year. Still, they may suffer another depressive episode later in life, so they must be given effective tools to help them through these times. CBT can be used to help teenagers and children by teaching them how their negative thoughts affect their emotions and behaviors. CBT techniques involve thought-stopping (a way of controlling negative self-talk) and thought replacement (a way of replacing negative thoughts with positive ones).

For example, a patient with lung cancer has never smoked, but she might believe that her cancer is caused by tobacco. This belief may make her feel guilty, depressed, and worthless (i.e., I am worthless because I gave in to smoking, my cancer is my punishment for smoking, and I will die because of it).

CBT would first try to assuage the patient's guilt with facts (such as tobacco causes certain types of lung cancer but not all types) and then challenge the patient's negative thoughts (such as if you didn't smoke, you wouldn't have this type of cancer anyway).

How to treat depression with CBT

Depression can be treated with CBT. First, it is important to understand that depression is a common condition, and CBT can be used to treat mild to moderately depressed people of all ages. However, CBT has become the go-to method for treating depression when it occurs in older adults. Studies have shown that older adults who received CBT were more likely to experience clinical improvement than those who received other types of treatment. However, once again, compared to the general population, older adults are less likely to receive help for their depression due to challenges in access and availability of services (such as financial challenges) and because they have a higher risk for misdiagnosis or medication problems.

CBT has also been used in treating anxiety disorders in children. Any individual with an anxiety disorder can benefit from this type of therapy, and recent studies have shown that it does help with the generalization of learned skills to everyday situations as well. It is not just useful for the treatment of children but also for the treatment of individuals who have panic attacks and other chronic anxious states.

For instance, CBT effectively reduced symptoms of depression and anxiety after a person experienced a traumatic accident that left them hospitalized. Other studies have found that certain techniques, such as stimulus control, reduce symptoms of anxiety disorders, including social phobia, generalized social anxiety, and panic attacks.

CBT is still used to treat people living with dementia, although it may not be the most effective approach. By increasing awareness of the symptoms and reducing exposure to negative social situations and the environment, CBT can help decrease the risk of depression and other forms of psychological distress. However, some findings suggest that depression significantly predicts functional decline for individuals with dementia. Therefore, treatment of depression in people with dementia requires careful monitoring for suicidality and other safety concerns.

Researchers have found that CBT may be a helpful tool as early as pregnancy for women who have or are at risk for experiencing depression during their pregnancy. CBT was found to improve the number of anxiety women experience throughout their pregnancies, and it also helps them to feel more prepared for their child's life after birth. It also helps them to understand the different types of depression and anxiety. This form of CBT can be especially helpful for families with a history of depression because it can make them more aware of their symptoms, which may help them recognize the signs earlier. Additionally, it also helps women to prepare themselves for postpartum experiences better.

In many cases, CBT is used in conjunction with medication or taken after some time on medication. CBT has significantly improved the outcomes of those receiving anti-depressant treatment when treating course one (moderate) depression. However, these findings must be interpreted cautiously because they only show an association between treatment and improved outcomes; this does not prove that CBT causes improvement by itself. For instance, other forms of psychotherapy also claim to lead to an improvement in depressive symptoms, yet research has shown that there is no significant difference between the different treatments.

This evidence suggests that CBT is not necessarily a better treatment for depression. Certain studies have compared CBT to other types of cognitive therapy or have analyzed the mechanisms behind CBT and have found that the improvements from CBT are mostly due to exposure and response prevention. This study found that exposure done systematically to expose people to feared situations without giving in to a coping mechanism (for example, exposure replaces avoidance) had most of the long-lasting effects on people suffering from anxiety disorders.

CBT for anger problems

Although every CBT therapist uses a different technique, here is a description of one approach.

Several techniques can be used to treat anger problems: cognitive defusion, here-and-now, and relaxation. Cognitive defusion is altering negative thoughts by using more realistic ones. Here-and-now techniques include empathic communication and compassionate responding. To help relieve anger in people with depression, it is important to teach them how to put their own needs behind those of others by criticizing or not accepting others' needs. Rather than focusing on how angry they are and how they want others to respond or behave, it helps them focus on what they want instead. Relaxation techniques, such as progressive muscle relaxation or guided imagery, are also quite effective in releasing pent-up anger.

People struggling with anger issues can try to follow healthy steps to avoid and de-escalate anger. One of these ways is avoiding certain people or places where they know they will get angry. Another way is by recognizing how alcohol or drugs can cause people to become angry and avoid them. In addition, taking a time-out from situations where people get angry can see them react more healthily than when they stay involved in the situation. Finally, people with anger problems need to avoid using violence or intimidation to respond when angry. These actions can lead to violence or bullying against themselves or others, especially children.

A clear expression of grief needs to be honored and attended to by the person grieving for a person's grief to resolve. People commonly express the grief they are experiencing without the conscious awareness that they are doing so. When there is a loss, often no one sees it coming, and when it happens, there is often shock and denial. This can lead to a difficult experience for the individual who has experienced this loss and those around them. Both individuals who have experienced a loss and those close to them may have difficulty understanding how someone can suffer such a traumatic loss. When grief is experienced, the individual who has experienced the loss will usually have strong feelings towards it and how it has affected them.

For someone to deal with their grief, it is common for people to try to avoid or distract themselves from their feelings. This can be very difficult for a person, as they may face many daily challenges that may cause them to become overwhelmed. People experiencing this kind of grief need to find ways to cope with these emotions healthily. One of the ways someone can cope with their emotion is by exercising or doing something physical. This activates the body's relaxation response, which helps someone calm down and understand what they are experiencing.

The grieving process can be very different for each individual. Some may want to express their feelings or talk about the loss, while others may not. While talking about it with someone who has experienced a similar loss, such as a therapist or family member, may help a person feel support and understanding for themselves. This can be very helpful in helping them work through their grief. In cases where people cannot say what they are experiencing, writing down their thoughts and feelings can help both individuals understand what they are going through and give them a way to cope with these emotions.

It is common for individuals who have experienced a loss to be angry with God during this time. Anger is commonly displayed when someone who has experienced a loss feels that there has been an injustice in the world. This difference can be an important way for people to express their grief, as they may feel angry toward God, but this anger is more directed at the world's injustice than towards God. Many people who have experienced a loss feel angry at God due to the unfairness of life and how unfair it can sometimes be. This anger will usually subside when people forgive themselves and others after experiencing such trauma as a loss.

How to overcome negative emotional habits with CBT

Changing negative emotional habits such as feeling stuck in depression can be challenging, especially if you are not used to doing so. However, if your negative emotions are closely linked to a habit that helps you cope with them and feel better about the situation, then it is likely that changing this habit will help you a lot. For example, if an individual is socially less active because they fear being judged by others, changing their social habits can make them feel better about themselves. The benefit of this approach is that the individual does not need to abandon their old habits completely but instead can move them into a new, more positive side instead of being stuck in the negative side. For example, if the individual is stuck in feeling stuck and worried that everything is going wrong, they can try to move this worry into a more positive emotion, such as being grateful.

In CBT, clients do not need to feel guilty about their emotions. It is the therapist who assesses what causes the client's emotional problems. The therapist helps clients identify their triggers, situations, or events that cause them emotional reactions. They also help clients recognize common misconceptions about emotions by explaining how negative emotions lead to destructive actions through patterns of thinking and behaviors. People can learn from their mistakes, develop new ways of coping with negative emotions, and become more effective at responding to them.

CBT helps clients identify the situations that trigger negative emotions and how these actions are linked to their emotions. CBT also helps people with anxiety disorders focus on the present moment because many are prone to worrying about the future or regretting the past. In addition, many people with depression tend to dwell on negative thoughts, which can lead to depression. Therefore, these individuals must focus on positive thoughts and things they enjoy to become more emotionally balanced. Psychologists have found that cognitive therapy can effectively treat certain disorders such as depression and can be used as an alternative or supplement to anti-depressant medications. CBT is also effective in depression, anxiety disorders, and other disorders.

A major advantage of cognitive therapy is that it can be used to treat a wide variety of different mental health issues and disorders. For example, people with mood disorders can experience a broad range of emotions and distress. Cognitive therapy helps individuals identify the situations that cause negative emotions and lets them know how they can use positive thoughts or behaviors to deal with these situations. Therapists also help clients recognize their irrational beliefs, which may contribute to negative emotional reactions. These irrational beliefs usually cause great distress because they interfere with the individuals' ability to make healthy decisions regarding their emotions and behavior.

How to treat sleep problems with CBT

In general, insomnia is a sleep disorder characterized by a chronic and recurring inability to fall asleep or stay asleep at night. However, insomnia may be characterized in different ways, such as difficulty initiating or falling asleep without other sleep apnea symptoms, frequent waking during the night or early morning, frequent daytime naps, and excessive daytime sleepiness.

Sleep deficits can negatively affect performance in various facets of life. For example, difficulty sleeping interferes with regular activities and responsibilities at school, work, and home. In addition to health-related problems (e.g., cardiovascular disorders) that may develop from insufficient sleep, poor sleep quality may cause a person to have negative feelings throughout the day (e.g., fatigue).

The cognitive behavioral therapy (CBT) technique must be used to treat insomnia. This involves helping the individual identify why they have difficulty sleeping and developing strategies to help them sleep. Many people with insomnia complain that they cannot fall asleep and think it is normal. However, this should not be normal for someone in good health since most people with healthy bodies can sleep well when necessary.

A treatment for insomnia consists of discovering what causes the person's thoughts about sleeping and how these thoughts cause them to feel physically tired. Some common causes of an inability to sleep are poor-quality sleep, anxiety, stress, and problems in social situations (e.g., having a job). As a result, insomnia is usually caused by a combination of different factors. More specifically, there are two types of insomnia:

CBT can be used to treat both types of insomnia. The difference between the two is that people with sleep initiation problems (difficulty falling asleep) tend to worry and think, "What if I fall asleep?" or "I can't do this," or even "What if I don't get any sleep?" while they try to fall asleep. This kind of thinking makes them anxious, negatively affecting their ability to fall asleep quickly.

To treat sleep initiation problems (not falling asleep), it is important to have the patient recognize that they can go to bed at a particular time with anxiety or stress. Then, they would tell themselves: "I am okay, I don't have to worry about sleeping, and I will be okay." This kind of thinking is called catastrophizing; many people cannot do it because they think it is impossible. However, this way of thinking is a matter of degree; all people are capable of doing something when they are stressed out and anxious.

In contrast, people with anxiety disorders that bother their ability to fall asleep (sleep continuity insomnia) tend to worry about their children, the health of a relative, or the details of the next day. They also worry about work or even their future and what will happen. These repetitive thoughts occur many times during the night and can prevent them from having a relaxing sleep. One of the main reasons for this kind of thinking is that people with anxiety disorders have difficulty when they are trying to go to sleep.

Treatment for these problems involves helping patients recognize how anxious they are when they try to fall asleep and how they can lower this anxiety by repeating positive statements that make them want to sleep.

How to treat panic attacks with CBT

Panic attacks are sudden intense fear in response to a nonspecific and highly personal threat. The attacks may happen without warning. They might begin with many feelings (e.g., chest pain, chills, numbness), followed by hyperventilation and a sense of suffocation. It is most common during physical exertion or roughly an hour before bedtime. Panic attacks are often experienced in the context of other panic disorders or phobias (such as obsessive-compulsive disorder). Although panic attacks may occur in isolation, they can also accompany agoraphobia and social anxiety disorder.

To treat panic attacks, therapists have focused on the cognitive behaviors that are often associated with the disorder. For example, people with panic attacks may feel overwhelmed by the presence of others. The therapist, in this instance, might ask them: "What is your perception of how safe you feel in social situations?" This is called distancing because the individual feels as if they are not involved in the situation. Furthermore, they may consider another person a threat while standing in line at a store and then fear any small movement or noise. As mentioned above, these thoughts also lead to hyperventilation; therefore, it is important to help clients recognize how their fear prevents them from breathing normally and leads to other physical symptoms (e.g., chest pain, chills, and numbness).

CBT also helps people recognize their feelings of panic. For example: "I am feeling fear, and I am breathing a lot faster." Furthermore, the therapist can help clients see the relationship between their feelings of panic and other life situations by asking them to recall why they have had panic attacks. For example, suppose a life situation is related to the anticipation of another anxiety-producing event (e.g., they might have a panic attack before going on vacation). In that case, they should be asked what would happen if they did not anticipate that situation anymore. In addition, more specific questions are often used to teach clients how to treat some of their symptoms (e.g., "What do you do when your heart races?").

CBT is sometimes used in combination with medications. There is strong evidence that CBT can help reduce panic attacks and the need for medication for people with a history of panic attacks (as well as agoraphobia and social phobia). The addition of CBT has been shown effective in those who are treatment-resistant to taking medications.

CBT is the most effective treatment for anxiety disorders. There are several ways it works, and it focuses on understanding why the person has anxiety disorders, what triggers them, and what makes them continue. Once a person understands their anxiety and its patterns, they can begin to take control of their anxiety.

Anxiety is a response to stress and a part of our natural defense system. The problem comes when the anxiety becomes excessive, occurs at the wrong time, or happens for no reason. When this happens, it is an anxiety disorder and can greatly affect one's life. It may be hard to do things that people usually do not think twice about: going to work or school, cooking, driving, dating, etc. Some people may also have physical symptoms associated with their anxiety, such as nausea or dizziness; these are called panic attacks.

How CBT works for obsessive-compulsive disorder (OCD)

Obsessive-compulsive disorder (OCD) is characterized by obsessions (obsessive thoughts) and compulsions (a compulsion to do something). Obsessions are thoughts that cannot be controlled and are often perceived as unacceptable. For example, people with OCD obsess about dirtying or infecting themselves or a loved one. As a result, they may wash their hands numerous times or lock the door repeatedly. The compulsions are behaviors the individual feels compelled to perform in response to the obsession; they usually bring temporary relief but only last for short periods. Compulsions include cleaning, counting, checking whether doors are locked, arranging objects in a certain order, etc.

Obsessive-compulsive disorder (OCD) is a more common disorder than people realize. It affects approximately 2.5 percent of the population, or 1 in every 40 people; however, this is often underreported because many individuals do not seek treatment. Furthermore, OCD is frequently accompanied by other disorders such as depression, anxiety, and eating disorders; these disorders are often treated with medication, leading to drug abuse.

OCD has several characteristics: obsessions (an obsessive thought), compulsions (a compulsion to do something), and resistance and avoidance of fearful situations. It is a type of anxiety disorder.

OCD often causes people to be anxious, depressed, and upset. It can also cause people to avoid things that do not need to be avoided, such as certain situations or people. People with OCD often have obsessions with contamination and germs; they may feel compelled to wash their hands several times throughout the day or avoid touching certain objects because they think they will get germs on them. Conversely, people with OCD may have obsessions about the wrong things (e.g., insects, hair) and compulsions that involve washing or checking those items over an excessive amount of time. For example, they may feel compelled to check the back of their eyelids, count certain things (e.g., the items in a drawer), or touch certain objects multiple times before performing a task (e.g., doors, doorknobs).

OCD is not always the same for everyone, but it can cause severe problems and may interfere with everyday functioning. People with OCD often do not want to seek help since they fear their obsessions are wrong; however, treatment can help relieve the obsessive thoughts and compulsive behaviors.

Many treatment options are available for people with OCD; however, CBT reduces symptoms. This therapy aims to help clients identify their negative beliefs about themselves, others, and situations and to modify those beliefs so that they are more realistic. In addition, therapists often use exposure and response prevention to help people overcome the obsessive thoughts that cause their compulsions. For example, when people worry about contamination, they may be asked to do a task involving contamination (e.g., touch paper for five seconds). The person may also be asked to perform the same task after their compulsive behavior; however, this time, they are told not to do the compulsive behavior (i.e., touching the paper). This process helps with desensitization, which helps people become less anxious about performing their compulsive behavior.

How to treat weight problems with CBT

People with obesity often report a variety of concerns, including fear of hurting their health, fear of gaining weight, fear of not being able to lose weight or keep the weight off, feelings of low self-esteem when they are overweight or obese, and concern about their appearance and how others will perceive them. Unfortunately, many people experience these types of worries long before seeking help. This can cause significant energy, concentration, and engagement problems at work or school. Studies have shown that CBT combined with medications is an effective obesity treatment; behavioral therapy (like CBT) and a structured diet plan improve outcomes.

Combining CBT methods with weight-loss strategies has proven to be successful. CBT aims to help people understand their eating habits and the underlying causes of obesity. When people develop an accurate view of the situation, they are in a much better position to make lasting changes. One study on obesity treatment showed that about 74 percent of participants experienced weight loss after undergoing CBT for six months. These results were similar regardless of age or gender.

This form of treatment is known to help people with eating disorders. CBT aims to help people understand their eating habits and the underlying causes of their disordered eating. When people develop an accurate view of the situation, they are in a much better position to make lasting changes. For example, one study on CBT for people with bulimia showed that about 56 percent of participants experienced weight loss after undergoing CBT for six months. These results were similar regardless of age or gender. Overall, after three months, patients experienced remission from symptoms, including binge-eating and purging behaviors and psychological symptoms; however, there were some fluctuations in symptom severity over time compared to pretreatment levels.

Some weight-loss strategies involve creating a diet plan and increasing physical activity; however, dieting often does not work in the long term. CBT focuses on dieting and exercise and overcoming negative weight thinking. CBT aims to help patients develop healthy eating and exercise habits. CBT therapists help patients identify and replace negative thoughts so that it becomes easier to make healthy choices. CBT techniques can be used in conjunction with any weight-loss method.

People who have undergone a concussion often experience headaches, dizziness, or problems with memory or concentration; however, these symptoms usually improve after one year. Unfortunately, many people do not recover as expected and instead continue to have abnormal brain activity, depression, and anxiety. In addition, treating concussions with medication can lead to drug abuse.

People who are overweight or obese should be given personalized treatment plans by their physicians and therapists. This involves working with people to find the underlying causes of their weight issues and setting a realistic goal appropriate for their health concerns, medical history, lifestyle, and current psychosocial situation. In addition, there should be a focus on self-awareness, healthy eating habits, and increased physical activity through exercise.

Weight problems can often be treated with CBT. However, this treatment cannot always resolve all of the individual's issues. Instead, treatment involves identifying the distorted thinking patterns causing the problem and replacing them with more realistic thinking. For example, a person may fear gaining weight because they believe that food will make them fat despite their size. Working with the patient to identify this distorted belief can lead to successful weight management.

Therefore, CBT can be used in conjunction with other types of treatment for these disorders. This can help people overcome the obsessive thoughts, feelings, and behaviors associated with their depression and anxiety disorders.

CBT, including cognitive behavioral therapy (CBT) and behavioral activation therapy (BAT), can be used to treat OCD. These forms of treatment include exposure, response prevention (ERP), and cognitive restructuring techniques. CBT is a form of psychotherapy that focuses on helping clients identify the negative thoughts and beliefs that cause their obsessions and compulsions and ways to change those beliefs.

How to treat bipolar disorder with CBT

Cognitive-behavioral therapy (CBT) effectively prevents or mitigates depression, anxiety, and overall distress in bipolar disorder. It is also used to help individuals manage their physical symptoms and reduce the number of relapses. In addition, CBT is often used to treat bipolar depression by improving sleep quality, reducing fatigue, and helping patients with problem-solving skills.

CBT is effective partly due to its ability to help patients change their emotions, thoughts, and behaviors to cope better with stressors in their lives. Therefore, CBT is regarded as an appropriate treatment for PTSD as it helps a person cope psychologically with their experience.

CBT is also used to treat trichotillomania (compulsive hair-pulling) and excoriation disorder (compulsive skin-picking). Treatment for these disorders can include attention, relaxation, habit reversal, and response prevention.

Although data on the use of CBT for substance abuse is limited, many researchers focus on individual CBT for substance use problems. People with Substance Use Disorders often have impaired decision-making skills, leading them to make poor choices about their drug use. In addition, people with addiction often have a poor self-image and feel weak-willed or out of control. CBT is designed to correct these issues by helping people modify their decision-making skills, identify negative thinking patterns, and relearn self-control.

Like substance abuse studies, the data on CBT for gambling addiction is limited; however, one study found that CBT combined with medications had a greater positive impact than medication alone or CBT alone. According to this study, people in the medication-only group were more likely to experience recurring thoughts of gambling than those in the group receiving both treatments.

CBT helps treat these disorders by targeting the thoughts and behaviors causing problems. After identifying the harmful thoughts or behaviors and replacing them with positive ones, individuals can effectively cope with their anxiety or depression symptoms. CBT also teaches clients to identify automatic thoughts or beliefs that trigger anxiety and depression and create alternate ways to cope with stressors.

In one study, CBT significantly impacted participants' emotional well-being, self-esteem, behavior, and job satisfaction two years after the treatment ended. Furthermore, people who completed the treatment were less likely to relapse into depression than people who did not receive the treatment. In addition, those who completed CBT reported less severe depression than people who received no therapy in follow-ups.

Bipolar disorder affects approximately 2.6% of the US population, with a lifetime prevalence between 5% and 10% in the general population. It is a severe psychiatric disorder that interferes with an individual's functioning and quality of life. People diagnosed with bipolar disorder are at risk for both depressive and manic episodes during which they may experience. These episodes of depression or mania can last days, weeks, or months.

The symptoms associated with both depressive and manic episodes are severe and interfere with an individual's ability to work and maintain relationships. Symptoms of depressive episodes include severe depression, weight loss, difficulty sleeping, fatigue, feelings of guilt/worthlessness, suicidal ideation/attempts, decreased concentration, and negative self-image. In contrast to this, CBT helps people with bipolar disorder by teaching them to monitor their moods; identify negative thinking; express emotions appropriately; problem-solve and make decisions; solve interpersonal problems; build on personal strengths; control over-thinking and avoidance behaviors; develop regular patterns for sleeping, eating, working and recreation activities.

In addition to the symptoms of depression, manic episodes are marked by feelings of euphoria and elevated mood, talking very rapidly and jumping from one idea to the next, increased activity; decreased need for sleep, racing thoughts; difficulty concentrating; grandiose beliefs/self-importance; impulsive behavior; sexual disinhibition.

How to eliminate procrastination with CBT

Cognitive-behavioral therapy (CBT) has been proven effective in treating severe procrastination by targeting the condition's cognitive, emotional, and behavioral symptoms. This therapy focuses on changing a person's automatic thoughts, irrational beliefs, and maladaptive behaviors that interfere with addressing important tasks.

CBT helps people with OCD identify their obsessions and how they relate to their compulsions. It then helps them develop coping skills by exploring the situations in which these thoughts occur and learning how to change their behaviors when they have an obsession. For example, one study focusing on people with OCD found that CBT reduced worry about negative events, improved mood, and increased overall satisfaction with life compared to a control group. The study also found that people in the CBT group were less likely to feel "stuck" or unable to control their symptoms and more likely to seek treatment after completing CBT.

CBT targets social, behavioral, and cognitive aspects of tics. It focuses on helping patients identify the thoughts and behaviors causing their tics and replace them with less disruptive ones. It also encourages patients to challenge irrational beliefs contributing to their tic symptoms.

CBT, especially in combination with other types of therapy, is an effective treatment for bulimia nervosa. CBT helps reduce binge eating and negative body image associated with this disorder. The treatment also helps patients identify irrational beliefs and worries about the weight that often contribute to binging episodes. In addition, it teaches them coping skills that enable them to eat more in moderation.

CBT can treat generalized anxiety disorder (GAD). Although the mechanisms by which it works are unknown, CBT effectively reduces anxiety symptoms and improves overall functioning. In addition, clinical trials have shown the benefit of CBT over medications when GAD is not severe enough to warrant medications.

Procrastination is a common problem that occurs in people of all ages. CBT is a psychological treatment designed to help people focus their efforts more efficiently and reduce procrastinating time. CBT teaches people how to break down large tasks into smaller ones and allocate their limited time to complete them promptly. This allows people to get more done in a shorter amount of time.

Some CBT techniques, such as rolling a ball back and forth between hands, or twirling a pen, can also help people with ADHD control their attention span. These techniques increase focus and reduce restlessness.

Cognitive-behavioral therapy is effective in treating ADHD. The treatment has been applied to children and adults with the disorder; it improves symptoms by teaching people how to monitor their symptoms and change unhelpful thoughts and behaviors that may be contributing to their ADHD.

Therefore, procrastination can be a major problem for people of all ages. It can seriously affect productivity and quality of life, making it very important to address it appropriately. CBT can help people suffering from procrastination to get more done in less time, improving their productivity and overall quality of life. CBT techniques, such as rolling a ball back and forth between hands or twirling a pen, can also help people with ADHD control their attention span to focus on the tasks at hand. In addition, better attention spans coupled with the flexibility to shift tasks keep work from becoming stale and make it more enjoyable for employees.

How to treat PTSD (post-traumatic stress disorder with CBT)

Cognitive-behavioral therapy (CBT) is effective for PTSD, especially when combined with exposure therapy, which can help people overcome their fear and re-inoculation to situations that cause anxiety. Exposure therapy is a CBT technique that involves confronting one's fear of being outside the safety of their home, like attending social events or playing games with children. Plus establishing new and more productive behaviors like initiating conversations and volunteering to help. CBT is also used to improve symptoms of OCD; this treatment has been proven effective in treating various disorders, including depression and phobias.

PTSD was first described in 1980 by psychiatrists and psychologists. It is an anxiety disorder caused by a terrifying event that overwhelms the person experiencing it. The person may not have been physically harmed during the event, but they believe they are in danger. This can lead to feeling emotionally numb, suicidal thoughts, nightmares, and flashbacks of the event.

CBT is a form of psychotherapy that anyone with PTSD can use to help them feel better and manage symptoms like anxiety or depression that may be related to their traumatic experience. CBT focuses on four components of treatment for PTSD: emotional regulation, maintaining healthy relationships and lifestyle, and learning new ways to cope with feelings.

Treating PTSD involves reducing or eliminating the anxiety caused by the traumatic event and helping the person cope with the symptoms. The goal of cognitive therapy is to help patients analyze their thoughts and change them in a way that helps them feel better about themselves and their ability to cope. Over time, this helps reduce triggers for anxiety or flashbacks related to the trauma, teaches people how to manage daily stressors, and gives them tools for managing emotions. Moreover, it improves their ability to have healthy relationships and helps them develop confidence in their abilities.

Therefore, PTSD is an anxiety disorder caused by a terrifying event that overwhelms the person experiencing it. The patient may not have been physically harmed during the event, but they believe they are in danger. This can lead to feeling emotionally numb, suicidal thoughts, nightmares, and flashbacks of the event. The goal of cognitive therapy is to help patients analyze their thoughts and change them in a way that helps them feel better about themselves and their ability to cope. CBT reduces or eliminates the anxiety caused by the traumatic event and helps patients with PTSD cope with their symptoms over time. In addition, it improves their ability to have healthy relationships and helps them develop confidence in their abilities.

How to use CBT to overcome Negative Automatic Thoughts (NATs)

NATs are common in people with depression. They are the unproductive (or negative) thoughts that people with depression habitually tell themselves, such as "I'm a loser" or "I can't do anything right." They can also include thoughts like "I am worthless," "everything is bad," or "I will never achieve anything in life." Cognitive-behavioral therapy (CBT) is a type of psychotherapy used to treat depression. The therapy involves changing unhelpful thoughts and behaviors to improve mood and overall quality of life. CBT helps people reframe their negative self-evaluations and harsh criticism of themselves to more positive ones. Furthermore, CBT can help people think about issues in new ways, and this can help them cope with stress and negative thoughts about themselves or the world.

Many people try to ignore NATs or even pretend they don't have them; however, this usually makes things worse because the problems continue to pile up without getting resolved. However, CBT offers a way to identify NATs and work on them to address issues and improve mood. CBT aims not only to change negative thoughts but also to change behavior patterns and overall outlook positively. Through CBT, people can learn what causes distortions or errors in thinking or behavior and the skills necessary for changing those thoughts and behaviors.

CBT helps people with depression identify the things that are causing stress in their lives. In addition, because depression is related to cognitive processes, including unhelpful thinking, CBT can help people with depression overcome their difficulties by changing how they think about themselves, other people, and situations. CBT also helps them develop strategies and coping skills to make them feel better in all relationships.

Anxiety Disorders are the most common mental disorders in the United States. Panic attacks, phobias, and generalized anxiety disorder are specific types of anxiety that have distinct symptoms among similar disorders. The center of treatment for these disorders is cognitive-behavioral therapy (CBT). CBT is a type of psychotherapy that can also be used to treat depression and substance use disorders. It involves helping people learn to identify negative feelings and thoughts while experiencing them to understand what triggers those feelings, prevent them from happening again, or change them when they occur. In addition, CBT helps people keep track of their symptoms and triggers for anxiety.

NATs are common in people with depression. They are the unproductive (or negative) thoughts that people with depression habitually tell themselves, such as "I'm a loser" or "I can't do anything right." They can also include thoughts like "I am worthless," "everything is bad," or "I will never achieve anything in life." Cognitive-behavioral therapy (CBT) is a type of psychotherapy used to treat depression. The therapy involves changing unhelpful thoughts and behaviors to improve mood and overall quality of life. CBT helps people reframe their negative self-evaluations and harsh criticism of themselves to more positive ones. Furthermore, CBT can help people think about issues in new ways, and this can help them cope with stress and negative thoughts about themselves or the world. Therefore, CBT is an effective treatment for anxiety disorders because it focuses on helping people learn to identify and deal with their fears and reduce the severity of their symptoms.

Cognitive-behavioral therapy (CBT) is a type of psychotherapy used to treat depression. The therapy involves changing unhelpful thoughts and behaviors to improve mood and overall quality of life. For example, CBT helps people reframe their negative self-evaluations and harsh criticism of themselves to more positive ones. Furthermore, CBT can help people think about issues in new ways, and this can help them cope with stress and negative thoughts about themselves or the world.

How to use CBT to solve common thinking errors

Various types of CBT are available for people with depression. The most commonly used type involves working on unhelpful thinking and problem-solving techniques. CBT works best when it helps people evaluate the situation, decide what to do, make a plan, and then implement their plan. It also helps people deal with difficult situations by modifying or changing their responses. These situations include dealing with anxiety issues, anxiety triggers, self-defeating thoughts or behaviors (such as smoking), and depressing emotions that lead to low moods. CBT helps people develop skills in working with stressful situations and their emotions, reduce stress, and become more effective at coping with the problems that make them feel less overwhelmed.

Thinking errors are the common, unhelpful ways of thinking or problem-solving that people with depression often use. These errors include negative self-talk, unrealistic expectations, negative reactions to stressful events, and mind reading. Using CBT, people with depression can learn and practice problem-solving skills, manage their distress after a stressful event, reduce their negative thinking patterns, increase the positive aspects of their moods (affect regulation), and help them be more effective at problem-solving. The cognitive part of CBT focuses on helping people identify treatment goals and determine what they need to do to achieve those goals to feel better. To determine treatment goals, people being treated with CBT must first identify problems causing stress in their lives. As part of this task, people should create a list of events that may have caused depression or other feelings, such as anger or sadness. The cognitive part of CBT is one way to accomplish this goal because it helps people identify their thinking errors and learn coping skills to deal with them. The behavioral aspect of CBT involves learning and practicing problem-solving techniques, which is another way for people with depression to improve their moods and manage stress.

CBT is a type of psychotherapy used in the treatment of depression. It can be considered a form of psycho-therapy that encourages people to change their thinking patterns, habits, and ways of acting to bring about significant changes in mood and behavior. The cognitive aspect of CBT focuses on changing unhelpful thinking patterns causing symptoms. These include thinking habits linked to depression, such as negative self-talk and distorted reasoning. The behavioral aspect of CBT is a way for people to develop skills to cope with problems and distress after stressful events. For example, this part of the treatment could involve learning how to begin problem-solving techniques, such as breathing to reduce anxiety, focusing on the positive aspects of life and helping other people, or reducing the effort to complete tasks. The behavioral aspect of CBT is also used to help people learn healthy and adaptive ways of coping with their distress, such as exercising to reduce stress or setting goals for stressful events.

CBT aims at changing distorted thinking; it encourages individuals to identify specific irrational thoughts causing negative moods and to begin changing these thoughts into more realistic ones. By identifying irrational thinking, cognitive distortions will be reduced, and one's mood will improve. According to the theory, the mood will improve if irrational thinking is reduced. However, CBT does not promote the idea of changing one's personality characteristics or behavior.

Cognitive-behavioral therapy (CBT) aims at changing distorted thinking and incorrect beliefs to reduce depressive symptoms. CBT attempts to identify erroneous, dysfunctional thought patterns that lead to negative moods and problematic behaviors to modify these thought patterns through cognitive restruc-turing in an attempt to alter behavior and manage negative thoughts. Cognitive restructuring has been observed as a therapeutic technique in treating depression, which involves the modification of cognition causing depressive symptoms. This process alters information processing to improve distorted cognitions and beliefs.

CBT aims to help people modify dysfunctional thought patterns to reduce depressive symptoms. Accord-ing to the theory, a dysfunctional thought pattern can result from a person's belief system. A person's beliefs are their way of perceiving, interpreting, explaining, and understanding their experiences; they are the basis of their thinking and behavior. Depressive thinking is usually based on the idea that something negative has happened or will happen. As a result, people tend to focus on these negative thoughts, which cause negative feelings and behaviors, resulting in a downward spiral toward depression. In cognitive therapy, people struggling with depression learn more appropriate ways of viewing situations, thus reduc-ing depressive symptoms.

A solution to common thinking errors for depression is to challenge beliefs and assumptions by question-ing and testing them instead of accepting them. By challenging these irrational, negative thoughts, new perceptions of the situations will be formed. These new perceptions can alter a person's mood or behavior. This is one way CBT attempts to help someone who has depression by challenging their irrational beliefs. For example, if an individual were to abandon the belief that they were less capable than others because they had not achieved as much in their life as others, this would result in increased self-esteem and a pos-itive change in mood. By changing the thought process that leads to a depressive mood, one can improve their symptoms and reduce the severity of their condition.

Cognitive-behavioral therapy is based on the fact that negative symptoms of depression are learned and can thus be unlearned. Based on this theory, depressive symptoms can be improved by addressing their behavioral manifestations. CBT, then, is a process of learning about the way one thinks and learns to cor-rect these negative thoughts that may result in depression. In this regard, cognitive-behavioral therapy can be seen as helping an individual understand how they think. If an individual already understands their thought process, they will have no problem correcting them if they become distorted or irrational.

How to treat infertility with CBT

This is a new approach to treating infertility. Infertility is a condition that affects about 6 of every 1000 couples. The most common reason for infertility is low sperm count or poor quality of sperm. This condition can also be caused by impotence, blocked fallopian tubes, and tubal blockage due to previous surgeries or infections. Some drugs and substances are also associated with the lack of fertility in men. Infertility can be difficult to treat as it is not always easy to identify the cause (low sperm count, poor quality of sperm, blocked system), and there is no reliable way to predict how long an individual will have bad results from treatment. One common treatment is Clomid which can result in multiple pregnancies after one cycle of treatment if used incorrectly with short-term alternate options available. The other methods include donor eggs (available in some countries) and long-term use of Clomid, IUI, and IVF.

Pregnancy is an important event in a woman's life, and her mental state should be considered during the entire process, from pregnancy to childbirth. Depression during pregnancy does not lead to childbirth complications but can affect the mother's mood and behavior. As there are many possible causes of depression that a woman may encounter during pregnancy, it is important to identify the cause of the problem before deciding on treatment options.

Clinical psychologists also have an important role in treating women who are suffering from depression while they are pregnant or when they are preparing to conceive. Some psychologists also use cognitive-behavioral therapy to treat women experiencing depression, especially during the perinatal period (during pregnancy). According to some specialists, cognitive-behavioral therapy is useful in "teaching women how to identify and reduce stress as well as managing their emotions and helping them to develop a healthy self-image."

When a doctor or psychologist diagnoses his patients with depression, he will recommend a specific treatment for each individual. For example, some may need anti-depressants while others just need simple psychotherapy. In addition, cognitive behavioral therapy treats people with depression because it focuses on improving self-esteem.

Therefore, CBT helps in the treatment of infertility in the following ways:

- Self-esteem improvement: CBT is used to help women gain self-confidence through various techniques such as relaxation training and positive self-talk. This way, a woman can deal with the stress of infertility and protect her emotional well-being.
- Stress regulation: Cognitive behavioral therapy can be used to stress regulation as it provides the tools for women to identify, evaluate, and change their thoughts that contribute to their anxieties. For example, CBT teaches women how to manage negative thoughts when undergoing infertility treatments, recognize anxiety symptoms, and then manage those symptoms to relax and reduce stress.
- Stomach ache and anxiety: Cognitive behavioral therapy teaches women how to recognize and deal with their symptoms of stress and anxiety. For instance, they can learn to identify their symptoms by asking themselves what they are feeling (anxiety, stress, or tension) and when did they feel this way (how long before the menstrual period), then learn different ways to relax or manage these symptoms without having negative effects on their mental health.

- Emotion regulation skills: Cognitive behavioral therapy teaches women to identify negative emotions such as anxiety, depression, or anger. This way, women can learn how to cope with these emotions when needed healthily by understanding them so that they will not lead to other harmful consequences such as drug abuse or suicidal thoughts.
- Coping skills: Emotion regulation is a coping skill used to help women cope with their stress and anxiety levels. Women can learn to solve healthily instead of being passive and then becoming aggressive, which usually leads to depression.
- Stress inoculation training: cognitive behavioral therapy can be used to reduce stress by teaching women how to adapt to and change adverse situations through various techniques such as realistic thinking, mental distraction, relaxation, increasing mastery, and catalytic thinking. The purpose of this technique is for women to recognize when they are feeling stressed, anxious or angry so that they can healthily manage these symptoms.

CBT and NLP for treating depression and anxious thinking

Sometimes this condition has been linked to the doctor's ethical pre-set choices that minimize risks for the patient in their treatment plan. However, when it comes to CBT and NLP, there seems to be a consensus that maybe these techniques can provide patients with a more effective solution when it comes to anxiety and depression by giving them tools at their disposal they never had before. Despite this, there is still much research and controversy surrounding these two psychological approaches to topics such as mental health issues.

CBT and NLP continue controversial because some people do not want to be treated with these techniques. This is a cause for concern because an individual that does not want to be treated with CBT or NLP will most likely default to medication and may be at risk for poor outcomes. Therefore, the conversation surrounding CBT and NLP must become more open and honest, especially when dealing with those experiencing anxiety or depression.

The greatest concern concerning CBT and NLP is that patients without depression but with anxiety can experience something referred to as "reactive depression." This form of depression is related in many ways to OCD, where the thought process is known as Ruminations or Rumination. The difference between the two is that they are moods. The thought process of Ruminations is often what goes on unconsciously, and if it's not addressed in time can lead to the development of depression. The term "reactive depression" is often defined as the depressive type that happens in response to a stressful life experience, such as losing a job, being criticized at work, experiencing family problems, or having to move. The good news is that CBT and NLP are among the most effective treatments for anxiety and depression because they can help patients confront and deal with these issues head-on.

A couple of different aspects regarding CBT and NLP effects on these disorders must be mentioned. For example, research shows that effective counseling interventions are one of the best ways to treat anxiety or depression and provide patients with a better quality of life. CBT and NLP are both effective in treating depression and anxiety. The one thing researchers must consider when dealing with CBT and NLP is that some patients may be more prone to these techniques than others, especially if they have a family history of mental health problems. The important thing to remember is that not every patient will respond to the same treatment. Still, finding what works for the individual will ultimately aid in improving their recovery.

Some patients may not respond well to traditional CBT and NLP because it does not meet their needs or because unique features are associated with their disorder. The good news is that researchers are studying other counseling interventions that may be more effective in treating anxiety or depression. Research on other treatments must continue, but so far, they are not as effective as CBT and NLP.

When it comes to effectiveness, there is solid evidence that CBT and NLP are effective when treating depression and anxiety. In one study, however, only 9 percent of patients improved with these therapies alone; in comparison, 50 percent improved with the addition of medications. The research must continue to be performed, but so far, it has shown that the combination of counseling and medication is the most successful method.

In many ways, CBT and NLP are two different techniques that can be used alongside each other to produce more effective results for anxious or depressed individuals. For example, CBT and NLP can be used simultaneously to help patients that have not responded well to either CBT or NLP because it gives them other options that were never there before. These two techniques will continue to be researched, but the consensus is that they offer an effective way of treating depression and anxiety.

Cognitive behavioral therapy and neurolinguistic programming can be used to treat anxiety.

The combined use of CBT and NLP will continue to improve since both techniques are effective for individuals that experience anxiety and depression. CBT alone may not be the most effective practice for treating this illness, but it is worth the effort because it can help people deal with these conditions and improve their quality of life. Therefore, using both CBT and NLP is something individuals should consider, especially if it has not helped them much.

A multi-modality treatment approach must be employed when treating anxiety or depression. With CBT, patients are often given homework or self-reflection exercises to continue treatment. For example, if a patient is experiencing anxiety, they may be asked to write down all the things they worry about and how they think these thoughts will play out. A patient may also be asked to identify times in the past when anxiety was present and what actions they took at that time. Likewise, when dealing with depression, patients may be asked to think about situations where they feel depressed and talk about this experience internally.

Another thing to consider is that there can be a lot of confusion in many cultures concerning CBT and NLP. Therefore, patients must be educated before they enter therapy or counseling concerning their diagnoses and how they will be treated during their sessions or sessions. There is a difference between psychotherapy and counseling, but when it comes to the latter, the patient's injuries should not be exposed, as this may lead to dismissal from treatment.

There are some other aspects to these approaches that may need more attention when it comes to the treatment of anxiety disorders.

Another example that causes people to become overwhelmed with anxiety is when a person experiences something known as "chronic worry." This is when one repeatedly thinks about a topic for days or weeks. It can be about finances, relationships, personal problems, or anything else that might need to be attended to in the future. This concept has similarities with OCD and is associated with the thought process known as Obsessive Compulsive Disorder OCD.

According to the book, "... the fact that there are still some persistent controversies about certain topics related to CBT and NLP has been a source of irritation for many researchers, who feel that instead of sticking to one specific approach to treatment, they should be able to draw from more than one theory when they start their sessions with patients. The idea is to avoid creating thought patterns in their minds that are rigid and inflexible, which is what seems to occur in people with anxiety disorder or depression.

The next chapter will discuss Dialectical Behavior Therapy (DBT). This therapy is based on the Cognitive Behavioral Theory. The theoretical concept behind DBT is that the therapist should focus on the patient's trauma history rather than symptoms. Rather than trying to eliminate these painful memories, DBT focuses on accepting and containing them so that they become manageable and less stressful. In addition to helping individuals increase their mental health and break free of destructive thought patterns, DBT is also focused on teaching individuals how to reduce their impulsivity, manage their emotions effectively, and improve relationships.

DBT includes several components, including relapse prevention skills training, acceptance skills training, mindfulness components, interpersonal effectiveness training, and safety planning. In addition, DBT aims to teach individuals how to reduce their self-destructive behaviors and increase their capacity for functioning.

Dialectical Behavior Therapy is based on multiple concepts used to treat Borderline Personality Disorder, Bipolar Disorder, and other mental health issues. This therapy teaches individuals how to manage their emotions effectively and improve relationships.

DIALECTICAL BEHAVIOR THERAPY

WHAT IS DBT?

Dialectical Behavior Therapy (DBT) is a treatment for Borderline Personality Disorder, which is characterized by emotions including anger, feelings of inadequacy or emptiness, difficulty controlling anger, and self-harm. DBT seeks to reduce these symptoms by using different therapeutic techniques, such as mindfulness skills and dialectics. Dialectical therapy can be particularly helpful for people who experience mental health problems that cause feelings of worthlessness. Dialectical therapy is effective because it gives people a sense of meaning in their treatment and control over their environment. People who experience Borderline Personality Disorder typically have trouble controlling their emotions due to how they perceive things. The way that they perceive "self" is often negative and always consuming, and they cannot accept parts of themselves that they do not like. In addition, these individuals frequently feel isolated when trying to understand their emotions or other people's emotions. Dialectical therapy can help individuals manage all these feelings by using dialectics as communication. People experiencing Borderline Personality Disorder often have difficulty understanding the need to expose and accept their failures. Still, dialectics are a way for them to understand that failing is an important part of life. Dialectical therapy is a helpful form of communication that emphasizes respecting and acknowledging others in the process of remembering to do so. DBT does not focus on symptom elimination but prioritizes effective risk management and core mental health improvement.

Dialectics can be defined as a method of solving problems involving contradictions or mutually exclusive positions. If two positions cannot be resolved logically or rationally, dialectics would help unite the two views into one unified perspective. This unified perspective is a process that helps individuals from any sort of conflict and problem resolution. Dialectics gives people a sense of meaning in the treatment and allows them to accept themselves. In other words, dialectics helps people feel better about themselves through understanding others' views and perspectives. This acceptance includes accepting failures because failure can be understood in relation to the context of one's life for failure to be meaningful. Failure is often understood as a way for people to grow, and dialectics allows them to recognize this reality by understanding what it means for those involved that something was wrong.

Dialectical behavior therapy applies this concept of dialectics to help people with Borderline Personality Disorder, characterized by experiencing problems with relationships and emotional dysregulation. People who experience Borderline Personality Disorder often have trouble understanding how their emotions affect them and difficulty being involved in relationships. Dialectical behavior therapy can also help people deal with strong emotions, particularly anger, and it can help them learn to avoid situations that are likely to cause problems. By teaching these skills through methods such as individual therapy, group classes on dialectics, and exercise groups, people can learn how to cope with their emotions effectively.

To understand how dialectics works in the subject of DBT, it is necessary to understand the way that DBT uses a system of four roles: the patient, who talks about how his or her problems began and are being treated; the therapist, who provides feedback and holds people accountable for their actions and behaviors; the therapist, who provides help regarding the patient's progress; and the therapist, who has a sense of meaning regarding treatment. As part of this system, therapists must be present throughout every session to provide useful feedback to patients.

Dialectics allows people recovering from conflict to have a sense of meaning and control over what happens during treatment. Dialectical Behavior Therapy can be particularly helpful for people who experience Borderline Personality Disorder because it allows people to understand the perspective of others, which helps them understand their own feelings. Dialectical behavior therapy recognizes the need for failure for anyone to grow and feel healthy. Dialectics are a powerful way for people to communicate effectively. DBT can be a highly effective treatment that allows people who experience Borderline Personality Disorder to have a sense of meaning in their lives and control over what happens during treatment.

In the past, dialectics was applied in a rigid form of analytical psychology. For instance, the general perspective on personality was of "the norm," who had no problems; it was all about getting rid of these abnormalities, which were believed to be caused by lack of nourishment, i.e., undernourishment. This kind of thinking made sense because many patients abused day-patient psychiatrists and other psychotherapists because they presented them with this rigid picture and expectations that seemed impossible to meet.

The role model that changed everything in this regard was Viktor Frankl. Frankl offered an alternative to the classical model of psychoanalytically-oriented psychotherapy known as "analysis", "psychotherapies," and "counseling" that focused on analyzing symptoms and then treating them.

In a way, Frankl was followed by some other great examples like Carl Rogers, Jean Piaget, and Erik Erikson. They were also all psychiatrists that applied dialectics in their specific therapy approaches. On the contrary, Theodor Reik devoted his life to developing dialectical psychotherapy. He spent time immersing himself in philosophy and created a comprehensive theoretical framework of his own concerning learning and experience.

Dialectics is based on the principle of "contradiction," a concept that describes how success and failure are interrelated. Frankl called his dialectical approach "process psychology". He studied the meanings and purposes of human life and looked at the experience of those with different types of problems. During his research, he noticed that people's reactions to certain situations were very similar. He found that these reactions came from a single common source in response to basic needs such as food, fear, pain, love, and sexuality. His theory explains that everything works according to social laws: contradictions do not exist due to personal circumstances; rather, they originate from universal law.

During Frankl's time in the concentration camp, he became acquainted with "alienation," which is a state of mind that happens when a person is disconnected from reality and self-identity. Instead, he came to believe that the following actions accomplished the destruction of an authentic life:

Frankl believed that the experience of personal responsibility was critical to overcoming his imprisonment. He reasoned that if humanity was to survive and prosper in this new world order, they must break free from the power of destruction by focusing on their ability to change situations in their lives and visioning themselves as able to take action.

Through his research and studies, Frankl developed a system that was a natural reaction to the contradiction of suffering and survival. This system focuses on how people react and how to resolve their conflicts. He believed there were two stages: the stage where individuals are treated as objects and the stage where they receive care as people.

Frankl believed that psychology should be viewed like an emergency room in a hospital. The patient has already suffered horribly, and now he needs assistance to survive psychologically. In this sense, psychologists need to not only treat the symptoms; rather, they have to use the same type of measures that are used in emergency medicine to restore normal brain function. So, in this respect, the priority is not to treat symptoms but to treat the "whole" person.

Frankl also realized that people have different reactions in their learning processes. When a human has a goal and finds something that contradicts his values, he will either search for compromise or change the goal to fit his values. But if he realizes something is an irreconcilable contradiction that he can't change or compromise on, he will resort to developing another value system. This new value system allows him to stand up when others would lie down and give up. He called this process "dialectics." Simply put, it describes how people deal with the process of change.

The following example demonstrates this concept:

For a person to improve his life and overcome a situation, he will have to go through four phases in his life:

These four phases are associated with eight basic values developed during childhood. By developing strong values, a person can find and express himself in the world; this is critical for a normal human existence and very important in improving one's quality of life.

Frankl's DBT, or Dialectical Behavior Therapy, is based on these concepts of change and values. The main idea behind DBT is that people with BPD have an intense need to control their lives. This is because they experience a sense of powerlessness in situations that would normally be experienced as positive experiences, such as: falling in love and marriage, ordinary jobs and responsibilities, and having children. On the other hand, people who have BPD suffer from intense anger and self-destructive behaviors.

These individuals tend to engage in self-destructive behaviors such as promiscuous sex with many partners or drug abuse. When a situation gets too intense for them, they tend to have suicidal thoughts and act on them. The main idea of DBT was to teach these patients how to deal with the world differently.

Therefore, DBT originated from the basic principles of Frankl's philosophy. The "values" that people respond to tend to be very simple:

People with BPD cannot learn from experience; therefore, they need the training to change their thinking and behavior. These individuals are usually very weak in self-management skills and find themselves wanting, especially when they have contact with people who can help them. This is why DBT tones down their emotions. It helps them learn how to cope with situations better by learning skill sets like impulse regulation, mindfulness, emotion regulation, and relapse prevention.

DBT has been proven to be effective for BPD patients. Its main purpose is to help improve the patient's quality of life and decrease self-destructive behaviors. It is also used as a preventative strategy as it aims to stop the patient from relapsing and allows him to be in control of his situation.

Despite being based on very different theories and clinical practices, both theorists agree that they must consider their clients' problems holistically. The main therapeutic approaches of both theorists center around encouraging their clients to integrate and accept themselves while practicing acceptance towards others, emphasizing the importance of personal responsibility, and teaching them how to take action effectively.

Frankl's chief influence on the current dialectical behavior therapy training is that there is a dualism at the very core of his theory. He believed there must be two aspects, "self" and "other," as separate and distinct entities but interdependent and mutually conditioning one another. This is not just for theoretical problems in psychology but also practical reasons. Because we all experience conflict from time to time, it makes sense to split the matrix of meaning into two parts: one part mediating the other. One of the ways he understands this is in terms of self-other and task-object distinctions, namely, that both are self functions that are required for survival (i.e., self-other differentiation).

This is a way of seeing the world that is very different from the classical one. He introduces this metaphysical issue by saying that we "must choose between competing values and [then] choose one." This dichotomy formula has three main components:

The basic concepts behind DBT are: "acceptance," "dialogue," "change," and "variability. "Dialogue" is tool therapists use to promote insight into reality in their clients. The most important characteristic of this dialogue is that it has to be non-judgmental. This means it should not have an objective tone; instead, the therapist should have a friendly presence that does not reject the client's behavior. The three main principles of being non-judgmental are:

By being more accepting of their actions and thoughts, clients can begin to accept themselves as they are and learn how to modify their behavior accordingly, for example learning to accept their emotions at certain times, such as when they experience low self-esteem or when they are feeling suicidal. The DBT focuses heal not only the client but also their families and friends. The focus of this therapy is to help their clients find their true self-esteem. At the same time, therapists should be prepared to help them change themselves and how they behave or think; they need to be intrinsically motivated to do these things.

One of the most important aspects of helping someone modify behavior is focusing on what they can do instead of what they cannot do. Therapists must understand that it's not always a matter of what can and cannot be done.

What are the components of DBT?

The goals of DBT are to help patients find their true self-esteem, change how they think about themselves and other people, and teach them how to cooperate with others. DBT uses tools such as differentiating self from others, acceptance, mindfulness, and relationship skills. It can be described by three main concepts: meditation, psychotherapy, and community involvement.

Today some dialectical behavior therapists use a combination of both therapies like DBT/CBT (as introduced in the book "Dialectical Behavior Therapy").

Psychoanalysis is one of the most controversial therapies out there because it creates a great deal of confusion about how it functions. It originated from the idea that our mental life is a continuous system of conflicts, for example, how we wish to master anxiety but not lose ourselves in an attempt to do so. This occurs where we are constantly engaged in a never-ending cycle of trial-and-error and constant adjustment. One major problem with psychoanalysis is that it assumes people can find the solution to their problems by looking inside themselves and talking to their therapists without any input from others (e.g., friends and family).

This therapy is based on the idea that all behavior can be explained by its hidden meaning, "the unconscious. " Unconscious thoughts are "anxiety-laden memories, wishes and impulses." Freud said: "In the unconscious, every motive finds its efficient force, every instinct its appropriate object and goal."

An unconscious mind is made up of three components: id (unpleasure reduction or basic instincts), ego (reality testing or method of regular behaviors), and superego (moral standards). The id works on the pleasure principle; it always wants what it wants when it wants it. However, if we don't get what we want when we want it, we go into a state of emotional turmoil. The ego tries to control these urges by coming up with rationalizations for why these urges are inappropriate. The superego is the conscience, whose function is to help us make moral judgments that hold us accountable for our actions. However, the superego also believes that we are not bad beings and want to care for others.

In "The Ego and the Id," Freud describes a theory of sexual development wherein infantile sexuality is set in motion as an act of aggression. The egotistical (ego) process represents adult sexuality coming into conflict with itself, resulting in motor disturbances because each part of one's personality is trying to express itself simultaneously. These conflicts are resolved through such methods of "defusion" as dreaming. The fantasy enables one to see the conflict without the discomfort or guilt that might otherwise be associated with it.

a.   Meditation

As a DBT concept, meditation is a form of self-treatment that allows the client to relax and focus on reducing anxiety. The meditation process is particularly helpful because it enables clients to develop "non-attached awareness." This means they are aware of the here and now without being attached to the past or future. Clients learn these skills by "recognizing their thoughts, focusing on their breathing, and turning away from their emotions." Meditation also helps clients understand how to respond differently to stressful situations when practicing this skill.

b.   Psychotherapy

Psychotherapy takes a variety of forms, such as individual therapy, group therapy, family therapy, time-limited therapy, and long-term therapies. DBT approaches therapy as a prevention and healing process by addressing the client's current problems. Individual therapy is particularly helpful because it helps clients learn how to deal with painful emotions with skill. The program may also suggest that clients seek psychotherapy from a therapist outside the DBT program.

c.   Community Involvement

DBT clients are encouraged to participate in a program called "community involvement." This process encourages them to get involved in the community by volunteering, working, going to school, etc. It is believed that being involved in the community will help them learn how to relate better to the world at large, which will enable them to make friends and grow as individuals.

Doing something different requires commitment and a willingness to try new things. As an approach, DBT is not easy. It is complex because it encompasses many treatment techniques and relies on collaboration between patients and therapists. It is also a very time-consuming treatment because its goal is to change clients' whole way of thinking, which can take years. Finally, DBT can be costly for patients and families. Unfortunately, most insurance companies do not cover treatment using this therapy, so many people cannot afford it.

DBT effectively reduces self-destructive behaviors and increases adaptive behaviors in people with BPD. DBT does not work for everyone, but it can help those for whom other treatments have failed. It appears to work particularly well when patients are highly motivated because they are committed to completing the treatment. It can be a very scary process for the patient, but they should try to take it one day at a time.

Therefore, DBT components include:

a.   Medication and Case Management

Medications are used to control symptoms of BPD. The most frequently prescribed medication for BPD patients is a mood stabilizer/anticonvulsant called lithium. Key to the management of this condition is early intervention before medication side effects have time to develop into a full-blown episode that may require inpatient treatment. The third element of the DBT program is case management, which stream-lines and coordinates the multiple services needed by patients with BPD who are eligible for treatment under Medicaid.

b.   Education, Therapy, and Psychoeducation

Psychoeducation is a major component of DBT; it includes reading self-help books and attending group and individual therapy. One of the main reasons that people with BPD engage in self-injury is to avoid their intense emotions. The "emotional regulation" (ER) skills teach patients how to cope with feelings without resorting to self-injury. During treatment, patients are taught four skill modules: mindfulness (reduces suffering by staying in the present); interpersonal effectiveness (helps patients communicate assertively without anger); emotion regulation (helps patients manage intense emotions without acting on them); and distress tolerance (teaches people how to be comfortable when they feel unhappy). It is believed that these skills change the brain.

c.   Family and Community Involvement

DBT therapists actively encourage family members and other important people in the individuals' lives to get involved in the treatment. This may be as simple as encouraging their attendance at group sessions if they are not already involved. It is also helpful to work with family members to learn how to help the person with BPD. DBT therapists often ask about the individual's relationships, such as how the individual feels about his or her parents, siblings, friends, etc., which helps therapists understand what barriers might impede treatment progress.

d.   Training

DBT therapists are required to take a specialized training program that involves 20 hours of training in DBT. Therapists can then attend one additional course and participate in continuing education (CE). These principles include:

a.   Assessing problematic psychosocial issues. This includes assessing the individual's interpersonal relationships, social skills, and other important issues contributing to their condition.
b.   Developing a treatment plan for the client. This entails identifying strengths and weaknesses and developing goals for treatment that will help them achieve optimal functioning.
c.   Identifying target behaviors related to their problems, building on strengths, and assessing readiness for change using outcome measures developed by the DBT team (e.g., act intended, frequency, intensity, etc.). These behaviors include self-damaging and those that interfere with social functioning.
d.   Treating the client using cognitive and behavioral therapy techniques tailored to the individual's needs and preferences.
e.   Working with the client to overcome obstacles to success, including therapy refusal, medication non-compliance, in-session behavior problems, and disruptions in therapy due to crises or self-injury.
f.   Following up with clients after they have been discharged from treatment by conducting telephone contact and evaluating treatment outcomes using a quantitative assessment measure (e.g., BPD rating scale or SIBRI).
g.   Developing written protocols for use by other providers.
h.   Advising and coordinating mental health services for the individual and their family members.
i.   Providing appropriate case management to patients under the supervision of a licensed mental health professional in collaboration with the individuals and families affected by their condition, as well as appropriate community resources and social service agencies.
j.   Ensuring that every client receives routine physical checkups, drug therapy, and medication education to maintain an optimum state of health during treatment and recovery from illness or injury

while under general medical supervision or on restricted medication that does not interfere with DBT training or practice.

Patients with BPD have an extremely high prevalence of social phobia. Social anxiety disorder (SAD) and psychosomatic illnesses are often associated with BPD. For example, people with SAD frequently have "attempted suicide because of rejection by others and had racing thoughts, feelings of terror, and physical symptoms such as sweating and blushing." Furthermore, research suggests that BPD patients often believe that they are physically weak compared to other people and therefore avoid social situations.

DBT aims to improve social functioning by teaching patients to control their emotions in stressful situations without externalizing their negative emotions or engaging in self-destructive behaviors (e.g., self-injury). The "Interpersonal Effectiveness skills" focus on helping patients communicate effectively with others and to listen more skillfully. The ultimate goal is to become emotionally independent and free from the various problems associated with BPD.

DBT has been tested in two RCTs conducted by psychologist Marsha Linehan and her colleagues. These trials showed that DBT could be implemented successfully in a psychiatric setting, producing significant reductions in suicide attempts, self-injury, and substance abuse among participants with BPD. The first trial compared DBT to treatment as usual (TAU), a practice that does not specifically target BPD but includes regular visits to a psychiatrist or psychotherapist and often hospitalization for severe crises.

Types of DBT

Some professionals have developed their versions of DBT. These variations are known as "off-label" applications of the treatment. This means they have modified the original treatment in some way to meet their own needs and the needs of their clients. An example is "Third Wave DBT," designed by psychologist Paul T. Mason, which in addition to the standard DBT program, also includes meditation, acceptance techniques, and cognitive therapy techniques.

Treatment costs depend on where treatment is administered and what kinds of treatments are available. For example, training a therapist to provide DBT could cost several hundred thousand dollars, but group sessions may be more cost-effective over the long term. Due to the nature of BPD and its co-existing disorders (depression and suicidal thoughts) and psychiatric and drug dependence, many patients cannot work during the acute phase of their recovery. As patients become healthier and more stable, they may join a part-time or full-time job to help fund future sessions.

The cost of DBT for an individual with BPD has not been determined, but the overall cost to society is high. BPD often goes undiagnosed or misdiagnosed, and patients are often in and out of mental institutions, hospitals, or jails. Although the disorder has a high prevalence rate, many people with BPD are never treated; thus, many go undiagnosed.

The name "dialectical behavior therapy" comes from dialectics and behavior therapy. It has dialectical elements in that it views the patient's difficulties as existing in a systemic and relational context.

Types of DBT include:

1. Individual DBT

This is where an individual, or the RT, works with a therapist to help them manage their emotions and regulate their behaviors to reduce self-harming and suicidal behavior.

2. Group DBT

Groups of 3-5 people dealing with BPD are designed to help build awareness about different situations/problems. A therapist leads the groups, but participants also take on leadership roles. "The broader goal of group DBT is not only symptom reduction but also the enhancement of the patient's quality of life."

3. Phone coaching (called "phone-DBT")

This is an element of individual DBT but also an expansion of the whole system of DBT. It involves training the patient to communicate better with the therapist by setting up appointments via phone, text messaging, or Skype video calls.

4. Functional assessment

This part aims to help the patient identify problems, feelings, and actions that are negative, painful, and irrational to help them change their thinking and behavior. Additionally, this helps them manage their emotions and regulate their behavior for those emotions not to trigger harmful behaviors such as self-harm or suicidal behavior.

5. Distress tolerance

This is another tool to help the patient better manage their emotions, which helps them avoid engaging in behavior that is unwanted and unhealthy.

6. Email coaching (called "email-DBT")

This part of DBT involves sending the patient helpful homework assignments through email. Moreover, email-DBT is the only part of DBT that the patient can receive via email.

7. Provision of services

This is a way to help the patient find employment or other ways to support their recovery and maintenance in DBT.

8. Modification of supervision

The patient's therapist can adjust the training between sessions as long as it does not cause harm to the progress made in therapy. Examples include giving additional homework assignments or discussing changes with the patient, but leaving it up to them on what will be discussed and how long should be spent on each issue.

9. Mindfulness

This is a technique used to help people better manage their emotions and regulate their behavior. The patients are taught how to develop an awareness of emotion without having strong emotions, which can lead to problems such as self-harm or suicidal behavior.

10. Acceptance

In this section, the therapist works with the patient to accept situations they cannot change or overcome.

This also helps them learn how to be more at ease with whatever is happening around them by learning to accept the situation and not take it personally.

11. Mindfulness of self

This is a way to help people overcome their internal dilemmas, such as emotional and behavioral abuse, by learning to be more aware of their thoughts and feelings. This also helps patients become more in control of their emotions and behavior.

12. Parenting

In this area, parents are taught how to communicate better with their children, talk about feelings instead of avoiding them, and teach the family coping skills at home.

Dialectical Behavior Therapy successfully reduces symptoms of BPD (e.g., suicide attempts, impulsivity). This has led many experts to endorse its application as an effective tool for the treatment of individuals suffering from BPD.

DBT VS. CBT

These are the two most common types of talk therapy, and they're both very helpful for people struggling with depression, anxiety, or addiction. Both types of talk therapy help you to express your feelings healthily, but DBT has one major difference. Unlike CBT, DBT helps you identify what is going on in your behavior and figure out how to change it accordingly.

If you are struggling with any emotional or mental health problem - especially if it's been ongoing for a long time - talk about your situation with someone specializing in DBT. It might not have worked for everyone else that tried it before; talking about your situation might bring up some new insights that were impossible until then. DBT is one of the most effective treatments for severe mental health disorders and can change your life.

DBT is one of the most effective types of talk therapy for helping people with chronic psychiatric or emotional problems such as depression and anxiety. It is a cognitive behavioral therapy that teaches people skills to cope with stressful situations and how to avoid using dysfunctional coping strategies (like self-harm). DBT talks about two different types of coping strategies: emotion-based coping strategies and problem-solving strategies.

Emotion-based coping strategies include talking yourself into being content or distracting yourself from your emotions. Problem-solving strategies are ways of directly addressing the problem, such as telling the person you dislike that you'd like them to change. DBT teaches people how to use emotion-based strategies because it's not always possible or even appropriate to try solving the problems that cause their emotional issues. Some problems just can't be solved, and helping someone to face that reality is necessary for long-term success in psychiatric therapy. Emotion-based coping strategies might seem like they're helping you, but they end up causing more problems. For example, when you're already feeling depressed, you might think it's a good idea to distract yourself from your emotions and distract yourself with something fun. So you go to the mall or do something fun with your friends. But when you come home and face the reality of what's left in your life, those distractions cause more depression instead of relieving it.

DBT is based on the work of psychologist Marsha Linehan and cognitive therapist David Tuller at the University of Washington. Linehan developed the program in the 1980s to help individuals with borderline personality disorder (BPD). Now, DBT is used to treat people struggling with eating disorders and depression and those at risk of suicide. The type of treatment often requires a certified DBT therapist to administer, so make sure to find one who is well-trained and experienced.

DBT's goal is to teach people skills that can help them shift how they think about their problems and increase their ability to cope with them. The goal is not necessarily a quick fix but a long one that works over time.

Why Choose DBT over CBT?

One of the main differences between CBT and DBT is that CBT is an external approach to handling mental health, while DBT has an internal focus. DBT does help clients identify things that are causing their behaviors, but it's not going to solve them for you. Instead, it's more helpful for people who need new coping methods to deal with their problems.

DBT creates a holistic approach to life management by teaching you how to handle stress better and how to deal with your emotions at the moment so that you can make smart decisions about the future instead of impulsively reacting without considering your options.

What are the main differences between DBT and CBT?

DBT is more focused on teaching clients problem-solving skills to improve their emotional state. CBT is more focused on identifying the symptoms of mental illness and improving outcomes.

This quote summarizes the primary difference between both treatments: "CBT seeks to change dysfunctional thinking, whereas DBT seeks to change dysfunctional behaviors."

Therefore, both therapies have been beneficial in treating people with a history of severe depression and anxiety. However, some patients may find that one approach works better for them than the other.

DBT, like CBT, also focuses on helping people recognize their symptoms and find the root of stress.

DBT attempts to help them build a healthier coping mechanism and reaction to everyday problems.

This process can take time, as different patients respond differently to treatments. The long-term goal of DBT is for people struggling with mental illness to cope with problems healthily when their negative or dysfunctional behavior patterns are triggered.

When you compare DBT vs. CBT, you need to remember that both therapies use mainly cognitive techniques to help patients develop a healthier thinking pattern that will gradually lead them out of their unhealthy cycle of depression or anxiety.

CBT is a "top-down" approach that requires patients to change their behavior and learn new coping mechanisms. DBT is a "bottom-up" approach, however, which teaches patients how to handle stress better in the first place.

One of the biggest benefits of DBT is that it focuses on helping people develop healthy behaviors from an early stage – instead of just teaching them to hold in their emotions until they feel better about them.

DBT does not focus on changing your thinking process as much as CBT does. Instead, DBT seeks to help people change their reactions to external stressors and habits instead of just changing their thinking patterns. The goal of DBT is for patients to "act" on the tools and techniques they learn instead of just learning them passively.

Cognitive behavioral therapy (CBT) often means psychotherapy that works by focusing on a person's thoughts, behaviors, and beliefs. The therapist will help you identify the thoughts and feelings that can cause or worsen your depression or anxiety, change how you react to those negative thoughts, and teach you how to develop positive alternatives.

CBT works to enable you to assess situations realistically and then take steps to change the way you feel and behave. This might include challenging your reactions, learning to relax and control your emotions, and changing how you respond to difficult situations.

It's not a quick fix, but it can give you the tools that allow lasting positive change.

When a person is depressed or anxious, they are often consumed by their negative thoughts and feelings.

Cognitive behavioral therapy teaches patients how to identify those thoughts and then let them go so they can focus on the present moment instead of being stuck in the past.

An example of this would be recognizing when you are using food to cope with anxiety, then identifying specific ways you could let go and find new healthy ways to cope.

CBT is focused on correcting the thoughts that cause symptoms of depression and anxiety, while DBT is focused on changing behaviors that create those same symptoms.

CBT makes sure you know how to recognize thought patterns that often lead to depression or anxiety becoming more severe. Then, DBT teaches people how to avoid these patterns in the first place.

This can be more challenging for some people since it's easier in the short term to just let negative thoughts and feelings flow through you, but it's not always healthy or sustainable in the long term.

Moreover, some more differences between CBT and DBT are:

a. Much like CBT, DBT uses the tools of Dialectical Behavioral Therapy.
b. In DBT, commonly used tools are homework assignments, a daily log, and an... "daily review" session.
c. Whereas CBT focuses on re-establishing a healthy balance between mood and thought patterns, DBT is more focused on maintaining a healthy balance in relationships as well as one's own emotions.
d. While CBT usually takes place in a room with other clients, DBT takes place in a private studio environment with the therapist but without any other clients present for confidential issues to be discussed.
e. CBT focuses more on the individual patient and their patterns of thought. At the same time, DBT focuses more on the relationships between family members and issues that might restrict individuals.
f. While CBT teaches patients how to identify their negative thought patterns and then let them go, DBT helps them recognize negative behaviors and then work to change them for the better instead of just identifying them as negative.
g. CBT focuses on helping patients find practical ways to cope with feelings associated with depression or anxiety. In contrast, DBT focuses on changing those reactions so that you can let go of depression or anxiety-inducing feelings in their entirety.
h. Therapists in CBT focus on helping a patient understand their issues and how those issues may affect other relationships, while therapists in DBT focus more on the person's interactions with others.
i. CBT aims to encourage patients to develop new coping patterns and behaviors that will help them maintain a healthy lifestyle and lifestyle balance by addressing negative cycles or patterns of thoughts or behaviors that often lead to depression or anxiety. DBT aims to address interpersonal relationships between family members and develop healthy behaviors for each family member.
j. CBT focuses more on teaching patient-specific patterns of thinking that cause depression or anxiety. In contrast, DBT focuses more on teaching a patient specific patterns of behavior that lead to depression or anxiety.
k. CBT is more heavily focused on cognitive behavioral therapy, while DBT is more focused on addressing the issue at the core of depression or anxiety.
l. CBT encourages a patient to recognize ways that depression or anxiety might affect relationships and

then work to strengthen them. DBT's goal is for patients to learn how to change their interpersonal relationships and improve their health.

m. CBT seeks to help patients recognize patterns in their thoughts or behaviors that lead to depression or anxiety and find healthier ways to cope with those feelings.

How Does DBT Work compared to CBT?

The acronyms DBT and CBT both represent terms that have become popular in the field of mental health. So what's the difference between DBT vs. CBT? Does one of them work better than the other?

Cognitive behavioral therapy (CBT) developed from a much older school of psychotherapy called rational emotive behavior therapy (REBT). The goal of REBT is to help clients recognize faulty, irrational thought patterns and replace them with more helpful, realistic ones. It was developed by Albert Ellis (originally trained as a psychoanalyst), who ultimately wanted to take REBT to more extreme lengths without losing its therapeutic effectiveness. So Ellis created a system that would allow people to identify faulty, irrational thought patterns and replace them with more realistic, helpful ones. The learning of this new therapy propagated quickly, and several other therapists invented their systems based on Ellis's model. The most well-known is probably Aaron Beck's cognitive therapy, which models Ellis's method but emphasizes behavioral therapy.

Cognitive behavioral therapy (CBT) is the more recent school of psychotherapy. It was developed by Aaron Beck, who envisioned it as an alternative to Ellis and other versions of rational emotive behavior therapy that were being practiced at the time. CBT is a form of structured therapy, not to be confused with psychoanalysis. It models several approaches and techniques to help clients achieve certain goals or work through specific issues. There are several different varieties of CBT, all of which have been developed based on Beck's initial model.

While cognitive behavioral therapy (CBT) can be seen as a subset of cognitive therapy (CT), dialectical behavior therapy (DBT) represents an offshoot from CT and REBT that has since been proven effective for patients with Borderline Personality Disorder (BPD).

Cognitive therapy is based on the idea that certain thoughts and behaviors can trigger negative emotions. Therefore, by changing these thought patterns is believed that a patient's problematic emotions can be reduced or eliminated.

Likewise, DBT teaches patients how to identify patterns in their thinking and then replace those thoughts with healthier ones. In addition, DBT emphasizes helping patients develop the social and life skills needed to deal with their emotions and change for the better.

CB therapists focus on minimizing a patient's tendency towards negative or unhealthy thoughts by addressing them head-on rather than just identifying them by name. However, DBT therapists are more concerned with the fact that those thoughts and behaviors often lead to unhealthy emotions and the ways those emotions may act on a person's relationships.

DBT therapists are concerned more with helping patients learn new ways to cope with their negative reactions rather than simply identifying them as negative. In this way, DBT is more closely related to cognitive therapy and REBT. Both forms of therapy focus on helping patients identify problems that recurring negative thoughts might have and then replace them with new ones that can lead to healthier emotional responses. But while cognitive therapy focuses largely on teaching patients how to change their thought patterns, DBT tries to teach them how to change their behavior patterns.

While cognitive behavioral therapy (CBT) is still seen as one of the most effective forms of depression treatment, dialectical behavior therapy (DBT) has also proven effective in treating patients with Borderline Personality Disorder.

From the 1960s, Ellis's rational emotive behavior therapy (REBT), inspired by the psychoanalyst Sigmund Freud and Albert Ellis, was originally designed to treat various psychological issues. Still, it was soon discovered that it worked best for treating depression. The method taught patients how to change their thoughts and behaviors to minimize their symptoms. However, Ellis later created a more extreme version of REBT called "rational therapy." Unlike REBT, rational therapy teaches patients how to change the world instead of their thoughts. The method was later renamed just rational emotive behavior therapy, but it was soon discovered that to change one's reality, one must first change their thoughts.

Rational emotive behavior therapy (REBT) is based on three different principles:

1. The principle of humanism: humans are responsible for their own emotions and actions at all times. No outside forces or events can cause you to feel or behave a certain way unless you allow them to do so.
2. The principle of environmentalism: You are responsible for making the world as pleasant and enjoyable as possible while still behaving morally.
3. The principle of the science of self-knowledge is that the only way to understand yourself truly or others is by applying reason and logic.

As REBT matured, it also began to develop several branches based on slight variations in technique and theory. Most notably, Albert Ellis developed rational emotive behavioral therapy (REBT) by removing the emphasis on changing one's external environment, which allowed him to focus more on helping patients change their thought patterns. He also emphasized that while a patient's feelings can be rational, the thoughts leading to those feelings are often irrational. Thus, REBT is a combination of cognitive and rational emotive behavior therapy (REBT).

It wasn't long before other therapists adopted Ellis's new method. Still, they soon began creating their treatment systems based on his system, and thus, various versions of rational emotive behavior therapy were created and developed. Included among these are:

Ellis' theory and practice influenced later theorists such as R.D. Laing, David D. Burns, Albert Einstein, and Carl Rogers. REBT theory and practice are also used extensively in self-help books, workbooks, and computer-based cognitive behavioral therapy programs.

Albert Ellis's Institute for Rational Living still exists in New York City, San Diego, and San Francisco. The institute offers free lectures on Thursdays at 8 pm, which anyone is welcome to attend.

REBT is seen as a more extreme form of CBT that views irrational thinking as the root cause of most human suffering. REBT therapists believe that almost every behavior stems from an irrational thought or belief held by the individual, which means that if you can change those thoughts, you can change their behavior.

Therefore, REBT therapists concentrate on helping patients identify the irrational thoughts that lead to irrational behaviors and then teach them how to change those thoughts and behavior to reduce their negative or unhealthy emotions.

REBT is sometimes called dialectical or Ellis method cognitive therapy. This is because it uses principles from cognitive therapy but also REBT. Both are based on the idea that people's problems stem from irrational thinking, and both use cognitive therapy techniques such as "logic" exercises, correcting thought errors, and challenging extreme beliefs.

Similarities between DBT and CBT

These similarities between DBT and CBT have led to the integration of DBT techniques in many current-day Cognitive Behavioral Therapy (CBT) types.

•DBT and Cognitive Behavioral Therapy (CBT) are founded on the belief that an individual's thoughts affect their feelings and behavior.

•Both therapies believe that it is important to understand your current situation, analyze the way you think, and learn new alternative methods to deal with problems.

•Both therapies attempt to help clients change their lives by changing their thoughts, feelings, or behaviors.

•Both seek to empower patients by giving them skills necessary for them to be successful in life.

•Both therapies use behavioral and cognitive techniques to accomplish this goal.

•Both therapies are meant to be a safe place to explore one's surroundings and acquire new skills.

•Both therapies recognize the importance of values or morals in everyone's life.

Reasons for integration of DBT into existing and newer CBT programs

These are the reasons why DBT has led to it being integrated into newer and existing cognitive behavioral therapy programs:

•DBT is a complementary therapy in many areas because it can help with issues such as suicidal thoughts, depression, anxiety, anger, addictions, co-dependency, interpersonal relationships, etc.

•DBT helps the patient learn many skills and ways of coping with their surroundings, which cognitive behavioral therapy can also do.

•The functional approach to therapy is based on the belief that patients with BPD can learn many skills which enable them to break out of their dysfunctional cycles, control their emotions and behaviors, and improve their quality of life.

•Overcoming your symptoms can be accomplished by teaching you how to regulate your emotions healthily.

•When working with clients, you focus on the present instead of worrying about the past or future. This therapy gives you a chance at life again, instead of having your life ruled by thoughts and feelings that keep you from living.

•DBT is based on the idea that all people's symptoms are due to their thoughts, feelings, and behavior. Therefore, DBT can help people with BPD make positive changes in their thoughts and feelings.

•	To treat clients, you must understand their symptoms, how they may occur, and how they got to be. This allows the therapist to help lead them through healing and recovery.

•DBT aims to teach clients a healthier lifestyle that works for them. This is accomplished by working with the client to create a life skills program.

•With DBT, you can help clients be aware of their strengths and weaknesses and teach them how to identify the negative influences in their lives. This enables them to begin working on themselves and their issues in the present moment.

•DBT aims to prevent suicide and self-harm behaviors that may be caused by emotional, cognitive, biological, or environmental factors.

•With DBT, you can also work on a client's mood swings and unstable emotions that may occur from time to time as part of BPD.

•DBT teaches clients how to identify the secondary gains they may experience from their symptoms and how to solve future problems by taking advantage of relationships or situations.

•In a DBT session, you can talk about emotional issues in the present moment with your partner in a very non-threatening, non-judgmental manner.

•DBT can target many different areas of functioning, including interpersonal functions, role functioning, family relationships, sexual intimacy, daily living skills, recreation activities, work and school achievement, and social interactions.

Therefore, CBT and DBT are similar in that they help with issues of emotion, relationships, and mood. They both also focus on working on all these areas simultaneously with a bigger goal in mind. Moreover, they use techniques to meet these goals, such as behavioral exercises, skills training, and exposure therapy.

Cognitive behavioral therapy is part of a broader cognitive behavioral therapy (CBT) approach. The other well-known member of this family is Dialectical Behavior Therapy (DBT). DBT was initially used for treating Borderline Personality Disorder (BPD), but it has now been validated for various psychological and mental disorders.

Because DBT adopts the same theoretical framework as CBT, many elements from the latter are also found in the former. In fact, by following the same principles and procedures, CBT and DBT overlap greatly in what they aim to achieve. Specifically, they both attempt to tackle the client's problematic feelings and behaviors by changing the way they think—albeit in different ways.

Regarding origins, CBT and DBT began their journeys in the 1960s and 70s, respectively. These two therapies are considered to be part of the second wave of cognitive behavioral therapy, along with Dialectical Behavior Therapy (DBT), Rational Emotive Behavioral Therapy (REBT), Interpersonal Therapy (IPT), Family Focused Treatment for Borderline Personality Disorder (FFT-BP), and Motivational Interviewing (MI).

Many similarities exist between these different therapies due to how they were initially developed. For example, all originated from the same group of therapists—those who originally developed Cognitive Behavioral Therapy (CBT).

Similarly, many of these therapies originated from the same source—Albert Ellis and Aaron Beck. These two influential figures developed Rational Emotive Behavior Therapy (REBT) and Cognitive Behavioral Therapy (CBT).

As a result, it is unsurprising then that both DBT and CBT are rooted in these two pioneers' work. In addition, both DBT and CBT stem from Albert Ellis' approach to psychotherapy, known as Rational Emotive Behavior Therapy (REBT).

Albert Ellis was one of the main people involved in developing CBT, particularly Rational Emotive Behavioral Therapy (REBT).

Is DBT Effective compared to CBT?

DBT is effective in treating borderline personality disorder compared to CBT. Therefore, a study was conducted in 2005 to compare the effectiveness of DBT, EMDR, and CBT treatments (jointly called ABT). Using a randomized controlled trial design, 80 patients were randomly assigned to one of the three groups. The participants were evaluated over six months: at the start of treatment, mid-way through treatment, and two weeks after completion. After this evaluation period, it was determined that both DBT and CBT were equally effective at reducing borderline personality disorder symptoms.

Since the widespread use of DBT is increasing in many countries worldwide, there is a need to determine its effectiveness as a treatment for borderline personality disorder. Therefore, the effectiveness of DBT was compared to individual and group CBT in a randomized controlled trial. The participants included 27 adults with borderline personality disorder (BPD) who participated in DBT and 27 adults with BPD who participated in individual and group CBT.

The participants were evaluated at the start of treatment, mid-treatment, and two-week after treatment ended. Both DBT and CBT significantly improved the participants who exhibited severe BPD symptoms and those with moderate BPD symptoms. However, individuals who received DBT had significantly fewer hospital days than those in the other groups.

Most studies focused on DBT have been conducted in Germany, as more DBT therapists have been located there. This country also has more psychotherapists trained in CBT than any other country in Europe. However, the same findings were found in other countries where DBT was used to treat BPD and other personality disorders.

The evaluation of treatment outcomes often includes measurements of improvement in mood, anxiety, and other areas of functioning. In addition, other measures like hospitalizations are sometimes included if severe disruptive behaviors or severe emotional distress are present at the beginning of the treatment period.

For one study, individuals randomized to psychoeducation (which could represent either DBT or CBT), in addition to their usual treatment, did not have an increased concurrent risk of hospitalization compared with usual treatment alone. However, this study was conducted in the Netherlands at a psychiatric outpatient clinic serving individuals with severe and persistent mental disorders; it did not evaluate DBT or test whether psychoeducation was an effective intervention for borderline personality disorder.

The effectiveness of DBT can be compared to that of CBT through a randomized controlled trial. This study was conducted in the United States on individuals with borderline personality disorder experiencing higher maladaptive behaviors (e.g., self-injury). Participants were randomly assigned to DBT, a version of DBT that included family participation or CBT. All participants underwent treatment for approximately two years, and all groups showed significant improvements from baseline to the end of the study. In addition, those who received DBT had fewer self-injury crisis days during and after treatment than those who received CBT.

Diversity has long been acknowledged as a fundamental premise in scientific research and practice. The role of minority groups in the development and future of DBT is worthy of special consideration. Many barriers need to be examined to reach diverse populations successfully. The therapist should distinguish between cultural diversity and individual differences when dealing with each patient's different needs. This differentiation is one-way therapists can increase their understanding of their patients and improve their treatment.

Cultural diversity can be defined as differences in thought, perception, values, and behaviors across different groups, especially ethnically diverse groups within a population. While most DBT specialists are Caucasian, therapists must recognize cultural diversity in individuals from different ethnic backgrounds.

THE BASICS OF DBT

Dialectical Behavior Therapy (DBT) is a form of psychotherapy developed to help people with chronic emotional instability, like Borderline Personality Disorder. DBT was designed to be an alternative to traditional talk therapy, which relied primarily on verbal communication between therapist and client.

DBT is based on the principles of Dialectical Behavior Therapy, which applies a scientific approach to eradicate and prevent emotional disorders in the individual by identifying and modifying distorted thinking patterns and behaviors.

The main distinguishing feature of DBT is the use of two core skills: Mindfulness and Distress Tolerance. These are combined with several therapeutic approaches and tools, such as behavioral exercises, mindfulness-based practices, and family therapy. These methods help people learn how to regulate emotions, protect themselves against disorder relapse, and lead more functional lives.

DBT can be implemented differently depending on the patient's needs and the available resources. Individual DBT (iDBT) is the preferred approach, but group DBT (gDBT) is also used. In addition, a Partial Hospitalization Program (PHP) or Intensive Outpatient Program (IOP) may be required. There are several standardized treatment manuals for each method of DBT.

Insurance coverage for DBT varies widely throughout different parts of the world and in different health care plans. Insurance companies often do not cover it; hence, this type of psychotherapy can be prohibitively expensive. In some cases, medication and psychotherapy have been used to treat depression and anxiety disorders.

The DBT approach assumes that the skills learned in therapy, including mindfulness, distress tolerance, emotion regulation, self-management, and interpersonal effectiveness, will help patients achieve more effective and adaptive behaviors and lead a more meaningful life. The authors of DBT note: "DBT is not limited to treating BPD; it has been applied successfully to a range of problems associated with chronically suicidal and parasuicidal behavior."

The origin of Dialectical Behavior Therapy can be traced to the philosophy behind Zen Buddhism. In "Zen and Japanese Buddhism" (1938), D.T. Suzuki posits that humans develop perceptions through subjective experiences. This corresponds with the "subjectivist" approach in Dialectical Behavior Therapy.

Several philosophical and therapeutic traditions have considered the concept of dialectics or dialectical thinking, including ancient Greek philosophy, Buddhism, and Taoism. Hegel coined the term. In practical terms, dialectic refers to an approach that refuses to accept a rigid dichotomy between two opposing concepts (e.g., suicidal vs. not suicidal), instead considering them as two extremes on a continuum that can be reconciled (e.g., less vs. more suicidal). In DBT, this dialectic approach applies to both clinical depression and BPD. John Rolland, a DBT pioneer, considered one of the fathers of DBT in psychology, wrote about how DBT applied dialectics to clinical practice: "Dialectical behavior therapy is rooted in dialectics. The person-centered approach grows out of the emphasis on seeing different parts as different aspects of an integrated whole. This perspective has yielded a style and set of inherently dialectical strategies."

Common Deficits of Behavior

Behavioral deficits are the observable behavior problems of a person. These deficits include, but are not limited to, problems with communication skills and behaviors that interfere with relationships and work productivity. Behaviors can either be aspects of a disorder or learned habits favored by the individual but may be disadvantageous or distressing to themselves or others.

Many behavioral deficits are associated with people diagnosed with a personality disorder, such as borderline personality disorder. Some of these deficits include impulsivity, self-harm, risk-taking behaviors, tantrums and mood swings (in the case of BPD), irritability, suicidality, self-neglect (e.g., hoarding), and reckless behavior (such as substance misuse). However, primary deficits are the behavioral problems present in the first year of a person's life before they develop a personality disorder. These primary deficits include emotional regulation and dysregulation, communication skills, and reward/punishment systems.

Borderline Personality Disorder is often characterized by several emotional dysregulation issues, including but not limited to impulsivity, affect dysregulation (e.g., explosive anger), self-harm/suicidal behavior, phobias (e.g., fear of abandonment), substance misuse, and risk-taking behaviors for pleasurable effects (e.g., sexual indiscretions). Most of these issues are very distressing for individuals with BPD, their family members, and their friends. Yet Borderline Personality Disorder is rarely formally diagnosed until the person is an adult. It is, therefore, a personal choice whether or not to seek professional help using a service such as the "Online Doctor" or an online therapist.

Therefore, common deficits of behavior in DBT include:

a. Impulsivity

In Borderline Personality Disorder, individuals present with several emotional dysregulation issues, including but not limited to impulsivity, fear of abandonment, and explosive anger. Therefore, common deficits of behavior in DBT include: Planning as a goal to set yourself and others up for success by weighing all possibilities when making decisions. In addition, tolerance for uncertainty can be achieved by developing skills such as perseverance and being willing to hold on to long-term goals. For example, e met. "I'll be punished if I don't keep pushing this project forward."

b. Communication skills

Individuals diagnosed with BPD often present with several emotional dysregulation issues, including but not limited to: difficulty initiating or maintaining relationships, conflict and irritability in the presence of others, and a tendency to sabotage relationships and work productivity. Therefore, common deficits of behavior in DBT include: "It's not that I'm bad at communicating; it's that I'm terrified of getting it wrong."

c. Mood swings

A person diagnosed with BPD may present with several emotional dysregulation issues, including affective instability (e.g., intense mood changes and irritability), self-mutilation, and suicidal behavior. Therefore, common deficits of behavior in DBT include: "I don't have a normal mood-swing cycle. I can be angry for no reason. They're just taking me as I am."

d. Suicidality/self-neglect

Individuals diagnosed with BPD present with several emotional dysregulation issues, including but not limited to: planning and monitoring their functions, difficulty with emotions and interpersonal relationships, suicidal ideation, and impulsive self-harm behaviors. Therefore, common deficits of behavior in DBT include: "I have to keep the house clean and tidy for my mother so that she'll feel comfortable."

e. Risk-taking behaviors

Individuals diagnosed with BPD present with several emotional dysregulation issues, including but not limited to: cutting, substance misuse, and risk-taking behaviors that are used to cope with anxiety (e.g., over-eating/binge eating, sexual indiscretions). Therefore, common deficits of behavior in DBT include: "I'm just identifying how I can use the coping skills I've been learning."

f. Irritability

Individuals diagnosed with BPD present with several emotional dysregulation issues, including irritability and anger in the presence of others, tantrums, and intrusive/intrusive behaviors (e.g., jealousy). Therefore, common deficits of behavior in DBT include: "I have to hold my tongue when I'm angry."

g. Anger

Individuals diagnosed with BPD present with several emotional dysregulation issues, including but not limited to: explosive anger, dissociation, and difficulty regulating emotions in the presence of others. Therefore, common deficits of behavior in DBT include: "It's not that I'm angry all the time. It's just that I can't control my anger."

Common Deficits of Behavior are defined as the observable behavior problems of a person. These deficits include, but are not limited to, problems with communication skills and behaviors that interfere with relationships and work productivity. "Impulsivity" is the most commonly cited deficit of behavior in DBT clients who present with an emotion dysregulation disorder. High impulsivity has important implications for treating emotion dysregulation because it can significantly increase the severity of associated symptoms such as aggressive behavior. Self-harm behaviors (e.g., attempting suicide) are also frequently present among people diagnosed with a personality disorder like BPD. Still, they are very difficult to treat, especially when they become a chronic behavioral problems like self-harm behavior (e.g., cutting).

Clients diagnosed with BPD present a variety of emotional dysregulation problems, including but not limited to: anxiety, fear, anger, impulsivity, and self-harm/suicide. "Emotions are not something you can control," Louis Swift said. "I think it is important for all of us to acknowledge that emotions are real and that they affect your behavior," he continued, "and that the solution isn't to push them away or try to suppress them." The ability to regulate emotions effectively in the presence of others has great implications for friendships or professional relationships.

The Relapse Prevention Plan

The Relapse Prevention Plan can be used to assist individuals in acquiring and strengthening adaptive behaviors. Relapse prevention plans are designed to prevent future relapses of the behavior problems that are the focus of treatment, which can significantly reduce suffering and improve quality of life.

Self-harm is a behavior problem associated with Borderline Personality Disorder.

Relapse prevention plans consist of three distinct steps: (1) setting specific goals and (2) planning how to achieve them, along with a list of possible situations that might trigger relapse; (3) observing emotions and generating coping statements and coping skills before you need them.

In the rest of this manual, the results of a relapse prevention plan for self-harm are used as an example of how a DBT client might use DBT skills to reduce aggression, harm, and self-harm risk.

The relapse prevention plan for self-harming is: (1) I will set specific goals, and (2) I will list hypothetical situations that could cause me to engage in self-harm. (3) I will observe my emotions, generate coping statements and coping skills, and decide on a course of action before I need them.

In DBT, "psychological flexibility" is the ability to be effective in various situations.

Awareness of thoughts and emotions in the presence of others, during physical activity, and when performing routine tasks can enhance psychological flexibility. The need for psychological flexibility becomes apparent when an individual's emotions do not support or contribute to constructive or proactive behaviors, such as goal-directed behaviors and healthy lifestyles.

How to do DBT

The key to using DBT successfully as a resident is to learn the skills and practice on your own to have some skills in place (as much as possible) when you start seeing a therapist. You can find free training videos on YouTube and go through the most basic ones to get an idea of how DBT might help you. You may also want to join the DBT online chat group to ask questions. A good therapist will not discourage you from checking out DBT for yourself if you are already thinking about it with or without a referral from them. Then, if DBT does seem promising, go ahead and do the full course of Mr. Linehan's recommended treatment (DBT-LITE). Ask a few therapist questions to assess if they will be compatible with you (how often they attend weekly therapy, how much of it is focused on skills, their goals for therapy, etc.). Ask about the target audience for DBT. Again, note that DBT is not just intended for people with serious mental health problems. It is also intended for people with moderate to severe chronic illness and substance abusers who voluntarily want to change their lives (which is why it can be so effective).

The DBT manual does not provide any specific implementation guidelines and does not prescribe a specific frequency or amount of individualized therapy sessions. At least some therapists do not follow this guideline. Before committing to DBT, find out how many individualized therapy sessions the therapist offers. Also, find out if DBT skills groups are available in your area or by phone, or at least an individual therapist who will do a telephone consultation. In some (but not all) areas of the US and other countries where DBT is used, a typical program will consist of a combination of individual sessions with a therapist and weekly support group meetings that are usually run by someone other than the therapist who works primarily with individuals.

Some people have a hard time getting into an individual therapy session. The therapist may offer telephone consultation sessions, or you may be referred to a DBT provider with a community-based practice. In addition, you can find good therapists via word of mouth. For instance, you might get a referral from your primary care physician or mental health providers, or by searching the internet for a "DBT Therapist."

Some therapists choose to combine individualized therapy with a weekly support group. Other therapists prefer individualized therapy and may not see others in their weekly support group meetings.

Therefore, these tips can guide how to do DBT:

a. Ask the therapist how often they attend weekly therapy to continue learning new techniques and skills.
b. Ask the therapist how often they have individualized sessions with clients.
c. Check internet reviews of therapists who are good candidates for DBT according to your needs and preferences, especially any that specialize in chronic mental health problems like BPD, depression, or

substance abuse that has lasted more than a few years (rather than short-term treatment of traumatic events or brief reactive episodes).

d. Check if therapists are available for a telephone consultation.

e. Find out what kind of support group meetings will be offered.

f. If a therapist may also be a good candidate for you based on your needs, compare their therapy style and goals with your preferences.

g. Note that a potential therapist's attitude toward medication may also be important to you since DBT is integrated with medications in some programs.

h. Also, note that your habits are also one factor determining how much progress you will make on your goals. Since many people's habits are not conducive to good long-term mental health, it may be important to try a new technique or form of therapy before committing to it.

i. Note that some people find DBT too difficult to do because of their personality or emotional difficulties, so it would make sense for you to seek advice from other therapists working with people with emotional distress before committing to DBT.

j. If DBT does not seem like a good fit for you, ask yourself why and reconsider if the goal is worth the hassle.

k. You can seek therapy from a therapist through insurance or by paying out of pocket. In addition, you can search the internet or ask friends and family for referrals to therapists. Your therapist will give you their credentials and recommendations concerning therapy sessions, support group meetings, and achievements in helping people with similar problems as yours and the eventual outcome of DBT in similar cases.

l. You may be able to find an individual therapist who has more flexible hours for people who work full time but want to attend therapy at times that are convenient for them (e.g., Saturday mornings).

m. You can also see if a therapist has other activities like exercise, hobbies, etc., which they can schedule into their busy schedules so that you will not feel overwhelmed by their high level of commitment to you. This is especially important if your therapist is part of a large community-based practice such as in cities.

If you can attend DBT, try to find one with whom both of you can openly communicate about the importance of your well-being and be patient and realistic about what can be done when people are still learning new skills in therapy.

The conflict between individualized therapy sessions vs. group meetings may be the most important issue (for people who need more social interaction).

Managing Thoughts and Behaviors

All of these techniques are designed to change one's behavior and thoughts. Because this is so important, it can be overwhelming to realize all the different behaviors involved. Generally, you can divide your thoughts into three groups:

a. Automatic thoughts

These thoughts stem from your basic beliefs. For instance, you start to think that you are worthless or somehow bad, even though this is not true. Or you think that "I always fail," even though this is not entirely true.

b. Emotions

You feel this way because of your feelings and reactions to automatic thoughts (e.g., shame). You feel bad, angry, ashamed, hopeless, etcetera because of how you interpret the meaning of these thoughts and their impact on your emotions and behavior.

c.   Behaviors

This is their behavior when people act in certain ways because these automatic thoughts get them into trouble (e.g., they drink or make sexual advances inappropriately, or they want to harm themselves). It can also be your thoughts that cause you to act a certain way and begin to feel bad.

You recognize these thoughts because they constantly pop up in your mind or tend to be recurrent themes that cause you trouble. You may not realize why you have these automatic thoughts and how they affect the emotions you are feeling and the behaviors you engage in (e.g., drinking alcohol). They may also seem meaningless and without any impact on your life. You may not notice that they cause you to do things that create more problems in your life. Therefore, it is important to figure out how these thoughts have gotten embedded in your brain, why they keep returning, and what kinds of things could trigger them (if you can find out what triggers them).

d.   Both automatic thoughts and emotions are associated with feelings. If people do not feel bad about themselves, they will not have these automatic thoughts. So, for people with BPD, emotions can run high, and they over-generalize how bad an individual feels about themselves because of their negative beliefs.

If you want to change the behaviors that you engage in (e.g., drinking alcohol), it is important first to identify why you are doing this (e.g., its effects on your behavior). This is called a functional analysis or behavioral assessment. It involves thinking about what happens when you act this way (e.g., using drugs or alcohol) and what triggers it (e.g., sadness, boredom, etcetera). It is important to notice that this kind of analysis of behavior involves paying attention to what happens before you act.

This helps you make sense of your thoughts and behaviors and helps get more clarity on your behavior (it forces you to take a closer look at things so that you can see that your automatic thoughts are not always true, nor are the conclusions about yourself that it draws). The behavior that results from these automatic thoughts is your response. For example, after an assessment, if you realize why drinking alcohol makes you think you are worthless or a loser but realize that it does not have a significant impact on your life or well-being (e.g., it does not affect your daily functioning), it is more clear-sighted whether to continue with this behavior or stop doing it.

Some of the main goals of DBT are to learn how to identify thoughts that lead to automatic behaviors, how these thoughts create emotions (e.g., negative emotions), and how they impact the behavior (e.g., drinking, binge drinking). This is done by:

a.   Having a functional analysis or behavioral assessment and realizing the impact an automatic thought has on your feelings and behaviors (note that there are many different ways to do this).
b.   Understanding which automatic thoughts cause problems in your life and who you are when you have these beliefs about yourself.
c.   Identifying when your automatic thoughts are coming from feelings (e.g., shame, anger) and who you are.
d.   Identifying which emotions come before you engage in behaviors that cause problems so that you can have a plan or have the skills to control your behavior (e.g., "If I feel bad and I think a thought like is true, I will do. This means identifying how negative beliefs (e.g., "I am worthless") influence your emotions and behaviors that create these problems (e.g., "If I feel bad, I will drink alcohol to dull my feelings.").

e.   Identifying when your automatic thoughts are coming from a part of yourself (e.g., "If I feel angry, I will do and being able to recognize these feelings and why they may come up.

f.   Identifying which thoughts trigger behaviors like drinking or other self-destructive behaviors (e.g., "If I think that I am worthless, I will go out and drink.").

How Can I Change My Automatic Thoughts relating to DBT?

Understanding the difference between automatic thoughts and emotions can be important in terms of your self-understanding now as you seek to achieve a better life.

a.   Automatic thoughts are the thoughts that result from all of how you interpret your pain and difficulties in life.

b.   You should be able to identify at least some of these automatic thoughts when you feel them (e.g., "I am not good enough, I am worthless," or "I always fail") or have an emotion that rises inside of you (e.g., about yourself being worthless). However, it may be that you have a lot more than these automatic thoughts and emotions floating around inside of your brain.

c.   You can work on changing these automatic thoughts by identifying the meaning you have about yourself concerning things that have happened in life, what bad things people have said about you (that are not true), and how this has impacted you.

d.   It is important to notice that your automatic thoughts may be associated with feelings (e.g., "I am a bad person" or "I am worthless"); this is why you are feeling the way you do (e.g., an emotion like sadness, anger, guilt, shame). It is helpful to know that these feelings will pass and not stick around forever. So, don't be too hard on yourself when you have negative feelings about yourself, as it may not be true.

e.   You can identify these automatic thoughts by reflecting on things you have done in the past or your behavior now. What meaning do you give to this behavior? (e.g., "I am a bad person for drinking alcohol when I know it is not good for me"). Consider this meaning and think about the thoughts you are having now. Concerning this meaning, what new meaning have you come up with that may explain why these automatic thoughts occur?

f.   Identify the emotions that come before your automatic thoughts (e.g., "If I feel sad, I will drink alcohol."). This means being aware of your emotions and how your beliefs may influence them about yourself (e.g., "If I feel angry, I will drink more than usual."). This awareness will help you think about what your automatic thoughts mean to you and how they influence your behavior.

g.   Being able to identify the thoughts that influence your feelings (e.g., "If I feel sad, I will drink more than usual"). This is knowing that these thoughts come from believing that you are a bad person, worthless, or stupid (these are only some examples). It is important to realize that this does not make sense concerning who you are and that it is not true (e.g., being a bad person or worthless is not who you are).

h.   You can start resetting your automatic thoughts by challenging them with other thoughts. See if you can come up with some other thoughts that are more accurate about you and how you interact with the world (e.g., thoughts like: "People don't think I am a bad person because I try my best, I have been sad lately, I am a good person,"). It is important to take time to think of what your new automatic thoughts are because your old ones may not be true.

i.   You can also question whether these unwanted beliefs are true. Repeating these thoughts may mean false (e.g., "I am a bad person if I drink alcohol even though it does not change anything").

Challenges and Difficulties with DBT

Many challenges and difficulties can arise when learning and implementing DBT.

Here are just a few examples:

a. DBT can be challenging because it requires you to change your thoughts about yourself and your life.

b. DBT can also be challenging because it is a very complex program of treatment that takes time and practice to learn and master.

c. DBT takes time and practice to learn since it is not one lesson you can learn immediately but a set of skills that need to be learned, practiced and reinforced to work correctly.

d. All these skills need to be taught simultaneously so that they become automatic and are always present in your mind whenever you are experiencing an emotion or a thought associated with one of these thoughts or feelings.

e. DBT takes time to learn. It is not something you can learn in a week or a few days and then move on with your life, but it takes time.

f. There are also a lot of questions one should ask oneself to understand the purpose of DBT (e.g., what is my purpose with life, why am I here, how do I live my life meaningfully, etc.) This can lead to many difficult feelings later when one is learning DBT and getting things wrong because they do not understand the true meaning behind their thoughts.

g. All of these types of questions that you will be asking about yourself and your life may lead to a lot of emotional pain and struggles.

h. DBT can also be challenging because it is quite difficult to accept the idea that you, who are reading this book, sometimes have thoughts that are not accurate about yourself or your life or may not be true (as opposed to the automatic thoughts that you may have). This can involve changing the way you think about and understand yourself and others concerning the world.

i. DBT can also be difficult because it involves accepting that there are things that do not make sense inside of your brain. In addition, these automatic thoughts influence your behavior which may lead to challenges in managing your emotions, thoughts, and actions.

j. DBT can also be difficult because it requires you to do things differently than you are used to. This will involve a lot of change for you to start thinking about yourself differently and accept that some of these automatic thoughts may not be true.

k. Since DBT is a complex problem-solving technique, it can get quite confusing if you are not paying attention or grasping the concepts behind what you are learning (e.g., why do I have these automatic thoughts which influence my behavior?).

DIALECTICAL STANCE AND STRATEGIES

Dialectical stance and strategies are a rare tool used to treat Borderline Personality Disorder (BPD). Dialectical behavior therapy was developed in the 1980s by Dr. Marsha Linehan. It is an evidence-based practice with well-documented efficacy for BPD.

Dialectical Behavior Therapy, also known as DBT, is a type of psychotherapy created in the 1980s by psychologist Marsha M. Linehan to help adults diagnosed with borderline personality disorder (BPD). The purpose of the creation of DBT was to allow those diagnosed with a borderline personality disorder to be capable of living an independent and functional life. However, symptoms of BPD were causing them significant distress and impairing their ability to function in society. Therefore, DBT is a type of behavior therapy known as "Dialectical Behavior Therapy" or DBT.

Dysfunction within self-concept, usually associated with identity disturbance, can be viewed as contributing factors determining the development and maintenance of behaviors controlling the individual's external world. In addition, dysfunctional patterns may also form due to other factors such as societal norms, personal history, and cultural influences.

Dialectical Behavior Therapy is divided into four major components typically implemented within a specific order during a course of treatment. The four components of DBT include individual therapy, group skills training, telephone consultation team, and psychoeducation to the patient's significant others (family, friends) who may be involved in the individual's treatment plan:

The fourth component of DBT involves psychoeducation for family members and loved ones on how they can best support the patient in their recovery. It is usually included at some point after the patient has been stabilized.

The goal of each component is to help the person effectively cope with their emotions.

A major aspect of DBT is the "Dialectical Behavior Therapy Skills Training Program." This program includes ten treatment modules that outline a series of skills that an individual must master to better cope with their symptoms and for the individual to be able to engage in everyday life.

Three initial modules instruct the individual on how to use their feelings, thoughts, actions, and behaviors to better cope with challenges that may arise in everyday life. There is also a more advanced module called "Flexibility," where individuals practice flexibly using their thoughts and actions as a form of self-regulation.

The individual therapy modules are designed to help individuals learn skills that can be used to overcome their emotional dysregulation. The skill is taught in a step-by-step fashion, which allows the individual to practice before moving on to the next skill with the hope that they will master it to help them function more effectively in their everyday life.

Currently, one module called "Acceptance and Commitment Therapy" has received great success within DBT. It is used for patients who suffer from emotional dysregulation and experience strong urges for intense emotions, such as rage, anxiety, and depression.

As part of the Skills Training Program, an individual will practice the skills they learned in an individual session with a trained therapist. The individual's therapist then reviews this training. In one study, on average, DBT therapists spent 17 hours per month with their clients.

Dysfunctional behaviors within self-concept can be viewed as contributing factors determining the development and maintenance of behaviors controlling an individual's external world. However, dysfunctional patterns may form due to other factors such as societal norms, personal history, and cultural influences.

What are dialectical stances?

Dialectical behavior therapy (DBT) is a form of psychotherapy that helps individuals with a borderline personality disorder. DBT is based on the idea that the person's personality has a split or two parts—that are usually in conflict with each other. The goal of DBT therapy is to help individuals learn how to manage their behavior and emotions to achieve a balance between these two parts. A dialectical stance is an approach that helps to understand and manage these conflicting forces within an individual. Dialectical stances help individuals recognize and understand their thoughts, feelings, and behaviors while simultaneously recognizing their relationship with their environment.

Marsha Linehan developed DBT as a treatment for individuals with borderline personality disorder (BPD). While the treatments for BPD are still being researched, DBT is an effective way to help clients overcome their symptoms.

Dialectical behavior therapy is based on the cognitive behavioral principle that most people have two mindsets (dialectical stance) or two opposing ways of thinking and feeling. These stances can be categorized as "more than" or "less than." For example, one could take the stance that life is generally good and enjoyable while simultaneously acknowledging that some aspects of life are more negative than others. These conflicting stances are referred to as dialectics because they frequently involve a change from one position to its opposite.

Individuals with BPD are believed to feel extreme emotional experiences in response to events around them or within themselves. This may lead them to feel intense emotional highs and emotional lows simultaneously. For example, an event could cause an individual with BPD to feel both happy and sad simultaneously, or the individual might feel depressed and angry at once. Research has found that individuals with BPD experience these emotions more intensely than what is considered normal by most people. Individuals with BPD may also struggle with controlling their impulses, which can cause difficulty managing their behavior.

Dialectical behavior therapy (DBT) is a form of psychotherapy used to treat BPD. DBT focuses on teaching individuals tools to help them cope with their emotions and learn how to regulate their behavior better. To help individuals with BPD learn these skills, therapists may assess clients' cognitive processes, such as their views on themselves, others, and the world. For example, therapists believe people with BPD see themselves as worthless or sinful while thinking they are better than others. Individuals with BPD may also think they are self-conscient or inherently have low self-esteem. Therapy will help individuals learn how to gain more self-esteem and develop healthier relationships. Therapists may also help individuals learn the skills to manage their impulsiveness and emotional dysregulation better. Improving these skills is expected to improve an individual's emotional life and help them become more effective in their everyday lives.

Dialectical stances, therefore, provide many benefits. First, dialectics allows individuals to acknowledge their internal and external worlds while recognizing the relationship between these two parts. They also help individuals who struggle with BPD recognize the difference in how they see themselves and others.

Dialectical behavior therapy (DBT) is a type of therapy that focuses on helping people who experience severe emotional dysregulation or suicidal urges. Because of its focus on helping people learn skills to regulate their emotions and behavior better, DBT is an effective treatment for people with BPD. In addition, the skills learned in DBT can help individuals form better relationships with others, make healthier decisions about their daily lives, and improve their quality of life overall.

Self-concept is an individual's perception of themselves. Self-concept can be divided into two categories, social self, and personal self. The social self is based on how the individual views their identity concerning other people. This can include their appearance, behavior, thoughts, and actions. The personal self category focuses on individuals' conception of who they are by themselves without being influenced by others. Self-esteem is the degree to which a person views themselves positively or the degree to which they value their abilities and traits (accomplishments). This is also referred to as self-concept. Self-esteem can be measured through self-report measures such as the Rosenberg Self-Esteem Scale and other measures of self-concept, such as the Multidimensional Scale of Perceived Social Support.

A person's self-concept can vary based on many factors, but its relationship with daily functioning is often linked. For example, people with high self-esteem tend to show more confidence in themselves and their abilities, allowing them to perform better socially and feel prouder. This can lead to higher performance expectations for themselves, which leads to the more frequent achievement of more desirable goals and positive experiences. On the other hand, people with lower self-esteem can experience sadness and unhappiness because they do not feel good about themselves. This can lead them to seek out negative experiences to validate their negative beliefs about themselves or avoid situations that may make them look bad to others.

People with a higher self-concept sense tend to have healthier relationships with others. They feel more comfortable with themselves and seek out healthy relationships (both platonic and romantic) more often. They also tend to be better at understanding the needs of others, which is likely because they can identify with those needs in a way that people with low self-concepts cannot.

Many people with borderline personality disorder (BPD) also experience low self-concept. This can result from their tendencies towards negative thinking, which makes it easy for them to focus on the negative aspects of themselves and their lives. People with BPD may also have experienced trauma or abuse during their childhood, which may affect their self-concept in a way that makes them feel like they are not deserving of love and care from others. Because BPD is associated with severe emotional dysregulation, many people with BPD may have difficulty controlling their emotions, thoughts, and actions, leading to negative social interactions that can worsen their self-concept.

There are many methods of dealing with low self-esteem, including therapy. Dialectical behavior therapy (DBT) focuses on teaching clients skills to help them positively cope with their emotions, allowing them to foster healthier relationships with others and themselves. DBT is based on the idea that an individual has a strong internal self, fully capable of making decisions and creating plans for their life, and an external self, which includes all of their social interactions. Therapists hope to teach clients how to use the "real" self (internal self) to better interact with others rather than falling into the habit of using their external selves (based more on their emotions).

What are dialectical stances used for?

Dialectical stances help individuals with BPD recognize their internal and external selves and how they are connected. They also help clients learn how to regulate their emotions, thoughts, and behavior based on these two parts. Dialectical stances are also used to help people with BPD develop better relationships with others. Dialectical stances can also help people with BPD improve their quality of life.

Dialectical stances are used in treating borderline personality disorder (BPD). Dialectical behavior therapy (DBT) focuses on helping clients learn to cope with their emotions and behaviors, which is BPD's main symptom. This can be done through dialectical training, which involves understanding the relationship between a person's internal and external selves. Dialectical thinking can help clients form healthier relationships with themselves and others.

Dialectical thinking also allows people who experience BPD to recognize that they do not need to rely on others for validation because they can validate themselves. They can also identify the thoughts and feelings they are experiencing, which allows them to understand themselves and their relationships with others. This can allow people to react more appropriately in social situations and develop more healthy relationships with others.

Dialectical thinking is also used in the treatment of people with BPD. It focuses on improving social skills, which is an important aspect of dealing with BPD. Dialectical training teaches individuals about the interpersonal relationship between internal and external selves (self-control) by teaching them that their "real" selves have a positive impact on their "false" self (social self). This allows individuals to recognize when they fall into dysfunctional behaviors that lead to poor behaviors, thoughts, or emotions.

The dialectical theory was developed by psychologist and psychoanalyst Wilhelm Reich (1897–1957). Reich realized that the full knowledge of human biology and psychology needed to include consciousness and unconsciousness, psychic and social factors, biological and social traits, logic, and illogic psychological laws. Furthermore, he informed therapists and patients that human beings are unique only in their ability to rationally experience and express emotional states, not in their competency to observe themselves.

Reich also believed that characterological development could not be understood without considering social and environmental influences on the individual's life and personal characterological makeup. He developed the psychosocial dialectic, a psychodynamic approach that uses mental illness to help explain systemic or societal conditions. The term "dialectical" derives from the Greek διαλεκτική (dialektikē), meaning "related to conversation or debate." The dialectical approach to psychotherapy services that any combination of opposing forces necessary to promote health and well-being

Reich used the concept of dialectics to explain how human beings can be egotistical and altruistic, suicidal and productive, hostile and open in their communication, or capable at times of contradictory behavior. In this view, an individual can be torn between characterological traits based on sensitivity or rigidity. By understanding how these opposites are linked, individuals can recognize the underlying motivations for their behaviors and actions. Reich believed that anyone who understands themselves would also understand social dynamics better.

Therefore, the roles of dialectical stances include:

a. self-attunement: a person acknowledges their passive and active role in social interactions.
b. self-regulation: a person is aware of their power to regulate the relationship between their internal and external selves, allowing them to understand the "true" self-better.

c.   conflict resolution: a person can use dialectic processes to resolve disagreements with others and maintain healthy social relationships determined by other people in their environment.

d.   altruism versus egotism: an individual recognizes that they can act altruistically or egotistically at different points in time or under different circumstances (i.e., emotional vs. adult).

e.   change of self-concept: an individual understands that their personality traits are not set in stone and the variables they can control change throughout their life.

f.   cultural diversity: an individual can recognize that many different cultures are based in different parts of the world, causing them to be more tolerant and accepting of other people's lifestyles.

g.   interdependence: an individual recognizes that they are inherently interdependent with others and can adopt a sense of altruism without being too dependent on others or having too much ego (i.e., dependency vs. independent).

h.   personal change: throughout their life, an individual recognizes that they are capable of developing different personalities, which gives them more options in their social interactions, relationships, and development.

i.   opposites are not mutually exclusive: an individual will find examples in the world where any given opposite is present at once (e.g., passion and coolness or illness and health). They acknowledge that there is no such thing as a mutually exclusive opposite. Individuals can recognize that they are capable of both simultaneously and will depend on how they perceive themselves (i.e., self-attunement).

j.   change in perception: an individual recognizes that change happens over time and that there are different stages to maturity (i.e., child, adolescent, adult).

k.   awareness of mind/body connection: a person understands that their health is intrinsically linked to their emotional health and vice versa (i.e., emotional and physical health). An individual understands the relationship between mind and body regarding emotional and physical issues such as illness or pain.

l.   awareness of social, cultural, and environmental influences: an individual can recognize that their upbringing, the people in their lives, and the environment can influence them (i.e., self-regulation).

m.   knowledge and understanding of various cultures: an individual understands various cultures based on where they are from, who they spend time with or where they come from in general.

n.   awareness of the external world: a person recognizes that certain things affect them emotionally and physically (i.e., physical health).

o.   awareness of others' thoughts and perceptions: a person can recognize the thoughts and perceptions others have about themselves and their reactions to those thoughts or perceptions (i.e., conflict resolution).

p.   awareness of the moods of others: an individual can recognize how they feel and what other people are feeling based on various situations. They understand how emotions can be contagious (i.e., interdependence).

q.   awareness of others' intentions: a person recognizes underlying motives and their effects on their thoughts and perceptions about others (i.e., altruism versus egotism).

r.   appreciation for differences: an individual acknowledges that different people or cultures have varying opinions about issues, beliefs, lifestyles, or values (i.e., cultural diversity).

Challenges and disadvantages of dialectical stances

Reich believed that the challenges or disadvantages of dialectical stances include:

a.   self-evaluation: an individual can become indecisive, non-resolved, or lose faith in their decision and what they believe to be true (i.e., self-attunement vs. rigidity).

b.   changing environment: a person may not be aware of the changes that are occurring around them and how their thoughts, perceptions, and moods are being influenced by those changes (i.e., altruism vs. egotism).

c. cultural diversity: an individual may become overwhelmed by all of the influences from other cultures and may start to conform to whichever culture is most similar to their own (i.e., cultural diversity).

d. failure to understand others' beliefs: an individual may fail to understand the motives or perceptions of others and make assumptions without fully understanding that person or culture (i.e., self-regulation vs. rigidity).

e. unrealistic expectations: an individual can expect others to act a certain way based on their self-perception rather than recognizing other factors involved (i.e., conflict resolution vs. rigidity).

f. limited awareness of one's personality: an individual may not be able to establish themselves as a separate and different person from the last person they were due to their inability to recognize the differences between themselves and those close to them (i.e., self-attunement vs. rigidity).

g. self-esteem issues: an individual's view of themselves may be lower than how they are and can be developed to meet their needs at the expense of others (i.e., self-esteem issues vs. self-service).

h. failure to recognize and adapt to change: an individual may not recognize the changes around them, which can cause them to become more rigid or indecisive (i.e., rigidity vs. change).

i. failure in perception: an individual may not clearly understand one's previous perceptions or changes in their current personality, which can lead to frustration and struggles in life (i.e., rigidity vs. flexibility).

j. failure to understand their strengths: an individual may not be able to recognize their strengths and weaknesses, which can lead to problems in relationships or understanding of one's goals in life (i.e., rigidity vs. flexibility).

Dialectical strategies

Reich defined these dialectical strategies:

1. Double-Sided Dialectical Strategies: This requires individuals to recognize their strengths and weaknesses and how others perceive them (i.e., sensitivity).

2. Dialectical Self-Regulation Strategies: a strategy that requires an individual to understand their current situation as well as their previous perceptions, moods, thoughts, or feelings to make appropriate decisions or avoid impulsive decisions (i.e., regulating).

3. Dialectical Awareness of Self Strategies: a strategy that requires individuals to recognize their self-perceptions, moods, thoughts, or feelings with others' perceptions of them (i.e., self-equalization).

4. Dialectical Accommodation Strategies: a strategy that requires an individual to recognize their strengths, weaknesses, and perceptions of other people to properly understand how each of them can be beneficial or hurtful to the relationship (i.e., altruism).

5. Dialectical Integration Strategies: a strategy that requires an individual to have an awareness of their strengths, weaknesses, and perceptions to acknowledge the impact on themselves and other people as well as how they can be beneficial or hurtful (i.e., understanding).

6. Dialectical Consciousness-Raising Strategies: a strategy that requires an individual to acknowledge the presence of other people and how their actions, perceptions, moods, thoughts, or feelings can be beneficial or hurtful for themselves and others (i.e., awareness of others).

Reich believed that the above strategies are not created by one's specific beliefs or behavior but result from life experiences. Those experiences can be changed to improve dialectical stances. For example, suppose an individual believes that people should always be accepting of everything. In that case, they will have difficulty in their relationships if they do not understand the differences between certain actions and emotions. They can then change their stance to understand better how people's moods or thoughts affect themselves and others.

Reich believed that dialectics could be used to understand what is happening inside people, such as their personalities or behaviors. He believed that this knowledge could help individuals better understand how their behavior affects others, allowing them to understand better other behavior and how they affect them. In this way, the individual can see their personality traits as something that is learned, not innate.

Reich believed that dialectics was a concept that could help people learn to act more effectively at work or deal with the problems they face at home or in relationships. He also believed that dialectics could be used to make decisions and problem-solve at work or change aspects of one's life to become happier.

Reich believed that dialectics is a "triadic philosophy of life" because it provided an understanding of life that was different from traditional Western philosophies. This is due to dialectics' ability to see the relationship between different influences, such as interpersonal and intra-psychic relationships. These two types of influences are referred to as "abstract ideas" since they are seen more than experienced and are not completely understood in their true forms.

Reich's belief about how individuals learn about their characteristics, such as gender or age, was similar to Freud's notion about how the mind and behavior were related. Reich's belief about how their surroundings and interactions with others influence individuals was similar to Gestalt therapy.

Reich believed that using dialectics could help individuals deal with people, such as coworkers or family members, who were critical of them. He believed that these people are not always critical of the individual. Instead, they may be being critical of the individual's situation or where they are in life. The person may not understand why they have these attitudes and behaviors, which can lead to an individual becoming angry or frustrated when dealing with them.

These strategies can be developed through mindfulness, which is engrained into the dialectical approach. Mindfulness is a process that involves being aware of one's internal and external environment. Moreover, it involves being attuned to the events that are currently taking place and being aware of how these events affect oneself and others. Mindfulness is said to allow an individual to be completely attentive to one's surroundings to understand better the relationship between their behaviors, thoughts, emotions, and other people.

Furthermore, mindfulness also involves having a non-judgmental attitude about the environment or current situation one is in. By not judging their surroundings or current situation, individuals can see it for what it is and not attach their emotions and thoughts to it. This allows them to objectively assess situations while remaining true to themselves and their feelings throughout any given situation. This can help them have less anxiety when dealing with critical people around them.

Disadvantages and challenges of dialectical strategies

Dialectical strategies can be an advantage for certain individuals to enhance their relationships and communication. Both professionals and laypersons can use them to achieve better outcomes that benefit themselves and others.

For the dialectic approach to work, the individual must have a "cooperative attitude." This means they must understand the concepts of their environment or situation being analyzed, accept it as an indivisible whole, and not try to change it by changing one variable in isolation.

The dialectic approach also requires a person to have adequate self-esteem, which is "the capacity of one's belief system, feelings, attitudes and behavior to cope effectively with environmental pressure." Moreover, their self-esteem should also be strong enough to allow them to be objective about themselves and their surroundings.

A person's approach to learning, the way they accept information, and what they believe in will determine whether the dialectic approach will benefit them or not. It also matters how receptive a person is to different views and opinions and if they are open-minded enough to understand and accept other ideas that do not follow along with popular views.

Reich's theory was developed from psychoanalytic theory by focusing on social issues to "rehabilitate character," which is comparable to the aims of other psychotherapists like Alfred Adler, who also were concerned with social problems.

Reich developed his character analysis theory from Freud's psychosexual development theory. This is why there are similarities between Freud's stages of sexual development (oral, anal, phallic, latency, and genital) and the different stages a person goes through during the character analysis process. Both are used to develop one's personality. However, Reich viewed the psychosexual stages as something a person goes through only once during childhood. In contrast, the character analysis process is something that a person can go through multiple times throughout their lives to understand better how they interact with others.

DBT STRATEGIES FOR AN INDIVIDUAL SESSION

DBT strategies for individual sessions can be used to address three different goals for individuals: mindfulness, emotional regulation, and interpersonal effectiveness. DBT strategies can be adapted to relieve any individual's problems. For example, a therapist might adapt DBT strategies for use with a person who engages in self-harm to reduce their need or urge to self-harm. Strategies that facilitate emotional regulation in an individual session might help them feel better within themselves after an episode of violence or harm. Finally, an individual session can focus on interpersonal effectiveness by teaching the person ways to avoid or reduce feelings that can lead to harmful behavior. In addition, the therapist might teach the person how to release pent-up anger and frustration "in a safe way."

Overall, the DBT model consists of three modules: The first is individual sessions, in which the therapist may focus on mindfulness, emotional regulation, and interpersonal effectiveness. The second module is group sessions, in which the therapist may focus on relapse prevention. The third module is phone calls to a therapist who specializes in DBT and can offer support and guidance. If a person fails to engage with basic modules after three weeks of therapy at a level one clinician would consider satisfactory; they will be referred to a more experienced clinician who conducts specialized training to treat those issues such as suicidal behaviors or severe reactions.

DBT is typically structured around more frequent core-skills group sessions with weekly individual 1-hour sessions and a support group. DBT uses four main strategies to address behaviors: situation-, emotion-, cognition-, and action-oriented. When a person has a behavior that disturbs them in some way, they bring it up at the next meeting of their therapy team. The team can then discuss how they will handle the situation based on different strategies. First, the emotion-oriented strategy involves choosing a nonjudgmental attitude by accepting one's emotions as one presents themselves without attempting to change them. Secondly, the situation-oriented strategy involves identifying the functional benefit of behavior for the person until they can achieve alternative ways to achieve that function, such as through DBT skills training. Thirdly, the action-oriented strategy involves choosing a behavior to replace the problem and learning to engage in that new behavior. Fourthly, the cognition-oriented strategy involves identifying how a person's distress interferes with their ability to think clearly and subsequently interferes with their ability to choose effective behaviors, leading them into more distressing situations.

Within each session, four main skills are worked on. The first of these skills is distress tolerance, which addresses a person's inability to tolerate high levels of emotional distress. The second is emotion regulation, which focuses on how a person can better control their emotions; this skill is used for distressing emotions that are hard to tolerate and for intense positive emotions. Thirdly, interpersonal effectiveness refers to developing relationships with others to improve the lives of the individual and those around them. Lastly, mindfulness refers to helping those who are depressed deal with negative thoughts without acting on them rather than reacting in response to these thoughts.

The focus in DBT therapy sessions is on "skill-building" so that clients can learn skills they will use between sessions. The skills that a therapist works on with an individual either in an individual session or during skill-building groups typically include the following:

There are four modules of DBT. The following outlines the typical approach to each module and an example exercise. Module 1 is structured around weekly one-hour sessions and includes skills training. Module 2, which takes place once a week, involves a more structured format than Module 1 and focuses on relapse prevention. In Modules 3 and 4, which occur once every other week, there is a focus on telephone consultations between sessions that can be done as needed or for help with recovery after self-harm and when individuals are considering suicide. Each DBT meeting consists of four major objectives. The first objective is to establish a foundation for the therapist and client. The second is to assess and modify any problems that the client may have. The third objective is to increase skills training session by session. A fourth objective is to create situations where clients can make errors with minimal negative consequences and learn from them.

The therapist will assess the person's problem behavior (e.g., depression, suicide) and then work on building up their ability to deal with distressing thoughts and any emotional struggles with both physical skills training in DBT and emotionally based therapy (EBT). The therapist will also assess the person's strengths and weaknesses and work with them on areas they are weaker in to help improve their quality of life. The therapist will also identify what type of attitude the person has towards other people and the person's general way of thinking to develop a better sense of how they relate to others.

The typical format for Module 1 includes three major parts, which are called "core-skills groups," "individual therapy," and "phone consults." Each part will be discussed in more detail below.

When working with clients in Module 1, there are 15 skills divided into four categories: distress tolerance, emotion regulation skills, interpersonal effectiveness skills, and mindfulness. Distress tolerance skills involve the person learning how to deal with their emotional struggles by gaining greater self-awareness and control of their emotions. Emotion regulation skills teach them to better deal with distressing thoughts by better identifying the connection between these thoughts and the emotions that occur as a result. Finally, interpersonal effectiveness skills focus on improving the communication between clients and their therapists. In contrast, mindfulness focuses on developing the individual's ability to think clearly and respond to negative thoughts instead of acting on them. In addition, two exercises are used during Module 1:

DBT strategies that facilitate mindfulness:

One of the Dialectical Behavior Therapy (DBT) goals is mindfulness, "which refers to an alert and nonjudgmental present-focused awareness."

The client is taught three skills: (1) observing with curiosity, (2) describing with equanimity, and (3) participating in activities mindfully. These skills help with regulating emotions both during and after triggering situations.

Mindfulness Skills in Individual Sessions: The focus of the present module will be on these mindfulness skills.

Observing with curiosity refers to staying in touch with the present moment and observing one's sensations and feelings without judgment.

Equanimity means letting go of judgments about one's feelings and just describing them with words.

Participating in activities mindfully refers to the daily activity as if it were being done for the first time, noticing every detail: sights, sounds, smells, tastes, and physical sensations. This skill may require a therapist to help refocus clients who get off track by judging their experience or comparing it with that of others.

Therefore, the DBT strategies for individual sessions include:

1. Observing with curiosity:

The present module teaches clients to stay present and maintain an active, inquisitive mind by using exercises. The skills required in this exercise include as follows:

Observing with curiosity in a way that helps clients realize they can be aware of what they are observing without judging it as good or bad.

Identifying the activities that cause suffering.

Mentally noting that when emotions arise, these feelings happen because something triggers them.

Recognizing these responses is not the same as wanting to change the situation or receiving comfort from others.

Learning how to be mindful of the sensations that come from within.

Remember that it may take time for them to understand these mindfulness skills and incorporate them into their daily lives.

The therapist should ask if they understand these skills and explain that they must practice applying them to improve their skills further. Challenges can occur when the individual believes they already have this skill or do not use it effectively. Therefore, the therapist needs to help refocus them on their goal of learning and practicing this skill. The therapist can also help identify triggers for emotional responses or a lack of mindfulness in daily situations so that clients can work on these areas.

2. Describing with equanimity:

The present module aims to teach clients to describe a difficult situation or experience without judgment. The skills required in this exercise include as follows:

Describing with equanimity in a way that helps clients notice their feelings and sensations with equanimity.

Identifying what they need and what they don't need, in an objective way, instead of reacting.

Knowing that expressing something can solve a problem rather than create new ones. Using "I" statements and describing the situation from their perspective is not based on what other people think or should say. Exercises consist of deep breathing exercises, meditation, and guided imagery.

3. Participating in activities mindfully:

The present module aims to teach clients to participate in daily activities with a new level of awareness. The skills required in this exercise include as follows:

Participating in activities mindfully by remaining present with everything they experience.

Identifying their feelings and sensations at that moment.

Including the feelings and sensations as part of their observations rather than ignoring or judging them. Exercises include walking, deep breathing, guided visualization, and mindfulness meditation.

4. Mindfulness exercises for daily living:

The present module aims to teach clients how to remain mindful during everyday activities that may evoke emotional responses or thoughts. The skills required in this exercise include as follows:

Resting the mind by practicing deep breathing, guided imagery, or mindfulness meditation for a short breather.

Reminding themselves to focus on their core values, especially those that help them manage their emotions and impulses, such as self-respect and other-respect.

Mindfully engage in a daily activity by practicing one of the above mindfulness skills.

Exercises include yoga, physical activities, and daily tasks like eating and bathing. In addition, they focus on observing without judging one's experiences while practicing self-care by taking time to heal. This can take time to accomplish because clients have spent years experiencing emotions and thoughts that have been unhealthy for them.

5. Behavioral exercises for daily living:

The present module aims to teach clients how to incorporate mindfulness into their daily activities and address barriers as they arise. The skills required in this exercise include as follows:

Identifying and addressing obstacles that may hinder their progress daily. In addition, they should use mindfulness skills, such as breathing exercises, meditation, and guided visualization.

Modifying behaviors or thought patterns can lead to emotional dysregulation or behavioral dyscontrol. They should allow themselves to experience their emotions without acting on them, even if it might be difficult for them. They should allow themselves to accept and explore their emotions while caring for their needs. Exercises consist of using Neuro-Linguistic Programming (NLP).

6. Interpersonal exercises for daily living:

The present module aims to teach clients how to remain mindful in social interactions and address barriers as they arise. The skills required in this exercise include as follows:

Modifying behaviors or thought patterns can lead to emotional dysregulation or behavioral dyscontrol. They should allow themselves to experience their emotions without acting on them, even if it might be difficult for them. Instead, they should allow themselves to accept and explore their emotions while caring for their needs.

Identifying unhelpful behaviors and how it makes other people feel. They should take responsibility for their behaviors and apologize, even if they cannot explain them. Often, this is the first step toward recovery for the individual because it helps create a more calm atmosphere in their relationships with others. Exercises consist of practicing NLP and educating clients on interpersonal skills.

7. The role of mindfulness in recovery and life:

The present module aims to teach clients how mindfulness plays an important role in their recovery.

They understand that they cannot return to old habits or patterns but must find a new way of living daily. This includes habits related to thoughts, emotions, and behaviors.

Understanding what mindfulness is and how it can be incorporated into their lives. They should continue practicing the skills they have learned throughout treatment to maintain their recovery from emotional dysregulation or behavioral dyscontrol.

The therapist will be able to find ways that fit the client's personality, goals, and style, as well as techniques that best suit them. The therapist will also be able to match the skills needed with what they can use to help their clients. Therefore, the therapist needs to assess their clients and then help them identify any personal characteristics they may have that would make certain skills more effective for these individuals. These characteristics include values such as respect or self-respect or learning styles like visual, auditory, or kinesthetic.

8. Discovery and formulation of a plan:

The present module aims to teach clients how to share their recovery plan with others and examine it regularly.

They know they must maintain recovery by staying present in their daily lives. They should continue practicing the skills they have learned throughout treatment to maintain their recovery from emotional dysregulation or behavioral dyscontrol.

9. Ongoing support:

The present module aims to teach clients how to maintain a lifestyle of mindfulness and how it is still necessary throughout recovery from emotional dysregulation or behavioral dyscontrol. They should continue practicing the skills they have learned throughout treatment to maintain their recovery from emotional dysregulation or behavioral dyscontrol.

This means they can seek relapse prevention techniques, such as setting boundaries, to avoid and repair unhealthy habits. They should also follow the structure or process that their treatment plan outlines and realize that it can take time for them to succeed in this way of living. Their therapist may ask questions about their daily behaviors progressing and guide them if necessary.

10. Life skills:

The present module aims to teach clients how to live a mindful life in every aspect of their lives, including relationships, self-care, work performance, and community involvement. In addition, they should continue practicing the skills they have learned throughout treatment to maintain their recovery from emotional dysregulation or behavioral dyscontrol.

These skills may include using relapse prevention techniques, assessing triggers, and recognizing when one is sliding back into old habits. They may also report trigger activities and engage in coping mechanisms that help them deal with emotions.

The mindfulness-based cognitive therapy program manual helps to understand the different and most effective strategies for treating individuals who suffer from emotional dysregulation or behavioral dyscontrol. Mindfulness-based cognitive therapy allows the individual to let go of distressful feelings that are often overwhelming by being self-aware.

Characteristics of DBT strategies

Mainstays in DBT include emotion regulation, social skills training, mindfulness, and interpersonal effectiveness (IPE). Although these components are common to several similar programs, they are particularly useful in DBT. Research supports the effectiveness of DBT for people with BPD. Findings suggest that people with BPD who participate in DBT may experience greater improvement than those who receive other types of treatment for their illness. One study examined the impact of DBT on patients with BPD and found significant improvements in interpersonal skills and psychotic symptoms over a 6-month follow-up period.

The main characteristics of DBT are as follows:

a. Emotion regulation skills: DBT for BPD seeks to improve emotional dysregulation and the relationship with the self by learning to identify aspects of emotions and thoughts. The therapist will teach clients to control their emotions by learning new techniques. These include mindfulness, emotion regulation, and ethical leadership.

b. Social skills: The therapist will use many different protocols, from social skills training, interpersonal problem-solving approaches, and cognitive-behavioral therapy (CBT) strategies. DBT for BPD embraces these methods but will also integrate other methods like dialectical behavior therapy (DBT) and motivational interviewing based on empirical research.

c. Mindfulness: Mindfulness, a popular new therapy method, is widely used in DBT. This technique is based on the mental perception that everything can be known. The therapist will use this technique to teach clients how to live in the present moment and understand their thoughts, feelings, and behaviors.

d. IPE: The improvement throughout treatment will eventually lead to recovery. The patient will learn how to relate to others as a person and not just with a diagnosis or illness. This way, they can utilize self-reflection, interpersonal effectiveness, and emotional intelligence (EI) skills. As explained in RFT tools, they can learn new ways of expressing themselves instead of using language as a weapon against others or themselves.

e. Problem solving: Clients will learn how to identify problems in their life and how they can find solutions to these problems. Strategies can also be used that help people work on their issues. Although members of the treatment team will assist with problem-solving, they are not therapists.

f. Negotiation and mediation skills: These skills are employed to solve disputes between others who may not be able to resolve their differences without intervention. Skills taught in these areas include the following:

g. Life review: Clients will begin to develop a sense of peace and find an inner sense of strength with the tool of life review.

h. Group therapy: As the patient's skills improve, they will be able to participate in group therapy. The therapist will help them use DBT skills such as dialectical behavior therapy (DBT) and cognitive behavioral therapy (CBT) in a group setting.

i. Medications: The team will continue familiarizing themselves with the therapist's medications. The patient's family, friends, or caregivers may also take these drugs during this period of intensive treatment as prescribed by their doctor.

j. Learning disabilities: People with mild or moderate learning disabilities or chronic BPD may need specialized assistance with social skills and cognitive restructuring to complete treatment.

k. Self-injury: One of the most difficult problems in BPD patients is self-injury. The patients may experience a sense of self-hatred and try to hurt themselves on their own or even at the hands of others.

m. Suicidal behavior: Another acute problem people with BPD can experience is suicidal behavior. Sometimes, a patient will present with a dangerous suicide attempt after completing treatment, as described above. In this case, ongoing treatment and support are imperative until this acute situation is resolved, as described in RFT tools.

n. Alcohol and drug use: People with BPD, who are of legal age, may be permitted to use alcohol or drugs according to their treatment plan. The therapist will monitor and supervise the patient's use whenever possible.

o. Relapse prevention: This is an important skill for the client who completes DBT for BPD. If these people stay in contact with their therapists and family, they are less likely to return to the previous unhealthy behaviors that brought them into treatment.

p. Recovering from bullying, violence, and abuse: These issues can be resolved by completing DBT for BPD treatment programs as described above with RFT tools as needed.

DBT for BPD is a revolutionary new way of treating BPD patients. Including old and new methods has created a whole new treatment incorporating many strategies for dealing with mental health problems. This treatment provides an ideal way for people suffering from BPD to manage their emotions healthily, strengthen relationships with others, and become better versions of themselves through self-evaluation, insight, and skill development.

Preparing for a DBT session

This process is different depending on the individual therapist. For example, some therapists may begin the meeting with a required script, and others will begin with a consultation. They may also ask for specific problems to be discussed in a session.

DBT therapists will often ask the client what they feel their goal is from therapy and how they think therapy can best help them reach that goal. The therapist may then frame it, asking how therapy can be used to address all elements of this goal in some manner; for example, using DBT skills to address self-injury or using DBT to address anger (your goals could be expressed as "I want to stop abusing myself" or "I want my anger to go away"). The therapist may then frame the discussion based on the client's answers by asking questions to help clarify why this is a problem for them (e.g., "how does self-injury make you feel?").

The therapist will then consider how this behavior affects other people in their lives and may ask what role other people play in perpetuating or encouraging the problem (e.g., whether there are thoughts or behaviors of others that serve to reinforce or maintain the difficulty). The therapist will also ask about things that help and support change in this area of life, as well as opposing points of view (e.g., what do they like about self-injury/anger?).

DBT therapists will consider the client's specific problems and treatment goals when preparing for these sessions. Some common goals may be:

* To become more aware of and manage emotions
* To build healthy relationships with others
* To establish a sense of self and identity
* To learn new skills to deal with life challenges.

These topics can be the focus of DBT sessions in combination with each other where appropriate.

A typical DBT session includes the following:

* Opening statements and general questions discussed with the client before beginning.
* A report on progress, including thoughts, feelings, behaviors, and relationships.
* Discussion of problems identified during the initial therapy session.
* Self-help materials based upon the client's goals are presented (e.g., coping skills, anger management skills).
* Behavioral experiments are discussed and planned.
* Implementation of behavioral experiments, including assignments given for homework to be completed between sessions.

DBT is intended to address the problems people experience through self-injury and other behaviors they consider unhealthy. However, therapy can help people identify the patterns of self-harm that lead to their problems and then form new, healthier habits to live.

Self-injury is a common problem for BPD patients. People with BPD may abuse drugs or have a compulsion to harm themselves at times of particular stress or unhappiness. They also may appear difficult to care for as they often have meltdowns that require medical attention and can leave family members and caregivers feeling frustrated, angry, or upset by the behavior of their loved ones.

Strategies for individual sessions include positive reinforcement in addition to RFT tools and skills. Therapy can also include discussing a similar problem that occurred in the past and using that experience as a teaching moment to help the client become more aware of their emotions and thoughts.

There are many healthy things that people with BPD can do in their lives. These include attending CBT, DBT, mindfulness, and relaxation therapy sessions and taking medication only as prescribed by a doctor. However, the tools for action and motivation to achieve healthy behaviors typically come from practicing the skills of change in DBT.

Key Points for Individuals

Important points for individuals who are undergoing DBT treatment include:

* Accepting that they have a problem with self-injury and abusive behaviors is an important part of recovery.
* Learning how to identify these behaviors or thoughts that lead to the need to harm themselves is essential to recovery.
* Working with a professional therapist who can help them identify the patterns in their thoughts, emotions, and behaviors that lead to harmful behavior is essential.
* Learning how to use cognitive behavioral therapy and mindfulness skills to cope with stress or incidents of self-injury are also essential.
* It is important to practice new healthy ways of handling situations that make them feel stressed or upset (e.g., take a walk).
* There will be times when people have urges for self-injury and abusive behaviors but can resist these urges before acting on them. This is just part of being human.

After a DBT session

It is important to note that in some cases of self-injury, the person experiencing urges may be unable to control their behavior. Therefore, it is important that therapy can also include a plan for learning different ways to get through certain problems. For example, people who have experienced self-injury or abusive behaviors may start taking medications prescribed by their doctor or therapist during DBT treatment. In addition, people may also begin medication for psychiatric disorders after undergoing DBT treatment (e.g., Xanax for panic attacks).

Many people who have experienced severe symptoms of BPD experience episodes of improvement and progress through therapy over months or years. During their time in therapy, clients can learn skills and strategies to help them with relationships, self-harm and abusive behaviors, emotions, and anxiety.

DBT treatment tends to be long-term in nature. The average length of treatment for BPD is about one year.

Although DBT was originally developed as a treatment for people diagnosed with borderline personality disorder (BPD), there is growing evidence that it can be effective for many disorders, including schizophrenia spectrum disorders, depression, bipolar disorder, and bulimia nervosa.

People with BPD are at an increased risk of developing mood-disordered psychotic symptoms, such as hallucinations and delusions, particularly during periods of high stress and low self-esteem. However, studies have shown that combining cognitive behavioral therapy (CBT) and medication may significantly reduce the number of mood-disorder psychotic symptoms experienced by individuals with BPD.

There is controversy over using CBT alone as a treatment for borderline personality disorder. In one study, many people who had previously been diagnosed with BPD did not respond to CBT alone and were not able to stabilize their emotions. CBT was also ineffective for treating some other psychiatric conditions experienced by clients with BPD (e.g., depression).

HOW TO USE DBT TO OVERCOME MAIN PSYCHOLOGICAL PROBLEMS

Dialectical Behavior Therapy (DBT) may be the solution if you struggle with a psychological issue.

DBT is an effective treatment strategy that can help people with various mental health problems, including depression, anxiety, addiction, eating disorders, and self-harm. It aims to manage these problems and improve one's quality of life by teaching mindfulness and emotional regulation skills.

The problem begins when one fails to manage their emotions appropriately in response to specific situations or events that trigger negative feelings. For example, if someone has an eating disorder triggered by food-related triggers or someone engages in self-harm due to past trauma, they may engage in compulsive behaviors such as cutting their skin without even realizing it. This happens because they cannot regulate their emotions.

Dealing with negative emotions using DBT involves four steps:

1. Identify the emotion(s) you are experiencing at the moment
2. Accept and acknowledge these feelings, noting them without judgment or thoughts of how to change them
3. Choose a healthy behavior to help you become less caught up in your emotions. This might include exercise, talking to a friend, meditating, or going for a walk
4. Repeat this process two more times throughout the day

To achieve healthy behavior change through DBT, specific skills, such as distress tolerance and mindfulness, must be used. Distress tolerance is the ability to cope with the physical and emotional effects of strong negative emotions. Mindfulness skills are ways of keeping yourself in the present moment without judging your current experience. The DBT therapist teaches these skills in a structured cognitive-behavioral treatment plan that combines individual, group, and telephone therapy sessions.

DBT was created as a treatment for Borderline Personality Disorder; however, it has since been modified to help with other psychological problems. It is used by psychiatrists, psychologists, social workers, and therapists who treat people struggling with anxiety, depression, and self-harm problems.

The most common treatment combines individual, group, and telephone therapy. This provides opportunities for the patient to practice new skills with the DBT therapist in an individual session and socialize with other patients in a group session. In addition, in telephone therapy, patient can call their therapist whenever they want to talk about something relevant to their problems.

In some cases, these three levels are unnecessary, and a combination of individual therapy, self-help materials, and weekly skills training groups may be sufficient.

Individual therapy sessions consist of a one-on-one meeting with the therapist at least once a week, usually lasting for an hour or more. The DBT therapist guides the patient in learning new skills for dealing with their emotions to achieve balanced and healthy behavior change.

Group therapy sessions are conducted in a very structured way, allowing the patients to work on the same skill step by step. For example, the group may work on reducing social anxiety by going out in public places. Previously, they avoided such places for fear of being judged or criticized.

Therefore, DBT can be used to overcome main psychological problems through:

a. Adopting a healthy lifestyle and feeling better with the right skills to help manage one's own emotions
b. Adopting a healthier, more physically active diet by learning to tolerate strong emotions and not engage in unhealthy behaviors
c. Learning to recognize and accept feelings without criticizing or acting on them
d. Taking more responsibility for one's life and looking after oneself without engaging in compulsive habits, such as self-harming or engaging in risky, impulsive behaviors that may lead to addiction
e. Avoiding reinforcing negative thoughts such as "I am not good enough," by avoiding any criticism or negativity in one's life, which can lead to self-judgment or shame
f. Maintaining a healthy social life by finding hobbies, making new friends, and developing the necessary skills to achieve and maintain long-lasting relationships
g. healthily dealing with negative emotions before they lead to addiction or other serious, harmful behaviors such as self-harm or eating disorders
h. Maintaining a proper diet while feeling better about one's body by learning to treat oneself with respect and love

Managing strong emotions is difficult; however, with the support and structured treatment offered through DBT, one can learn to manage their emotions in healthy ways. DBT is a comprehensive treatment strategy involving many different therapy sessions.

For example, through mindfulness exercises, one learns to be aware of their thoughts and feelings without judging them or engaging in compulsive behaviors. In individual therapy, the therapist encourages patients to look at their destructive behavior and develop new skills to deal with difficult situations.

By practicing these new skills, patients can find healthier ways to handle strong emotions and addictive behaviors while living a more balanced life. Therefore, DBT can help overcome most psychological problems through adopting a healthier lifestyle and learning to cope with one's negative emotions in positive ways that are not harmful to oneself or others.

How to use the skills

DBT skills can be used in all kinds of situations. Some skills help deal with a specific situation, while some are general properties that can be used repeatedly regardless of the situation. Skills are also used through different mediums. For example, skills can be practiced in therapy and used in real-life situations. Skills can also be practiced through self-help material or journaling.

Three primary skills are used in DBT, and each can help deal with specific situations. These three skills are Mindfulness, Distress Tolerance, and Emotion Regulation.

Mindfulness is "learning to observe your thoughts, emotions, and experience, non-judgmentally" (Linehan). Through mindfulness, people can recognize their thoughts for what they are and not act on them. It is also a great example of acceptance because through mindfulness, one accepts the way things are rather than trying to change them or make them different from how it is. DBT patients can practice several types of mindfulness exercises to practice mindfulness. Mindfulness can be used for all aspects of life, so it is an important skill to have.

Distress Tolerance is a skill that helps the patient confront their feelings and not give in to them. It also involves the patient learning to accept and tolerate strong emotions without engaging in compulsive behaviors such as self-harm or eating disorders. In addition, this skill can help a person empathize with different feelings and learn how to respond appropriately in different situations.

Emotion Regulation is a skill that helps the patient learn how to deal with their emotions in healthy ways. It also involves the ability to reflect on one's behavior when dealing with emotions and to take responsibility for one's actions. The main idea is not to let emotions control your behavior but to take control of your negative emotions. For example, suppose someone is angry instead of physically lashing out at someone or through smart remarks. In that case, the person should be responsible and find a better way to express their anger, such as punching a pillow or talking to themselves about their feelings.

Dialectical Behavior Therapy Skills can be practiced in group settings, individual therapy sessions, and in self-help material.

Therefore, these DBT skills can be implemented through:

a. Group (supportive) therapy

This is a good way to practice DBT skills because the other group members can help support, motivate, and encourage each other. Patients can also learn about the different issues others are facing, such as their struggles or what they have been able to overcome. This is also a good opportunity for patients to talk about their problems with others who know how they feel and understand what they are going through. Therefore, group therapy sessions could be used to discuss problems in a supportive environment and learn new skills that could be applied in real-life situations.

b. Individual therapy

Individual therapy helps identify the patient's behavioral patterns and work with them directly. For example, the patient can discuss problems, and the therapist can work with the patient to help them deal with those problems in an effective way. Sometimes, individual therapy sessions prevent the patient from engaging in impulsive behavior such as self-harming or abusing drugs or alcohol.

c. Self-help material

This is another good way to practice DBT skills because it encourages patients to learn how they can apply these skills in their everyday life. Patients also avoid behaviors that could lead to addiction if they start engaging in them on their own and then find a problem that will develop if they stop doing so, resulting in a serious situation where they need treatment. Self-help material is beneficial because patients can use their time to help themselves improve and learn new skills to apply in real-life situations.

Thus, DBT skills can be effectively used in individual therapy sessions, group therapy, and self-help material. Through these practicums, one can learn how to accept themselves and overcome their problems rather than continuing down a path of self-destruction that is harmful to both themselves and others.

d. Journaling exercise

This exercise allows patients to reflect on their feelings and apply the skills they have learned through therapy or self-help material. For example, patients can reflect on a situation or a feeling they have been having and then use that as an example of how they want to handle similar situations in the future. They can also respond differently to their past behavior to learn from their mistakes and change for the future. Furthermore, patients can organize their thoughts in a way that is easier for them to understand the problem at hand because putting things down on paper allows you to see things more clearly and put your thoughts into words instead of keeping them bottled up inside your head.

e.   Journaling on the diary sheet.

The diary sheet allows patients to take their thoughts from therapy sessions and organize them into a written format that they can reflect on and learn from in the future. In addition, the DBT Diary Sheet contains spaces for multiple types of therapy, including mindfulness, distress tolerance, emotion regulation, and interpersonal effectiveness. Therefore, all these different aspects of DBT skills can be effectively taught through all these different mediums to help patients develop new skills and apply them to real-life situations to improve themselves as people.

There are several stages in DBT for targeting the treatment of patients. First, Transtheoretical Model (TTM) is used to adjust the treatment intensity level based on the patient's progress, which is determined by surveys and assessments. These stages are Stabilization, Early, Intermediate, Advanced, and Termination or Relapse Prevention.

Stabilization is a step that takes place within the first three sessions with an individual. The therapist will decide how many sessions they would like to have with that specific patient and what goals they want to accomplish in those sessions. The patient and therapist should establish a stabilization contract with goals for each session.

The early stage comprises the first 6 to 12 sessions with the individual. All patients will go through this stage, and it is here where they will work on establishing trust in their therapist and build a relationship with them. During this stage, there will be an emphasis on improving self-esteem and building more skills based on depression and anxiety. Patients here can learn how to recognize their feelings as well as how to deal with them. They can also learn how to accept themselves for who they are, let go of negative thoughts, and take control of their actions rather than letting those things control them.

The intermediate Stage is the next stage after the early stage, and it occurs when the patient has learned some more skills and mastered the ones they had before. During this stage, patients are encouraged to take a more active role in their treatment and keep track of their progress. In addition, the therapist can give patients more freedom by asking them to balance different aspects of their life, such as work, family, or self-care. Patients are also given homework assignments to continuing practicing what they have learned in sessions.

The advanced Stage is for the most severe cases of patients who need intensive therapy and extra support from the therapist and other professionals throughout treatment. During this stage, the therapist will work on improving skills further and provide more structure to the patient's daily life. In addition, the patient is encouraged to continue taking care of themselves by exercising, eating correctly, and working on their overall health.

The termination or Relapse Prevention Stage is a way that patients can look back through the treatment process and evaluate their progress and effectiveness in therapy. In this stage, patients are encouraged to take responsibility for their own lives to learn how to approach new situations to help them reach their recovery goals instead of just avoiding them or letting things worsen.

The main goal when practicing mindfulness is to help patients learn how to deal with their emotions by being aware of them and learning to confront them in healthy ways. To work with these skills, therapists need tools that can be used in DBT sessions, such as a DBT worksheet or the Mindfulness Journaling & Meditation for Emotion Regulation Seminar available online. Likewise, the main goal when practicing distress tolerance is to help patients manage their emotions without engaging in harmful behaviors, such as self-harm or eating disorders.

Setting up a DBT skill plan

This can play a significant role in establishing a treatment plan. When implementing skills, the therapist will need to utilize the treatment manual, which is available online, and describe the skill set. Resistance skills, such as mindfulness or distress tolerance, are described in the individual therapy manual and are used to create an emotion regulation contract. For example, if a patient were to ask for immediate reassurance from their therapist during their session instead of working on the skill at hand, it would be considered a resistance skill.

The therapist can give patients a DBT worksheet to help them organize their thoughts and put them into words. This helps the patient apply what they have learned in previous therapy sessions and implement change in their behavior. The therapist should also use their assessment tools to determine if the patient is ready to master the skill or if they need more time to practice it. For example, if a patient has recently had an episode of self-harm, they may not be ready to work on new skills, and their therapist will have to allow them some time in this situation.

To explain the use of DBT as a complement to standard treatment for eating disorders, it is helpful to review its origins. Linehan originally developed DBT for patients with chronic suicidality; these patients were typically diagnosed with borderline personality disorder (BPD). However, later studies indicated that DBT could also be effective for patients with other life-threatening behaviors, such as self-injury or eating disorders. It was the first approach shown to be effective in both groups. As a result, Linehan recognized the potential for DBT to be used with other forms of self-injurious behavior and eating disorders.

Linehan's original focus on treating suicidal and self-injurious behavior led people to speculate that DBT would not be effective for bulimia nervosa (BN). Still, she did not initially consider this. Linehan has since begun a trial with BN patients, demonstrating that DBT, which includes acceptance and commitment therapy (ACT), is an effective treatment for BN improving body image and disordered eating behaviors. Several other studies have also demonstrated that DBT may be effective for BN.

Linehan initially created DBT as a treatment for self-injurious behavior based on her work with chronic suicidality. In her original manual for DBT, she stressed that DBT was a treatment for suicidality, not bulimia nervosa. Despite this disclaimer, Linehan later acknowledged that BN might be an appropriate population to use the skills in a behavioral therapy program. In addition to Linehan's acknowledgment of BN as an appropriate population, several other studies have also demonstrated the efficacy of the skills in treating BN.

Therefore, DBT skills can be set up through a treatment plan to include a bulimia nervosa-specific skill set. For example, if a patient were to use the skills in a way that directly impacted their bulimia, the therapist would need to intervene and teach different behaviors or explain how the patient was misusing them.

Linehan's original DBT skills were designed for borderline personality disorder (BPD) patients. She believes BPD patients are uniquely vulnerable to self-injurious and suicidal behavior. The skills incorporate principles from ACT and mindfulness therapies; these two therapies have already been validated as having benefits for BPD patients.

How to stop self-harm thoughts and behaviors in DBT terms:

Linehan indicates that any self-harm behavior must be addressed to challenge it. This technique can reduce the rate of self-harm or remove harmful behaviors entirely. However, it should not replace traditional treatments for eating disorders and self-injurious behavior because it will have minimal effect on improving body image and reducing disordered eating behavior. The therapist should not get overly frustrated with the patient's repeated self-harm behaviors; instead, they should remain calm throughout this process. The therapist should convey empathy to the patient and accept them, even when they are engaging in dangerous behavior. They should also help the patient develop a food journal to record their feelings about food, eating, and hunger. This will help the patient identify their disordered eating behavior and the triggers that prompt them to engage in self-harming behaviors.

The therapist should measure the patient's rate of self-harm behaviors and continue to observe them throughout treatment. If they see these behaviors increasing, they can use specific techniques to reduce them. For example, by using a rule such as "I will give myself one minute without cutting" or "I will think of something else for one minute," the therapist can increase pause periods and remove painful imagery; this has been shown to decrease self-harm behavior. The therapist should also use a block schedule where they stick with their scheduled time frame no matter what happens during the session. The therapist should also help by encouraging the patient to tap into their emotions around their eating disorder or self-harm.

Linehan describes how these techniques can be implemented to help patients change their body image, reduce self-harming behavior, and ignore feelings of guilt that prevent them from engaging in healthier behaviors.

For example, if patients were struggling with weight gain and anorexia nervosa, they may have thought they were gaining weight or were not losing weight fast enough, prompting them to engage in self-harm behavior. Their self-harm behavior, in turn, would result in more guilt and anxiety.

To help them change their thoughts and behaviors surrounding this problem, the therapist must work with the patient to find a way around it. First, they should carefully listen to what the patient has to say and validate their concerns that there is extreme emphasis or too much focus on being thin. They should also help them find a way of accepting things they cannot change instead of becoming preoccupied with things they cannot control. The therapist can also help them explore their feelings about weight and eating using paradoxical intention; this involves agreeing with the patient that life would be easier if they were thinner, for example. The patient then has to do things opposite to their goals to learn more about themselves and gain awareness of things that bother them.

The therapist should then help the patient identify their self-harm behaviors and help them by teaching new skills or ways to deal with these behaviors. For example, they should encourage the patient to develop new exercises focusing on physical activity, such as walking or jogging, instead of engaging in harmful behaviors. They can also teach them to focus on "physical" sensations like breathing and their feet touching the ground instead of negative body image thoughts. They should also encourage the patient to practice these exercises in between sessions. If patients continue to engage in harmful behaviors, they should observe them throughout treatment and remind them that they are there to support and work with them. They should also help the patient identify their feelings around body image, eating disorders, self-esteem issues, and emotions surrounding this problem. The therapist can then use behavioral experiments to help the patient identify behaviors associated with positive or negative feelings and target those specific behaviors.

For example, if a patient struggles with self-harm behaviors because of depression and suicidal thoughts, they should learn new ways to cope with negative thoughts and reduce overall stress. These techniques will reduce their urge to self-harm. The therapist must help the patient break things down into smaller parts so it is easier to tackle their problems in a manageable way. They should also be sure that the problem is not due to medication issues or any other condition or disorder that may impact them negatively. In some cases, they may need new medications or supplements to help manage the symptoms of the disorder or illness they are struggling with. The therapist should examine their options, including medical treatment and other options, such as therapy.

To help patients change their disordered eating/body image habits, they can do behavioral experiments where they try to challenge their negative body image thoughts. Negative thoughts typically correlate with bad behaviors and self-harming behaviors. Linehan suggests that patients use an "A" list (Positive) of positive thoughts and associate these thoughts with a negative or frightening emotion so that it is easier to remember them. They should then use a "B" list (Negative) of negative thoughts and associate these with a non-hostile/non-fearful emotion so that it is easier to remember them.

What are some examples of how people use DBT in their lives?

They may find it useful in assisting them with building a more positive and intimate relationship with their significant other.

They may find it useful when struggling with self-esteem in the workplace or school. In addition, it can be helpful for people who do not feel they are getting the recognition and feedback they deserve.

They may find it helpful when they have a bulimic or anorexic relationship with food, which is common among people with BN, for example. It can help them learn more about what triggers these behaviors and how to cope better if they want to avoid relapse.

It can also be helpful for people who have a history of having trouble with alcohol and drug abuse. It is believed that by using DBT, they will find it easier to achieve and maintain sobriety.

They may find it useful when they are trying to develop better communication skills. This can be useful in helping them become more effective communicators at home, school, and work.

It can also help people with anger management problems because it teaches them new ways of coping with their anger, such as trying not to get angry in the first place or finding better ways of managing their anger rather than engaging in self-harming behaviors or engaging in an unhealthy relationship.

It is also believed that it can help people with eating disorders who are struggling with depression, substance abuse, self-harm, and

Dating violence can also be prevented and healed using DBT.

It can also be helpful for people who have a history of struggling with interpersonal relationships.

Although all of the above examples benefit many people who struggle with various issues in their lives, it is important to note that this therapy is only available to those who meet certain criteria. It may be useful for some time, but in the end, there may not be a good fit between you and your therapist. Don't be afraid to break away if the fit is not there. It may be the best thing for you, or it may just be that you are not a good fit for DBT treatment.

A great analogy for this technique is the road map of a city. Following a map set, routes allow you to arrive at your destination safely and quickly. Knowing which roads to take and in what order, you can reach your intended destination efficiently and effectively. Likewise, in DBT, you must know your landmarks to achieve your recovery goal.

DBT is a cognitive, behavioral, and dialectical approach to treating numerous mental health disorders. Dr. Marsha Linehan developed it in the 1980s at the University of Washington. Despite its development more than thirty years ago, it is still considered one of the most effective and innovative therapies available today for treating Borderline Personality Disorder BPD, as well as other mental disorders such as depression, eating disorders, and substance abuse. In fact, in 2006, the United States Department of Health and Human Services, Substance Abuse and Mental Health Services Administration Research Division awarded Dr. Linehan a $1.9 million grant to research DBT treatment for suicidal adolescents.

HOW TO USE DBT TO TREAT BORDERLINE PERSONALITY DISORDER EFFECTIVELY.

Dialectical Behavior Therapy (DBT) is a treatment for Borderline Personality Disorder that effectively reduces the symptoms of borderline personality disorder. DBT was developed by Marsha Linehan and was originally used as an application for cognitive behavior therapy to reduce the symptoms of chronic or suicidality among individuals with a borderline personality disorder. Given the high mortality rate among individuals with borderline personality disorder, this therapy has proven so successful in ameliorating symptoms that it has expanded into other areas like substance abuse treatment and anger management. Although DBT is by no means a cure for Borderline Personality Disorder, it is possible to use this form of therapy effectively to minimize the symptoms of borderline personality disorder.

Most people with borderline personality disorder who suffer from depression are unaware of the intense amounts of pain they are experiencing daily. When emotions become too painful or difficult to manage, individuals will often attempt to repress them through addictive behavior such as substance abuse, risky sexual behavior, and suicide attempts. For many individuals, this process often continues for many years until the person realizes that they have a serious emotional disorder that is destroying their quality of life. The symptoms of borderline personality disorder are so intense they often feel impossible to manage daily.

The first step in treating a borderline personality disorder is identifying how intense the person's emotional pain is and how they manage it. Individuals with borderline personality disorder typically tire themselves out by repressing all their emotions and attempting to control them with addictive behaviors such as substance abuse, risky sex, and suicidal behavior.

This condition is characterized by extreme instability in moods and interpersonal relationships, as well as an intense fear of abandonment. Because of this instability, borderlines are often very self-conscious and anxious. They often feel that people judge or condemn them for their feelings and behavior. As a result, they may become angry or depressed when these feelings arise because they believe others should never feel the same way they do.

Research suggests that borderline personality disorder is genetic (inherited) but isn't caused by a specific illness or brain injury since symptoms can be found in people with a family history of depression and those without one. Instead, research suggests that it is a combination of genetic and environmental factors contributing to the development of borderline personality disorder. However, researchers are still trying to understand exactly what causes this condition.

It has been suggested that personality disorders like borderline and dissociation manifest a single underlying process or psychological pathology. However, researchers aren't quite sure what this process is. This would mean that the cause of borderline personality disorder may not be a single thing but instead the result of various unconscious processes interacting with each other and external stimuli. In addition, research suggests that borderline personality disorder occurs more frequently in men than women.

Symptoms of borderline personality disorder

Most people with borderline personality disorder struggle to control their emotions, feelings, thoughts, and behavior. They often experience intense fear, anger, or guilt when they feel out of control. Four major symptoms associated with borderline personality disorder include:

Over time, these symptoms will become more and more extreme as the person with borderline personality disorder struggles to cope with the pain they are feeling in reality and their minds. This will cause them to continue to push away those who try to reach out to them or help them cope. Borderlines may also make attempts at suicide as a result of the stress they are experiencing.

Individuals with borderline personality disorder can exhibit a wide range of symptoms. Some of these symptoms are:

a. Frantic efforts to avoid real or imagined abandonment.
b. A unstable and intense interpersonal relationship pattern characterized by idealization and devaluation (sometimes called "splitting").
c. Identity disturbance: markedly and persistently unstable self-image or sense of self.
d. Impulsivity in at least two potentially self-damaging areas (e.g., spending, sex, substance abuse, shoplifting, reckless driving).
e. Recurrent suicidal behavior, gestures, threats, or self-injuring behavior such as cutting or burning oneself.
f. Affective instability due to a marked reactivity of mood (e.g., intense episodic dysphoria, irritability, or anxiety usually lasting a few hours and rarely more than a few days).
g. Chronic feelings of emptiness.
h. Inappropriate, intense anger or difficulty controlling anger (e.g., frequent displays of temper, constant anger, recurrent physical fights).
i. Transient, stress-related paranoid ideation or severe dissociative symptoms.
j. Markedly disturbed function of identity: markedly and persistently unstable self-image or sense of self (e.g., fragmentation of identity).

A borderline personality disorder is often associated with negative social consequences, as it can lead to unstable relationships, problems with addiction, and sometimes self-harming behaviors. Because of this, many people suffering from this condition have difficulty maintaining stable employment. Many also have legal issues or other problems in the workplace due to their behavior.

However, research has shown that treatment with psychotherapy and medications for borderline personality disorder helps alleviate symptoms and improve daily functioning.

The underlying cause of borderline personality disorder is still unknown. The following theories are just some researchers' ideas about what might maintain or exacerbate borderline personality disorder symptoms.

a. Social learning theory suggests that specific environmental factors contribute to the development of borderline personality disorder. This would mean that even children born with a predisposition towards this condition could be helped by changing their environment, though they may still have to deal with the pain caused by it.
b. Cognitive processing theory suggests that people suffering from this condition interpret certain situations in a way that causes them to feel extreme emotions and behave in ways that don't always benefit themselves or others.
c. Object relations theory suggests that patients with borderline personality disorder have a distorted view of themselves and others in their lives that may cause them to behave in ways that are self-destructive or harmful to others.

d. The biological model suggests an imbalance in certain chemicals like serotonin that affect brain functioning, which can lead to symptoms of borderline personality disorder. This does not mean, however, that the condition is cured by simply correcting the chemical imbalances.

e. The psychoanalytic perspective suggests that this condition can result from an unresolved childhood conflict between a child and their parent and other family members, which can lead to serious issues throughout adulthood.

Since many people with borderline personality disorder go undiagnosed for a long time or are diagnosed with other disorders, it is important to use an effective and efficient method to identify and treat those suffering from this condition.

a. The most effective way to diagnose borderline personality disorder is by using one of the diagnostic manuals utilized by mental health professionals in hospitals and clinics. These diagnostic manuals will have lengthy questionnaires that can be used to assess a patient's symptoms to determine whether or not they have a borderline personality disorder and other possible conditions that might be causing their symptoms.

b. If a patient has a borderline personality disorder, it is crucial to find a therapist who has experience treating people with this condition. This will ensure that the patient receives the most personalized and effective care possible.

To minimize cognitive distortions, patients can be taught to recognize them by their therapists and then reframe them in more positive ways.

Other techniques used for BPD include Dialectical Behavior Therapy (DBT) and Mentalization-Based Therapy (MBT). In addition, emotion regulation therapy teaches individuals with BPD how to regulate emotions, so they remain in control of themselves, whereas general psychotherapy uses individual, family, or group approaches to help patients learn basic skills such as communication and problem-solving.

Society's distorted view of BPD can result in overgeneralizations, misconceptions, and other negative attitudes, which may worsen an individual's symptoms. One reason for the stigma surrounding BPD may be that it is commonly associated with violence and aggression. It is important to understand that while patients with this personality disorder are at a significantly greater risk of having violent moments than others, they are far more likely to be the victims of physical and mental abuse. Recognizing risk factors such as childhood abuse, substance abuse, homelessness, unemployment, or living alone can help individuals avoid placing themselves in potentially dangerous situations. A common issue for borderline personality disorder patients is dealing with abandonment issues. The fear of being rejected is intensified when people suffering from BPD have relationships, jobs, or any other aspect of their lives end abruptly.

It is also important for individuals without BPD to understand that the disorder does not mean a person can't be helped. There are effective forms of treatment for borderline personality disorder, and those with the disorder can lead healthy, functional lives with proper help.

The main symptoms of a borderline personality disorder usually begin in adolescence or early adulthood and continue throughout a person's life. People with this condition can have intense mood swings, impulsive behavior, lack self-control, and struggle to make decisions about their lives.

The following symptoms may be present in people with BPD:

Impulsivity – individuals with borderline personality disorder are sometimes impulsive and make decisions without considering the consequences. This can cause issues with relationships, jobs, school, and other aspects of their lives.

Somatic blame – patients with a borderline personality disorder may feel that everyone else is responsible for their problems and has no control over what happens to them. This can lead to depression and anxiety.

Unstable relationships - These disorders can often lead to an unstable relationship with significant others because of their impulsive behavior, mood swings, and other problems with self-control.

Intense periods of sadness or distress – a person with a borderline personality disorder is likely to have constant feelings of sadness, anxiety, or other forms of intense emotional distress.

Self-harming behavior - Some people with BPD may engage in self-harming behaviors to cope with their internal pain and other problems. As a result, many people suffering from BPD may be at risk of being suicide bombers or committing terrorist acts.

Suicidality - Individuals with borderline personality disorder can be at extremely high risk for committing suicide because of their unstable moods and tendencies towards impulsive behavior.

Lack of emotion control - a person with a borderline personality disorder, may find themselves unable to regulate their emotions and may engage in dramatic emotional outbursts such as rage, sobbing, and other forms of emotional distress.

Emotional numbness – Often, a person who has borderline personality disorder will have to struggle for years before they can express feelings that are stronger than feelings of emptiness.

Anxiety - the feeling of constant fear is often present throughout a person's life with borderline personality disorder, making them susceptible to anxiety disorders such as OCD, panic attacks, or general anxiety.

Depending on the patient's needs, your sessions could vary anywhere from once a week to once every couple of months.

Cognitive Behavioral Therapy (CBT) is an essential part of DBT. This can include skills such as calming oneself down when faced with emotional or threatening situations. The DBT therapist and the patient work together to learn ways to calm one's emotions and feelings down to a non-destructive point.

For DDT to be effective, patients must have had some therapy prior so that their therapists may properly diagnose their disorders and treat them accordingly.

The goal of a therapist is to help patients learn how to form healthy relationships by using behavioral and cognitive techniques.

In addition, the therapist helps patients work on their emotions and provide support in self-care, coping skills, and communication.

Despite the reality that people with BPD can be helped through DBT, we all must understand that this condition cannot be helped if not treated properly at an early age.

Similar Treatment Approaches From Other Mental Health Specialties For Borderline Personality Disorder

Another important aspect of treating borderline personality disorder, specifically for children with this disorder, is family therapy.

One such therapist who has found success with families around the country is Dr. Jill Myra Henningsen, a licensed clinical social worker and family therapist from Wisconsin.

In an interview with The National Association of Social Workers, Henningsen stated that families often are in denial about their borderline children's issues, so it takes time to work through their problems together.

She also said that children struggling with a borderline personality disorder might have other issues, such as eating disorders or previous trauma, that must be addressed.

In another interview, Henningsen stated that "borderline parents often have loveless relationships with their children because they don't know how to express their love and rage in healthy ways."

Henningsen has used her expertise in family therapy to help families get through difficult times and help families through transition.

When it comes to teens and young adults, there is far less research on borderline personality disorder than there is for adults.

This means that fewer experts specialize in treating this population of patients. Therefore, it is crucial for teenagers struggling with these disorders to seek help as early as possible if they want treatment to be effective.

DBT is a form of psychotherapy that has been used with a variety of disorders, such as PTSD and eating disorders.

Because these disorders have very similar symptoms, including outbursts and mood swings, it was assumed that DBT would effectively treat borderline personality disorder patients.

DBT is used to help patients in therapy practice skills that can help them learn how to control their feelings and reduce the impact that negative feelings may have on their lives and relationships.

Most people suffering from BPD find themselves in therapy with a therapist who specializes in cognitive behavioral therapy.

These skills can be taught to patients in therapy over six to twelve weeks. If a patient is not doing well with this therapy and does not feel their symptoms are adequately treated, the therapist may elect for DBT instead.

While DBT is effective for treating BPD, it is important to know that some experts recommend against this form of treatment for borderline personality disorder altogether.

This stems from the fact that DBT does focus on changing the dysfunctional thoughts and behaviors associated with BPD, which can cause unwanted changes in mood, outbursts, and honesty issues on a day-to-day basis.

This can harm the patient suffering from BPD and the people they are close with.

DBT is an effective form of therapy for a wide range of disorders and illnesses. However, as some illnesses can be treated differently, so can borderline personality disorder.

The reality is that there are few studies available regarding how effective DBT is when it comes to treating patients who have borderline personality disorder.

This means that the truth about whether or not this therapy is effective for BPD may not be known for quite some time.

DBT is a form of psychotherapy that has been used with a variety of disorders, such as PTSD and eating disorders.

Because these disorders have very similar symptoms, including outbursts and mood swings, it was assumed that DBT would effectively treat borderline personality disorder patients.

DBT is used to help patients in therapy practice skills that can help them learn how to control their feelings and reduce the impact that negative feelings may have on their lives and relationships.

Most people suffering from BPD find themselves in therapy with a therapist who specializes in cognitive behavioral therapy.

These skills can be taught to patients in therapy over six to twelve weeks. If a patient is not doing well with this therapy and does not feel their symptoms are adequately treated, the therapist may elect for DBT instead.

While DBT is effective for treating BPD, it is important to know that some experts recommend against this form of treatment for borderline personality disorder altogether.

This stems from the fact that DBT does focus on changing the dysfunctional thoughts and behaviors associated with BPD, which can cause unwanted changes in mood, outbursts, and honesty issues on a day-to-day basis.

This can be harmful to the patient suffering from BPD and the people they are close with.

DBT is an effective therapy for a wide range of disorders and illnesses. However, as some illnesses can be treated differently, so can borderline personality disorder.

The reality is that there are few studies available regarding how effective DBT is when it comes to treating patients who have borderline personality disorder.

This means that the truth about whether or not this therapy is effective for BPD may not be known for quite some time.

One of the reasons experts believe that DBT may not be recommended for borderline personality disorder is because the patient's partner influenced their recovery.

The partner may feel afraid to seek treatment for themselves because they worry that their partner will leave them if they receive treatment.

This, in turn, can cause the patient to continue suffering from a borderline personality disorder and draw out the period in which therapy may be ineffective.

If a therapist or family member believes that a patient's behaviors indicate borderline personality disorder, getting them help as soon as possible is important.

The earlier patients seek help, the sooner they can start working on changes to their behaviors and relationships with others.

The longer a patient suffers from BPD, the more likely they feel out of control and hopeless.

If they can seek help early in their disorder, they are much more likely to be able to improve the way that they feel and start showing signs of remission.

It is important not to wait until your loved one's symptoms become unmanageable because this can lead to a breakdown in your relationship with them.

Doing everything you can to get them help is the best action if you believe they may have a borderline personality disorder.

Even if a patient can continue being in therapy and successfully practice the skills introduced, it is still important for them to develop other skills for managing life after therapy.

It is possible for patients with borderline personality disorder who experiences a change in their symptoms from BPD to take these skills with them for the rest of their lives.

This will allow the patient to be able to control their emotions better and able to deal with issues on a day-to-day basis.

The long-term effects of DBT depend on certain factors but can help patients live happier lives.

This depends on the patient's willingness to learn new habits and desire to improve.

This may not be necessary for patients who feel their life is already in chaos and that they cannot make any changes.

If patients have difficulty learning new skills, they may want to look into other options to help better them control their lives and emotions.

The long-term effects of DBT depend on certain factors but can help patients live happier lives.

This depends on the patient's willingness to learn new habits and desire to improve.

This may not be necessary for patients who feel their life is already in chaos and that they cannot make any changes.

If patients have difficulty learning new skills, they may want to look into other options to help better them control their lives and emotions.

Various treatments for a borderline personality disorder are available, including DBT and cognitive behavioral therapy.

The main difference between these two therapy forms is the therapist's approach.

This can have very different outcomes because the symptoms of BPD tend to change daily, making it difficult for a therapist to predict how a patient will respond in treatment sessions.

A borderline personality disorder is characterized by instability in mood, self-image, relationships, and impulsivity. Dialectical behavior therapy (DBT) was introduced in the 1980s to treat people suffering from borderline personality disorder's debilitating symptoms by teaching behavioral skills. This therapy is based on the belief that people with borderline personality disorder and their families are stuck in an "emotional conflict loop," in which they feel helpless and often act out in destructive, self-destructive ways. The goal of DBT is to help patients move out of this negative cycle by supporting them with healthy coping skills, improving communication skills, and building a relationship with a therapist that encourages patients to take charge of their own lives.

There were two main components of DBT that Marsha Linehan, Ph.D., identified. These two parts included individual psychotherapy and group skills training. The individual psychotherapy techniques included psychoeducation and mentalization-based treatment. Psychoeducation helps patients learn to accept their emotions without fear of consequences. Mentalization-based methods helped patients develop the ability to observe their behavior, as well as the behavior of others.

The other part of DBT was the behavioral training groups that focused mainly on safety behaviors, emotion regulation strategies, distress tolerance strategies, and interpersonal effectiveness strategies.

Though DBT effectively treats people with various emotional issues, it focuses on social and interpersonal skills such as emotion regulation and mindfulness. This book will explore how DBT is used to treat borderline personality disorder specifically and share some tips for successfully incorporating DBT into your treatment regimen.

The main goal of DBT is to help patients regain control over their emotions and behaviors.

This therapy has a lasting effect because most people who complete it continue to practice the skills introduced.

Therefore, if you believe that your loved one should consider therapy for borderline personality disorder, you can introduce them to DBT now so they can start practicing these skills immediately after the therapy session.

Although many people believe that there are only two possible outcomes of therapy: cure or death, this isn't always the case. Various therapeutic methods can be used to treat patients with borderline personality disorder, and each has its advantages and disadvantages.

You may want to consider DBT if you believe your loved one needs these skills to improve. The best thing you can do is research the therapy and decide based on what's best for them.

If you decide DBT may be the best option, a few things need to happen. First, your loved one must attend at least five therapy sessions before resuming their everyday lives.

This lets the therapist evaluate their progress and implement new strategies if necessary. If patients cannot attend therapy regularly, it may be difficult to learn how to manage their behavior and emotions effectively.

The next chapter will discuss Acceptance and Commitment Therapy. This is a type of therapy used to help the patient feel at ease and cope with their emotions. Moreover, this therapy helps them be more aware of the issues associated with their borderline personality disorder. Sometimes, people with this condition feel anxious and worried about their physical health or what others think about them. This is sometimes referred to as being emotionally dysregulated.

Emotion regulation is the ability to adapt to your environment accordingly. Unfortunately, many people with BPD often have difficulty doing this because they feel trapped by their emotions; any change in emotion feels like a double-edged sword.

Various techniques can be used to treat borderline personality disorder, but CBT, DBT, and ACT are the most effective. After a patient is diagnosed with BPD, individual therapy may be necessary to determine how their symptoms affect daily life. One of the simplest and most effective ways to treat borderline personality disorder is through acceptance and commitment therapy (ACT).

ACT was developed by Steven Hayes, Ph.D., who recognized that patients with BPD have difficulty recognizing and dealing with their emotions. This is often done unconsciously, so it is difficult for them to make rational decisions about their behavior as emotionally dysregulated patients tend to engage in excessively risky behaviors.

ACCEPTANCE AND COMMITMENT THERAPY

WHAT IS ACT?

Acceptance and Commitment Therapy (ACT) is a psychological intervention that introduces mindfulness and acceptance-based techniques. The ACT's goal is to help people become more aware of their thoughts, emotions, fears, and physical sensations to make changes that bring greater well-being.

Acceptance and Commitment Therapy is based upon the work of Steven C. Hayes, Ph.D., a clinical psychologist; Kelly G. Wilson, Ph.D., a behavioral/cognitive psychologist and researcher; Russ Harris, Ph.D., a clinical psychologist who introduced ACT to the general public through his book "The Happiness Trap," and their colleagues at the University of Nevada Reno. The name "Acceptance and Commitment Therapy" was initially proposed for what was then called "behavior therapy" by Charles Swenson in 1978 and later published in 1979. ACT was then identified as "therapy in which clients practice accepting the present without judging it as good or bad, right or wrong." The first full-scale ACT program, based on Hayes and Wilson's acceptance-based model of psychotherapy, was a university-based clinical program at the University of Nevada Reno. ACT became fully accredited in 1992 under the name "Acceptance and Commitment Therapy: An Experiential Approach to Behavior Change" by the American Psychological Association.

ACT is based on several principles. Most significantly, ACT aims to help people live rich and meaningful life. The ACT model is mainly used for treating problematic areas of human functioning, including clinical depression, chronic pain, bipolar disorder, eating disorders, substance abuse, and personality disorders. ACT also promotes applied research on human functioning related to health, educational attainment, occupational performance, and other quality of life indicators.

Hayes and colleagues developed a 6-level hierarchical model (or "hexaflex") describing the process individuals may undergo in resolving psychological problems. This level model has been applied to various psychological and behavioral difficulties such as depression, generalized anxiety disorder (GAD), borderline personality disorder (BPD), psychosis, and pain-related issues.

In the model, difficulties can be categorized into low, moderate, and high-intensity categories. The goal of ACT is to help people accept and work through their problems with the hope that they will move to higher levels of functioning.

ACT uses mindfulness techniques in both the treatment and mediation sessions. Mindfulness is defined as paying attention in a particular way: non-judgmentally, on purpose, and for the duration. Mindfulness techniques focus on bringing awareness to the current experience without judging it as good or bad, right or wrong. The first step in the ACT is usually cognitive defusion: identification of internal thoughts (cognitions) attached to negative emotions (feelings).

ACT is founded upon the premise that we all can create our own experience of the present moment. For example, suppose a person can believe they can experience happiness even when it may be difficult or that they can accept themselves even when they do not feel good. In that case, they will feel safer in making decisions and being with others in the present moment. The belief in one's ability to shape one's experience, called self-efficacy, is critical in the ACT. In this way, people are more likely to take risks and be willing to explore new possibilities for how their life may unfold rather than staying stuck in pre-existing patterns of behavior.

The formal development of ACT started in 1978 at the University of Nevada, Reno, where Steven Hayes was a psychology professor and Kelly Wilson was a doctoral candidate. After reading "The Power of Awareness" by Viktor Frankl, Hayes and Wilson developed "behavior therapy." This early form of ACT involved patients identifying their problems and then actively trying to solve them.

In 1979, Charles Swenson read an book by Hayes about this work. He was impressed with Hayes' work and knew he wanted to replicate it more comprehensively. Swenson discussed his ideas with Kelly Wilson, and a more comprehensive ACT version was conceived. This new approach would be called "ACT" by its first practitioners.

In the 1980s, the first formal ACT program was developed by Hayes, Wilson, and their colleagues at the University of Nevada Reno. This program used a treatment manual that detailed Hayes' model of psychotherapy as well as practical exercises for clients to learn how to develop self-acceptance and "habituate" thoughts and emotions toward acceptance. The program began in 1982 when there were only seven clients; now, there are over 1,300 annually.

Over the next decade, ACT was refined and developed through exposure by word of mouth, journal books, and papers presented at professional conferences. ACT was presented in Swenson's book "The ACT Works" in 1993. This book helped popularize the practice of Acceptance and Commitment Therapy.

ACT was established as a formal course at the University of Nevada Reno in 1995 and eventually became a doctoral program in 2000. In 2002, the first non-residential training was offered for practicing clinicians and started an increasing interest in Acceptance and Commitment Therapy. In 2006, the university formally approved acceptance and commitment therapy as a Ph.D. program in Clinical Psychology with Dr. Russ Harris as director of graduate studies and Dr. Kelly G Wilson as chief supervisor of students.

In 2000, the first accredited ACT certification training was developed by Russ Harris and Douglas E. Hart at Flinders University in Adelaide, South Australia. The European Association for Behavior Analysis International Conference held in Budapest in 2003 included a particular track on acceptance and commitment therapy (ACT). This conference provided an opportunity to present and discuss the evidence for the ACT as a viable treatment approach. The International Association of Behavior Analysis (IABA) has been promoting interest in the ACT since then. The American Psychological Association approved Acceptance and Commitment Therapy as a third-wave CBT approach in 2006. The National Institute for Health in the United Kingdom funds a network of ACT practitioners and ACT training organizations.

Theresa Summerford, a University of Nevada Reno student, developed a new model in 2006 that would lead to increased emphasis on mindfulness and acceptance exercises in clients' work. This resulted in a therapeutic approach that involves both cognitive defusion and behavioral practices aimed at facilitating client acceptance of unwanted thoughts and emotions. This approach has become the basis for Acceptance and Commitment Therapy.

ACT is a relatively new approach to therapy and has been subject to much debate. Proponents of ACT claim it can be used as a treatment for difficulties such as depression and anxiety, whereas some cognitive behaviorists have challenged the evidence for these claims. A review of available studies found that results regarding the effectiveness of ACT for anxiety reduction are somewhat mixed. Some studies show positive results, whereas others do not. Similarly, research on depression treatment with ACT has varied as well.

The following are characteristics of those who might benefit from ACT:

Certain people with specific traits seem to benefit from ACT and vice versa. However, the following are general characteristics that can include ACT users and benefit recipients.

ACT uses an acceptance-based approach that focuses on how clients can become aware of any unwanted thoughts or feelings, pay attention to them as opposed to reacting to them, and then let go of these thoughts and feelings. This process can be accomplished with a variety of exercises.

The first step in the therapy is called self-disclosure. The therapist starts by asking the client if they would like some time to talk about what is bothering them. The therapist then discusses with the client the difficulties they are experiencing. During the self-disclosure, the therapist helps identify the client's strong thoughts or feelings and then coaches them through three critical acceptance exercises.

The first exercise of accepting thoughts is called defusion. The therapist asks a client to repeat their negative thoughts out loud. The client should then focus on these statements and try not to judge them as good or bad but instead focus on what it would be like if these thoughts were accurate and accept them as a fact. The next step is letting go of these feelings. In this exercise, the therapist might start by asking clients to acknowledge that they feel this way without reacting emotionally or judging themselves.

This process is continued with the third exercise, which involves focusing on positive thoughts, then accepting these thoughts without resorting to judging oneself.

The ACT goal is to help clients become aware of the source of their emotions and worries and then let go of those thoughts or feelings. So often, a person experiences difficulty in controlling their emotions and worrying about events that may not occur. This is because humans are born with limited knowledge about the world and tend to have preconceived ideas about what others or imagined circumstances might be like. ACT addresses this by teaching clients how to accept uncomfortable states so that they can relax in them instead of getting caught up in them. This can ultimately reduce unwanted and excess emotions that may have been causing distress in clients.

ACT uses a similar approach to CBT as its third-wave counterpart but differs in its use of mindfulness practices such as low focus awareness, acceptance, and defusion to evoke change. ACT has been adapted into over 20 languages.

ACT works by focusing on the difference between internal and external events. Individuals have thoughts and subjective evaluations of their environment and behavior, but they also have beliefs about those same thoughts. For example, the view that I am a bad person is an internal event, while the idea that I am bad is an external event. ACT has four steps that help to identify the differences between these events and then change them:

The goal of this therapy is not to get rid of all unwanted thoughts or feelings but to notice them when they happen so that they can be accepted as part of life without being judged as positive or negative by a client. This process helps clients to get themselves without trying to control others. This process is carried out through a series of exercises.

The first exercise in the ACT is to become aware of negative thoughts and not try to control them or change them into something else. This can be done by repeating the sentence, "I'm a bad person," for thirty seconds without reacting emotionally.

The second exercise involves noticing thoughts and feelings in your body during stressful situations. The goal is to enhance awareness of self, with acceptance towards whatever is taking place at that moment. It can also help you accept rejection if you strive for a goal.

The third exercise in the ACT is to notice your thoughts and then gently try to let go of them. A client is asked to repeat a negative thought or feeling (for example, "I'm stupid") for thirty seconds and then stop thinking about it. This allows them to become more aware of their thoughts without judgment.

The fourth exercise in ACT focuses on noticing internal experiences, such as feelings and bodily sensations. Instead of focusing on the thoughts or events, the goal is to allow participants to see these without reacting. This can be used by those who have trouble accepting their problems or being alone with these thoughts.

The fifth exercise in ACT involves noticing one's thoughts and feeling, acting on them, and then letting go of them. This includes taking a few deep breaths and noticing thoughts and feelings during this time.

The last exercise in ACT aims to notice one's thoughts, feelings, and bodily sensations without trying to change or control them. The client then pays attention to the present moment for thirty seconds without reaction. This allows one to become aware of the present without being caught up in their thoughts or feeling.

Sanderson and Bolen (1982) conducted a study in which they followed eight people through the course of the therapy. Six months later, they were interviewed to see how their thoughts had changed since the treatment. They found that all participants remembered more thoughts than could be accounted for by chance. However, overall, they did not notice significant changes in other mental health variables, such as mood and behaviors.

While there is some evidence that ACT may be effective for anxiety disorders and depression, it is unclear how well it works across differently-identified populations like children or adolescents with anxiety disorders or obsessive-compulsive disorder (OCD). Research on the effectiveness of ACT is limited to randomized studies and has not been consistently replicated in controlled studies.

Basics of ACT

Acceptance and Commitment Therapy is a proactive approach to problem-solving that uses acceptance, mindfulness, and values-based decision-making. ACT focuses on the change process rather than being fixated on the outcome. The goal of ACT is to increase psychological flexibility and improve self-awareness.

ACT encourages experiential learning through mindful inquiry to examine one's reactions in challenging situations. This allows for an increased ability to commit and adjust behavior accordingly due to increased awareness of one's feelings, thoughts, intentions, values, and behaviors related to these feelings/thoughts/intentions. While ACT can be applied in many ways, three fundamental principles are openness, responsiveness, and values-based decision-making (VBDM).

a. Relabeling: Identifying a problem as a "thought" or "feeling" reduces focus on managing the problem as a threat, while it can also help disengage from the problem.
b. Reattribute: Disentangle and disidentify from thoughts and feelings by recognizing their transient, subjective and psychological nature and how they are conditioned by an individual's history of experiences, perceptions, and culture.
c. Refocus: Act differently rather than thoughtfully to calm remaining thoughts and feelings that may lead to maladaptive behavior. This may include distraction techniques or acceptance of one's experiences.
d. Revalue: Appreciate the usefulness of values-focused decision-making to make decisions that can be very effective during difficult situations.
e. Replot: To make plans to commit and circumvent the problem while maintaining one's values
f. Values-Based Decision Making (VBDM): This involves choosing a practical behavioral course of ac-

tion by examining values in various situations, with emphasis on living a life that is consistent with these values and behaving in ways that contribute to living a valued life

g. Self as Context: A sense of self as compassionate, non-judgmental, and consistent when responding to others, rather than an individual that acts based on internal reactions or thoughts.

The treatment of depression has been well studied using Acceptance and Commitment Therapy (ACT) as a model for psychological treatment. One study found that ACT may be as effective as Cognitive Behavioral Therapy (CBT) in treating depression over eight weeks, with a more significant number experiencing remission in both ACT and CBT than in a waitlist control condition after 16 weeks of treatments.

ACT process

The ACT process may be divided into five elements:

a. Reflective Listening
b. Relabeling
c. Emotional Freedom Technique (EFT)
d. Values-based Decision Making (VBDM)
e. Commitment Therapy (CT) or Commitment Practice (CP).

Reflective listening is the first step in the ACT and is also known as self-observation. It requires the client to recognize and name their thoughts, feelings, intentions, and actions related to a situation. This allows more profound insight into their mental processes that may lead to unhelpful behavior or thought patterns. Reflective listening helps the client examine their thoughts and feelings concerning how they are engaging with the situation, rather than simply engaging in a "fight or flight" response by either defending themselves against an inappropriate thought or trying to distance themselves from an uncomfortable feeling.

This is followed by relabeling, where a problem can be re-defined as being more meaningful than it initially seemed based on one's values. This involves individual values and how to live with these values in everyday life. Relabeling also examines how thoughts and feelings are formed from conditioning through one's experiences, perceptions, and culture. Once this is accomplished, the client must learn to refocus on the value that is important for them in the current situation and commit to acting in accordance with it.

EFT involves tapping on acupoints that can be accessed through the client's body, often while experiencing some form of emotional reaction or conflict. This allows access to positive emotions, which can subsequently enhance self-awareness and dynamic flexibility by allowing one to recognize their thoughts and feelings as being subject to change by choice.

Values-based Decision Making involves examining values in various situations, emphasizing living a life that is consistent with these values, and behaving in ways that contribute to living a valued life.

ACT also teaches clients how to make commitments. Commitments are made by the client deciding on how they will commit each day and then taking action according to the commitment. This is known as commitment therapy or commitment practice. This therapy is effective in many different areas, including criminal behavior, social relationships, and substance abuse.

Davies and Howson (1994) investigated the effectiveness of ACT in teaching a range of people to form new mental health beliefs about their symptoms based on their values for self-care. They also examined its effectiveness as a treatment for depression. The main focus of therapy was to help people better understand why they have become depressed and try to change how they thought about themselves and their lives.

The results showed that after treatment, depression was reduced, and participants had significantly better scores on all measures of psychological health, such as life satisfaction.

ACT is an evidence-based treatment for depression that is effective for individuals with depression. It teaches clients about their thoughts, feelings, and behaviors contributing to their symptoms of depression and negative thinking patterns while teaching them how to work through those patterns in a values-based way.

Additionally, ACT helps clients understand that their symptoms are not "who they are" but rather the result of conditioning (fear of failure and low self-esteem) based on their history (past experiences), perceptions (how they judge themselves), and culture/environmental factors (what society tells them). It teaches clients how to understand this conditioning better. Finally, ACT teaches clients that their symptoms of depression can be changed by changing how they think about and view themselves, which in turn allows them to change how they relate to other people.

The fact that ACT treats negative thinking patterns based on conditioning is essential because it shows us how our thoughts are not as permanent or "true" as we may think.

ACT has also been used as a therapy for post-traumatic stress disorder (PTSD). ACT has shown success in treating PTSD by helping clients to understand their thoughts and behaviors better, recognize and accept their fears, identify the meaning of what happened in their traumatic events and learn how to respond well to stressful situations. ACT has also been shown to be as effective in only one hour of treatment sessions as in 20-hour sessions.

The Four Principles of ACT

1. Acceptance

This principle teaches people to accept the thought, emotion, or behavior they are currently experiencing instead of fighting it or making it go away. In addition, this leads the person to experience their thoughts, emotions, and behaviors in an anon-judgmental way, without trying to change or escape from them.

2. Presence

Presence is centered on being mindful and present in every moment as much as possible through accepting what is happening and not focusing on the past or future. This helps people engage with their experiences more thoroughly and helps them find meaning in those experiences.

3. Values-based action

This principle is used in conjunction with the other guides to help people engage in behaviors consistent with the values and beliefs necessary to them. ACT teaches people how to self-regulate by identifying their values and how they can live a valued life. This helps people accept themselves as they are and make better choices about how to behave in their lives, as well as assisting them in better understanding their relationships between values and chosen actions.

4. Acceptance and Commitment Therapy

ACT uses this acceptance principle, followed by a committee process that involves making daily commitments to act according to those commitments. This helps the client stay focused on the present and make choices that align with their values instead of just fighting how they feel or trying to make it go away.

ACT is mainly used as an approach for depression, substance abuse, and PTSD. This is because these three conditions are the subject of research that has shown ACT to reduce symptoms effectively. However, ACT can also be used for anxiety, stress, and any condition brought about by negative thought patterns, such as low self-esteem and negative self-talk.

Acceptance and commitment therapy (ACT) focuses on helping people accept their emotions, thoughts, and behaviors at the moment instead of fighting anything or wishing it would go away. Studies have shown that ACT has been effective in helping clients to create new ways of thinking, which leads to them being less depressed. They also found that learners showed improvement in their symptoms of depression, with 94% showing a significant reduction in their symptoms after treatment.

Similarly, studies have also shown that ACT is effective in reducing symptoms of PTSD. However, PTSD makes it difficult for people who have experienced trauma to make sense of their experiences and get beyond the traumatic memory. Although people can learn a lot about what happened to them through ACT, it is not yet clear how this might reduce the effects of PTSD on an individual's life.

ACT can be used for many other conditions besides depression and post-traumatic stress disorder. For example, people with eating disorders have found success with ACT and have been able to overcome many obstacles that had previously prevented them from getting better. The antithesis of acceptance for people suffering from eating disorders is the need for control. By learning to accept the way, they feel in the moment, even if it is uncomfortable or painful, they can let go of that need for control and begin healing.

ACT has been found to be as effective as other therapy approaches to treat anxiety. ACT reduces anxiety symptoms by teaching clients about their thoughts and feelings, identifying underlying concerns about those thoughts, and being aware of triggers for anxiety symptoms. ACT has also been used as a treatment for anxiety disorders and symptoms of PTSD.

Studies have shown that ACT produces similar outcomes to CBT by focusing on people's thinking. In addition, studies have found that ACT is as effective as CBT in treating depression and better than CBT at reducing anxiety symptoms. ACT has also been shown to be an effective treatment for substance abuse. For people with co-occurring depression and substance abuse, there are "complementary" benefits, with both treatments working together to get the most use of each therapy approach.

ACT is a relatively new form of therapy, developed in the 1980s, so more research needs to be done about its effectiveness for other conditions and long-term results.

There are no specific conditions that ACT should not be used for. However, there are some limitations to the treatment. For example, in studying the effectiveness of ACT for PTSD, researchers found that it is helpful for people who have had mild to moderate PTSD symptoms to improve their symptoms. However, for people with severe PTSD, ACT did not prove as effective. This could be because severe PTSD is more debilitating than other types of anxiety disorders and has many different causes that require specific treatment plans.

ACT was developed to treat clients with "widespread pain" – negative thoughts and emotions that significantly impact a person's life. This includes the symptoms of depression, anxiety, stress, and substance abuse. As such, ACT is less effective for people with a personality disorder. However, this does not rule out the possibility that ACT will work for those individuals. For those clients, therapists can consult with a psychologist who specializes in personality disorders to determine if this therapy would be helpful for that client. Research has shown that ACT is effective in reducing symptoms of depression and PTSD and can be used as an alternative treatment to CBT and other therapies used to treat these conditions.

What makes ACT different from CBT

Acceptance and Commitment Therapy is a type of psychotherapy that focuses on acceptance, mindfulness, and values-based decision-making. Steven Hayes developed it in the 1980s. ACT has many similarities with Cognitive Behavioural Therapy but also includes skills from Gestalt therapy, Transactional Analysis, and Dialectical Behavioural Therapy.

ACT is based on the belief that emotional pain derives from a lack of acceptance of reality and is often directly connected to past experiences. People learn to accept their situation in the present by becoming more objective about it, thereby managing their emotions. Acceptance is based upon a shift from control to awareness. One can experience different ways of being present, including being detached from pain (as in mindfulness), separated from issues that create suffering (as in values clarification), and open to change (as in acceptance); each way implies an acceptance experience. Acceptance may be combined with value clarification techniques depending on the client's needs, goals, and resources.

ACT provides a method of self-discovery that enables the client to increase their level of personal responsibility. By accepting the present, a client can develop more willpower, self-esteem, and positive emotion, thus preventing negative moods such as anger or depression.

ACT is based on acceptance, choice, and values. ACT emphasizes that people often have a limited amount of control over their lives and that they are ultimately responsible for their problems. Therefore, individuals should seek to develop greater personal power by accepting the past experiences that have led them to be where they are today (past events), clarifying their values around what is essential (choices), and taking action in line with those choices (values).

The goal is to develop the skills to "act" and "not react" in line with one's values and create a more satisfying life for the individual. ACT also emphasizes the importance of "having a life worth living." In other words, the goal is to live a meaningful and purposeful life.

ACT is considered an "experiential therapy," meaning it focuses on the present moment. Unlike Cognitive Behavioral Therapy, ACT does not use homework. Instead, it aims to focus on "here-and-now" issues and use mindfulness skills during therapy sessions to prevent automatic thoughts from taking over.

ACT is based on acceptance and mindfulness as an alternative to more traditional forms of CBT, which may be seen as too directive by clients. ACT does not administer direct advice to clients, as is common in CBT, but rather provides a resource for clients to learn more about themselves. The goal of ACT is to develop a more accepting attitude towards behavior and emotions that may be experienced. By being open to these experiences and observing them with greater awareness, individuals can commit fully and freely to whatever activity they are undertaking.

ACT also emphasizes committed action, which means doing what is essential to the person in the context of their values instead of intense inner struggle about whether or not to do it.

ACT treats several conditions, including chronic pain, anxiety disorders, depression, and substance abuse. ACT is also effective in treating stress and burnout. A recent meta-analysis concluded that ACT was significantly more effective than control groups on various measures.

Acceptance and Commitment Therapy has also been used to treat chronic pain. A 2006 study demonstrated that Acceptance and Commitment Therapy was a promising treatment for chronic pain. In this study, patients were randomly assigned to 12 weekly sessions of either Acceptance and Commitment Therapy or Cognitive Behavioral Therapy for Chronic Pain. This study showed that Acceptance and Commitment

Therapy resulted in significantly more significant reductions in pain-related emotional distress when compared to those who received Cognitive Behavioral Therapy for Chronic Pain. The authors concluded that treatment based on acceptance effectively reduces emotional distress while increasing clients' engagement in meaningful activities associated with their values.

Cognitive-behavioral therapy (CBT) is a well-established posttraumatic stress disorder (PTSD) treatment. CBT was first developed as a treatment focused on the past. But researchers now know that focusing on history is not as effective as focusing on the present. The theory of ACT suggests that negative emotions and troubling psychological problems are caused by people's attempts to control things in their lives that they cannot control. They experience these attempts to retain as stressful, and managing leads to emotional pain. The goal of ACT, therefore, is not to control anything but rather to face what exists in the present moment and make peace with it. ACT theory suggests that people can make peace with themselves in the present through acceptance.

CBT focuses on changing thoughts, but ACT does not focus on how someone thinks about things. CBT focuses on how a person feels about things, but ACT does not focus on what a person thinks or feels. CBT emphasizes the "circumstances" of the patient's problems, which is the source of their suffering. But one of the aims of ACT is to develop an attitude toward present circumstances that has value to the individual. For example, if someone experiences stress in their life at work, an ACT therapist might help them find new meaning in their job by helping them clarify their values and commitments in this context. ACT emphasizes the importance of committed action, a conscious choice to do what is essential to the person. CBT focuses on the present moment and makes cognitive changes to keep people in control, while ACT focuses on committed action and values.

CBT uses a more direct approach to solving problems. CBT therapists believe that clients must figure out what happened in their past, even if they will not be able to change it, so they can "figure out" how to live their lives appropriately. They believe that people have a responsibility for their behavior and emotions and must take responsibility for them. ACT therapists use minimal conversation regarding how clients were raised or how they are responsible for their lives' problems that may be difficult to overcome. They believe that working toward behavioral change will help people feel better and that changing thoughts or feelings can only result in increased suffering. ACT does not believe that a lack of willpower causes symptoms caused by unconscious beliefs about oneself. In other words, it does not matter if a person has poor self-control if that person's unconscious thoughts lead to poor behavior and pain.

ACT also emphasizes learning more about what values are essential to the person, which is why it is necessary to clarify one's values before embarking on any treatment plan. If a person does not know what is truly important to them and does not know their values, then it is doubtful that the therapist will be able to provide the treatment plan that the person needs to improve. On the other hand, if a person knows precisely what their values are and how they can best be used in conjunction with one another, then it is more likely that they will be able to move forward with their therapy goals.

ACT treatment focuses less on changing people's thoughts and feelings but on changing how they feel about themselves. In this way, people become more accepting of who they are as they grow and change as adults. ACT focuses on growing and what a person can do in life. It is often said that acceptance of who you are at this moment is the first step to change.

ACT treatment does not use the same methods as CBT because the two therapies do not focus on the same things. While CBT focuses on changing thoughts and feelings, ACT focuses on changing behavior and helping people develop meaningful lives by clarifying their values and making commitments based on those values. The goals of ACT and CBT also differ, which results in different therapeutic approaches. CBT focuses on the past to change the present, while ACT focuses on the present and on who a person wants to be in the future.

CBT is most effective when working with more specific symptoms. ACT is most effective when working with broad lifestyle changes. CBT helps people develop more positive behaviors and attitudes. In contrast, ACT helps people improve their lives by improving their relationships with others, increasing their feelings of acceptance of themselves, and helping them be more creative in finding solutions to problems they face in life.

ACT emphasizes acceptance of thoughts as they occur, but acceptance and surrender do not mean passivity or giving up. For example, a therapist who uses ACT might encourage a client to change their behavior and take action rather than waiting for external conditions to change. It is possible for the person to accept the situation but at the same time work toward changing it so that they may feel better.

ACT works best in people over 40 and who have experienced many losses and disappointments in their lives. It is best used by people who have become frustrated with CBT treatment, which focuses on past events. The goal of ACT is to help a person come to peace with their life and find enjoyment in it, rather than trying to live up to unrealistic expectations of how life should be or should have been. A person frustrated with their past will not be able to make meaningful changes in their life.

The present-centered therapy of ACT helps people make decisions based on their values rather than the circumstances surrounding them. It allows people to accept who they are without changing anything about themselves. ACT teaches you how to experience life fully and find meaning in your experiences rather than trying to avoid or change your thoughts and feelings.

ACT helps clients learn how to live a whole life regardless of adverse situations. This type of therapy is most effective when working with depression and anxiety. CBT focuses on acceptance, but it does so in terms of thoughts and feelings rather than behaviors and actions toward others.

ACT focuses on present moment problems and changes actions based on those thoughts, while DBT focuses on the person's current situation and plans to help them manage their problems. ACT helps a person accept their ideas as they come, while DBT helps a person change their thinking.

ACT is more passive in its approach to changing the client's thought patterns to manage pain. DBT is more active and encourages clients to step forward and face their feelings head-on before learning how to manage them effectively.

The goals of ACT are very different than those of DBT, which diverges from ACT in the treatments offered. For example, ACT focuses on the client's feelings of well-being, while DBT is focused on helping the client avoid situations that result in negative emotions.

ACT wants the client to be present with those thoughts and to accept them regardless of their content, while DBT encourages clients to change their ideas to improve their lives. ACT uses acceptance as a means for moving forward with life and managing pain, whereas DBT uses acceptance to control anger, improve relationships, and increase self-respect.

The link between ACT, CBT, and DBT

In this chapter, we will discuss the connection between Acceptance and Commitment Therapy (ACT), Cognitive Behavior Therapy (CBT), and Dialectical Behavior therapy (DBT). The theory behind these three therapies is to help people learn how to accept the things they cannot control while committing to actions that serve their well-being. Although CBT and DBT have different goals and applications, all 3 share the primary mechanisms of behavioral change: Exposure and Acceptance, Mindfulness, and Value-based living.

These therapies are used as interventions for a variety of psychological disorders. ACT effectively treats depression, anxiety disorders, chronic pain and other physical ailments, addictions and substance abuse issues, anger and aggression problems, borderline personality disorder (BPD), post-traumatic stress disorder (PTSD), and burnout. CBT focuses on helping people cope with emotional issues by identifying negative thoughts and replacing them with positive ones. CBT treats problems like depression, anxiety, grief, loss, eating disorders, pain management, addictions, and more. Marsha Linehan developed DBT to help people with Borderline Personality Disorder (BPD) cope with their emotional problems.

The three therapies also share similarities in the way they function. ACT and CBT are primarily goal-directed, while DBT emphasizes acceptance of the patient's current situation. All three use methods of exposure therapy, which involve exposing the patient to a condition that causes their suffering to help them decrease their fear of the situation and change their reactions to it. They also use mindfulness techniques which involve concentrating on what is happening in the present moment without judging or evaluating that information. Mindfulness helps patients see things as they indeed are. Finally, all three therapies focus on helping the patient develop a set of values or what is most important to them. These values can help guide choices and decisions that lead the patient toward their long-term goals.

ACT has been shown in clinical trials to be effective in treating anxiety, depression, and chronic pain on par with other behavioral interventions like CBT and DBT. ACT focuses on teaching patients acceptance of painful experiences in their present moment while also helping them commit to valued behaviors that can better their life. The therapy starts with exploring the client's current reality and the resulting values these create. This allows them to identify which values are essential and make deliberate choices for the positives that come from the negatives. ACT looks to create a therapeutic environment where patients can accept the present moment without trying to control it.

Cognitive Behavior Therapy (CBT) is a behavioral intervention used to treat depression, anxiety, anger, and other emotional disorders. CBT is designed to help people see how they perceive negative events and how this perception affects their feelings and actions. In the later phases of CBT, patients are taught methods of changing their thoughts to change how they feel. These thoughts can be negative or positive depending on the context and can be identified as realistic or unrealistic.

Definition of ACT, CBT, and DBT

Understanding how these therapies differ helps to understand what they are. Acceptance and Commitment Therapy (ACT), Cognitive Behavior Therapy (CBT), and Dialectical Behavioral Therapy (DBT) all fall under the umbrella of behavioral therapies. These therapy methods involve exposing a patient to their negative emotions, thoughts, and behaviors to help them accept the present moment as it is while committing to healthier behaviors. These may be behavioral or cognitive challenges that can be defined as difficult but not impossible to complete. By practicing these three therapies over time, patients can learn more about themselves and their behaviors and identify new ways of reacting to situations that allow them to act more positively toward themselves, others, and life.

Now that you know that ACT, CBT, and DBT are all related to behavioral and cognitive therapies, it is essential to discuss how they differ. The first similarity these therapies have is the goal they share: to help the patient learn how to live more positively with the negative events or experiences in life. This goal is the only treatment-specific element in each of these therapies. The techniques used by each treatment are different but equally effective when properly applied. A therapist can use many methods, but if there is no goal for achieving change, changing behavior towards positive action will not succeed.

ACT and CBT involve using behavioral approaches to help the patient develop a set of values they can live by while simultaneously addressing any mental or physical problems they face to help them achieve those values. This means that the therapist needs to take a non-judgmental approach with each patient to correctly select which therapist's techniques will work best for that patient.

CBT is similar to ACT in this way. However, CBT uses cognitive and behavioral techniques to help patients identify negative thoughts like "I don't deserve this" or "This is horrible. How could they do this to me?" Then, they are taught to replace these thoughts with positive ones. CBT's non-judgmental approach means that the therapist is not allowed to tell patients what they should think. Instead, the therapist works with each patient to help them make more conscious decisions about how they react and behave while also choosing behaviors that bring only positive feelings.

DBT differs from ACT and CBT in its focus on treating trauma and related disorders, such as PTSD (post-traumatic stress disorder) and borderline personality disorder (BPD). It is primarily designed to help patients with these disorders identify and express their feelings healthily. This can be done by following a set of guidelines, including being aware of the present moment, staying in contact with their body, and maintaining mental flexibility. These guidelines help patients act in a positive way that is aligned with their values rather than reacting to situations with behaviors that are unhealthy.

DBT does not involve traditional psychoanalytic therapy but action-oriented treatment approaches such as exposure therapy, cognitive restructuring, and emotion regulation training. This means it may be more time-consuming than conventional psychoanalytic treatments, which include more verbal sharing of thoughts and feelings. In addition, to be effective with patients with trauma disorders, DBT must focus on helping them behave differently than they did during the traumatic event(s). Therefore, DBT does not focus on the patient's past and instead looks to move them forward.

DBT was initially developed to treat borderline personality disorder and has since been adapted from its original format by researchers and clinicians. The most notable adaptation is mindfulness-based DBT or M-DBT, which includes a component of mindfulness training. Mindfulness is a specific form of meditation used in CBT treatments. In M-DBT, patients are taught to notice their thoughts, feelings, and sensations without judgment. This helps patients become aware of their emotions, ideas, and behaviors while accepting them as part of themselves. This heightened awareness allows patients to behave more positively towards themselves and others while treating any underlying mental health conditions.

It is essential to recognize the differences between the behavioral theories because they are used by different practitioners and may have other goals. For example: while a therapist may use ACT in a social work or psychology practice, CBT is usually done in more traditional primary care practices. As such, the goal of each therapy will vary depending on how it has been adapted for use by that therapist.

Cognitive Behavior Therapy (CBT) grew from the work of Albert Ellis and Aaron Beck. Ellis developed Rational Emotive Behavior Therapy (REBT) which is based on an individual's thoughts and how they interact with their emotions. REBT was created to treat depression but has since been used for many other emotional disorders like anxiety, phobias, panic attacks, and substance abuse. In the 1940s, Beck expanded on this therapy, creating Cognitive Therapy to treat depression by focusing on identifying negative thoughts that led to negative actions. These two therapies eventually evolved into what we know as Cognitive Behavioral Therapy (CBT). But CBT was not the only therapy that grew out of these early works.

General Discussion about ACT, CBT, and DBT

As previously stated, ACT, CBT, and DBT all work to accomplish the same goal of helping patients achieve mental and emotional balance. However, the therapeutic techniques and plans are different for each. ACT focuses on developing a core set of values while identifying one's emotions and how they affect behavior during stressful times. CBT focuses on changing negative thoughts or beliefs into positive ones while identifying faulty cognitive processes contributing to these negative thoughts. DBT works with trauma disorders like BPD or PTSD by helping patients become more aware of their thought processes, emotions, and behaviors. To accomplish this goal, DBT will use mindfulness techniques to help patients recognize when they are being triggered and how these trigger responses affect their behavior.

ACT, CBT, and DBT also differ in the techniques they use. ACT is based on the philosophy that people should be aware of their feelings while simultaneously being aware of their present moment surroundings (action orientation). It focuses on teaching patients to develop their core values and use this information to direct how they respond to situations. As such, ACT focuses on helping patients identify and express feelings healthfully. This can be done through anxiety-reducing techniques like breathing exercises or learning cognitive techniques like focusing on positive thoughts rather than negative assumptions.

CBT is primarily used for patients with anxiety disorders or depression. CBT focuses on helping patients change their negative thinking patterns and beliefs into positive ones. However, this is not a magical process and must be maintained over time. CBT will also teach how these thoughts affect moods, behaviors, and emotions. To do this, the therapist will work with the patient to identify negative thought patterns and how they affect emotions, behaviors, and moods. Once this is done, the therapist will help the patient learn new ways of thinking that can lead to positive feelings like happiness or contentment. CBT may include exposure therapy (a behavioral treatment) to help patients face their fears, even though it does not focus directly on doing so as DBT does.

DBT is similar to ACT in that it focuses on an individual's core values but with a very different emphasis. DBT is designed to help patients with trauma disorders, like PTSD or BPD, become more aware of how their environments affect their thoughts, feelings, and behaviors. It also teaches patients to respond to situations differently than they did during the traumatic event. DBT teaches patients how to regulate their emotions and develop healthy coping strategies to manage the effects of these traumatic events better.

DBT was initially developed as a therapy for borderline personality disorder (BPD) but has since been adapted by researchers and clinicians in other mental health fields.

Determining which therapy will be most effective depends on what you try to accomplish with treatment. For example, suppose you need emotional support or guidance through a rough time in your life. In that case, all three therapies can be effective since they provide non-judgmental advice through difficult situations. Suppose, on the other hand, suppose a specific mental health condition (like depression or anxiety). In that case, it is best to seek out a therapist who has experience using any of these therapies with patients who share that diagnosis. As stated previously, these therapies are not the same and can be effective for different goals.

If you are interested in learning more about how one of these therapies can benefit you, it is best to consult with a therapist who has experience using one. An efficient way to find a qualified therapist is by using a phone book or asking your primary care provider for recommendations.

How to develop willingness and acceptance

Willingness is a decision to act and is described as a will to do. Conversely, Acceptance is the acknowledgment of what is, characterized by recognizing that someone has no control over the situation. It is quite paradoxical that people often want to live in a world free of suffering yet insist on being part of it.

Willingness is a response to a challenge, whereas acceptance is a strategy for coping with life. We've all heard that "willingness is what it takes to make a will, and acceptance is what it takes to keep one." Both willingness and acceptance are necessary if one is to achieve goals and resolve conflicts, yet the relationship between the two is not very clear.

Will means to make a decision or to act. In the context of ACT, willingness refers to the conscious decision "to initiate and persist in goal-directed action despite obstacles."

For example, you might have the goal of finishing your thesis on time, but due to illness or procrastination, you are unwilling or unable to do so. To overcome this challenge with willingness is characterized by consciously deciding to put aside personal preferences and needs (e.g., social engagement, health) to accomplish your goal even if you're not feeling well.

One of the most frequent symptoms is "Willingness vs. Acceptance." It may be the case that people want to work with a therapist, but they are not willing to make any changes. On the other hand, it may also be the case that people don't want to see a therapist at all. The latter example is often the case for people experiencing intrusive thoughts due to trauma. They may recognize that their behavior is not optimal, but they don't want to make any changes. In such cases, willingness is lacking.

Acceptance refers to the conscious acceptance of reality, focusing on feelings. For example, suppose you are unwilling to think about your mother dying or contemplating how liberating it would be to quit your job. In that case, you may experience discomfort with these thoughts, yet you may accept that this is a healthy part of human existence.

Understanding the difference between willingness and acceptance

The first step in developing willingness is realizing there is a potential conflict between those who want change and those who don't. This can occur when one group wants to use therapy as part of their regular treatment, and the other group doesn't think that therapy or treatment is necessary or helpful.

The second step is realizing that a willingness to change must be nurtured and supported through acceptance. Knowing something needs to change in your life is not enough. You have to accept that something is going to change, but it's up to you whether you want out of this situation or not.

In particular, accepting that you want therapy may mean accepting the reality of your past experiences with anger and hostility, so they can become part of who you are now rather than destructive parts of your past.

Acceptance also involves recognizing how good it feels (relaxation) and how bad it feels (fear). Acceptance of negative emotions and thoughts allows you to develop new behaviors that encourage acceptance when change is wanted. For example, if you are willing to set a goal to quit smoking but are not anxious about how hard it might be, this can help you align your will with your actions.

Some research has also shown that acceptance of negative emotions and thoughts is related to emotional well-being, whereas willingness to these feelings was linked to emotional distress. Therefore, supporting people in developing a willingness to face their problems or considering the possibility of changing their lives may not always be the best strategy. For example, one client reported that his wife often told him: "You should go out more often; people will think you're antisocial."

In contrast, acceptance is characterized by the following symptoms: Curiosity, trust, and humility are essential characteristics of acceptance. In the case of a living situation with an abusive person (such as an alcoholic or a person with an autism spectrum disorder), curiosity and trust can be developed by exploring what it looks like to accept this type of person in one's life without judging them. Humility is necessary because it ends all judging, including self-judgment. When someone lives with such a person, they realize that it is essential to be open, not to judge, and not to blame oneself. It is positive in that it makes one see what is good in one's life, and this attitude can lead to an awareness of the "real" problem.

Acceptance can enable a person to have a more useful life. This means that acceptance helps people overcome their limitations and flourish. Acceptance facilitates a more engaging, creative, and meaningful relationship between self-concept and actual reality, as well as between self-concept and other people. The quality of life within oneself will also be apparent instead of being clouded by anxiety or frustration.

The process of achievement of acceptance within oneself goes in two directions. On the one hand, they accept that their condition is fixed and cannot change (acceptance as a kind of fatalism). On the other hand, they accept to change their lives and make them better or change themselves (acceptance as an attitude of willingness). The latter approach requires a certain amount of courage, but it may determine a person's quality of life.

Willingness can also be developed in one's life. When people accept what they are, they are willing to change themselves. This attitude is an essential step in therapy and leads to a new beginning.

Two factors predict the individual's reaction to a problematic situation: (1) pre-existing tendencies to react in a certain way and (2) potential for the person to react differently. The first factor is called "a tendency," while the second is called "potential."

When a person is confronted with an ambiguous situation, they tend to determine which strategy will allow them to maximize their advantage and generalize from this result. In cases where one's reactions are predictable, the individual may be identified as having a particular personality type. For example, suppose someone has no tendencies about what reaction to take to various situations. In that case, they may be regarded as having no or an average stable personality.

Predicting the reaction to a difficult situation is also important for therapists. Therapists may find themselves in situations with little information about a person's personality. However, even in such cases, it is possible to catch an individual's tendency to react in a certain way. For example, therapists can predict which patients are likely resistant or compliant based on their characteristics.

It is essential to consider the following points:

1. Acceptance is not an act of resignation but courage.
2. Acceptance can be developed by considering one's situation as one would if one had to live with the situation permanently.
3. People may not be prepared to change themselves, but they are prepared to change their behavior and make it acceptable for others.
4. People often develop a sense of "false self" in difficult situations that can prevent them from being honest with themselves and others.
5. Learning begins when people realize they have some control over their lives (even if it is not much).
6. Difficult situations have the potential to cause great suffering, but the ability to experience suffering is essential to achieve a greater sense of truth.

An overview of factors associated with willingness has already been presented in this book. Briefly, willingness can be described as follows:

These characteristics characterize willingness:

1. Readiness for change Worry about how others might judge oneself. People who are not willing to change themselves often worry about how others will respond if they make changes in their lives (e.g., how family members might react if they change their behavior).
2. Ability to learn from experience People who are unwilling to change themselves do not want to learn from their mistakes and are afraid of making changes.
3. Ability to make decisions People who are unwilling to change themselves often don't know how to decide what to do during difficult situations.
4. Ability for self-reflection People who are unwilling to change themselves may have difficulty being aware of how they feel and think about a particular situation.
5. Ability for empathy People who are unwilling to change themselves may have difficulty recognizing what others think and feel during difficult situations.
6. Ability to experience pain People who are unwilling to change themselves may not be able to experience the pain that comes with a painful decision or difficult situation.
7. Ability to act People who are unwilling to change themselves cannot act and make changes in their lives.
8. Willingness is developed by becoming more aware of what one can change in their life, the costs and benefits of any changes, and the actualities that one accepts about oneself and other people: what one can accept about their behavior, how one might react differently under challenging situations, etc.
9. Willingness is developed through the process of willingness: the actual decision to do something different and then making this new behavior a permanent characteristic of oneself.
10. Success requires a person willing to make changes, a problematic situation that can be made more manageable, and an environment that allows for some change and growth.
11. Willingness is developed by having goals in life, being able to take risks, being confident in one's abilities, and anticipating success.

Therefore, willingness and acceptance can be developed through:

a. Being willing to make changes in one's life.
b. Choosing goals and making them a part of oneself.
c. Having confidence in one's ability to find solutions and make decisions.
d. Understanding that one can only be successful if the environment supports them.
e. Being aware of who, what, and where one is being successful and not being successful at each step in life.
f. Developing a way of thinking that allows accepting difficulties encountered along the way (acceptance as a kind of fatalism).
g. Having a way of life-based on confidence and preparation (pre-planning in advance or pre-training).

Therefore, having the mind of a person who is willing to change and accept would:

a. Readiness for change by understanding one's situation and acting accordingly.
b. Ability to learn from experience by selecting accurately good situations (and not insignificant difficulties) that can be mastered.
c. Ability to make decisions by anticipating situations that need to be changed or adapted, assess the actuality of these situations, and choose a strategy based on this thought process (e.g., what is best in terms of success, reasonable compensation, etc.).

d.   Ability for self-reflection by thinking about how one feels and what they think about a particular situation during difficult times in life (e.g., what is one is doing wrong?).

e.   Ability for empathy by understanding other people's thoughts and feelings during difficult situations (e.g., what happens when I lose my job?).

f.   Ability to experience pain by recognizing that not everyone is happy in difficult situations, but being able to decide what causes this and how one wants to cope with it when the person is no longer there (i.e., accepting the loss).

g.   Ability for action by being able to implement changes that are useful or necessary in the long run (e.g., making new friends so as not to feel lonely).

h.   Willingness is developed by being reliable, having an optimistic attitude towards others, and being a problem-solver (i.e., having the mind of a person who is not lacking in confidence or abilities).

i.   Willingness is developed by thinking more about what one can do rather than what one cannot do and assessing situations in terms of actuality without exaggerating.

j.   The mind willing to change and accept can be developed by having a positive attitude towards oneself, other people, and the world at large (optimism).

k.   The mind of a person who is willing to change and accept can be developed by using strategies that are based on the way things are and not on ideas that are based on romantic notions (e.g., thinking realistically)

l.   The mind of a person willing to change and accept can be developed by accepting that there are things one cannot do and does not want to do (e.g., giving up smoking).

How to help patients define their value directions

Acceptance and Commitment Therapy (ACT) is based on well-supported psychological research in humanistic psychology, cognitive-behavioral therapy, and behavioral medicine. This therapeutic approach is time intensive and requires considerable skill to administer. However, ACT offers therapists an efficient clinical tool that they can learn relatively quickly to help patients define their value directions—what they want in their lives—and create a plan for achieving those goals.

One of the core principles of ACT is based on valuing one's emotions as opposed to suppressing or being consumed by them. Suppression of emotions, significantly negative feelings such as fear, anger, sadness, and shame, often leads to long-term distress. In addition, people will likely emerge in other inappropriate contexts if they suppress these feelings. Thus, it can be helpful for people with mood disorders to learn to experience the full range of their emotions without acting on them or suppressing them.

ACT therapists will typically ask their patients to create "values lists," which help a person define their life goals and values. Then, the ACT therapist will have the patient evaluate the degree to which these goals are based on each of these values. For example, if someone values personal relationships, the therapist would ask what assurance there is that people can be trusted and can be counted on in different settings. In terms of money, what evidence exists that money brings more happiness than sorrow? To the extent that a goal cannot be supported by evidence, it is not likely to have much value for the person concerned.

The ACT therapist will then ask the patient to identify the things that would enable them to achieve these goals. For example, those who want financial security in life might list some of their resources, such as savings and investments.

Although this point sounds somewhat obvious, it is often overlooked. Without being too technical, money can be thought of as a resource that gives one particular opportunity of which one may not be aware should come up in this way or at this time. In other words, one could have specific opportunities they would be happy to experience at some particular time without necessarily having any idea when or where they will appear.

The ACT therapist will then ask how important the patient considers each resource to be. The patient may be asked to give a number, on a scale of 1-10, indicating their importance. In this example, the patient might say that savings and investments are an 8 (highest).

ACT therapists encourage patients to understand what they have done to make successful changes in the past. They then ask them to evaluate whether or not they have achieved any of their values in life or have made any financial gains. If they have made such gains, some of their values were likely being met at the time.

Therefore, the following tips can help patients define their value directions:

1. Encourage self-evaluation and goal setting

Self-evaluation is essential and can help people develop self-awareness. It is also important to set goals that one can achieve. For example, suppose a person values family relationships. In that case, they may achieve this through setting up and maintaining a network of close friends, showing kindness to their children and partners, or visiting their parents or siblings regularly. Likewise, they may benefit from watching the stock market's gains or managing an investment portfolio if they value money.

2. Prioritize values

Each individual has several core values in life. Each core value often points to one or more overarching goals in life—one's "ultimate values. These ultimate values may be expressed by words to the effect of "health, wealth, love, and so on.

Importantly, patients are asked to rank their overarching goals in life regarding their importance. So, for example, if someone values being healthy and being wealthy as significant goals in life, they would ask themselves: "What evidence is there that I am meeting both of these goals?"

3. Create an action plan

ACT therapists will encourage patients to create an action plan to achieve their ultimate values by identifying specific outcomes or changes that would enable them to achieve those goals. For example: "I will demonstrate kindness and generosity toward my family this week. I will try to be more caring and thoughtful toward my children." "I will work on improving my fitness by exercising three times per week. I will also try some new recipes this weekend to have more healthy meals available during the week."

The problem with asking patients to make specific changes in their lives is that they may not know how to do this, especially if they are not used to making specific changes. Therefore, ACT therapists often help them by giving them examples of what the first step might be. For example, if someone has a goal of being healthy and is overweight, the therapist might suggest that they begin exercising by walking for 20 minutes after dinner each night. If a person wants to be wealthy, the therapist might suggest that they start saving and investing monthly money.

4. Give these steps some time

ACT therapists will encourage patients to be patient with themselves and not get too frustrated if they do not achieve their ultimate values or goals straight away. Doing essential things in life takes time and a lot of practice. In this sense, moving toward your goals often involves "baby steps" or "baby steps" forward that are each small enough for people to accomplish them without feeling overwhelmed.

The mindfulness aspect of ACT, which is present in most forms of CBT, contributes to general awareness development; thus, it can help people notice how they feel while moving toward their values. However, some people have difficulty identifying or describing their feelings. In these cases, an ACT therapist might encourage them to use a rating scale (for example, from 0-10) to rate how they feel throughout the week. This can help patients become more aware of their feelings and why they feel them.

5. Be flexible

ACT therapists are aware that, although many of our goals have been with us for quite some time, they may sometimes need to be revisited, changed, or refined. For example, if patients notice that they are not consistently moving toward some of their core values, they may need to re-evaluate their purpose in life by asking themselves: "What is important to me? What goals can I achieve? What is the evidence that my life is moving in the direction I want it to?" It is also essential for patients to remember that not achieving one goal does not mean that other goals cannot be achieved if a person stays committed to them.

ACT therapists usually encourage people with chronic illnesses or who have experienced significant trauma in their lives (e.g., abuse) to work toward achieving specific steps toward their core values. These include people who have had the following conditions:

ACT aims to help patients develop self-acceptance and learn to value themselves as they are, in the here and now, rather than pursue particular values or goals that may or may not be attainable. This is based on the idea that people often have many goals and values they want to achieve. However, people sometimes hold onto these ideals without the hard work needed. For example, people may say to themselves, "I want to be rich" or "I want to be a good person," without recognizing that achieving these goals requires specific actions.

Some people may have goals that are out of touch with their core values. For example, it is unlikely that someone who values close relationships and has few friends would pursue becoming a TV celebrity if it meant sacrificing time spent with loved ones. ACT therapists will encourage patients to re-evaluate their goals by first asking what the patient wants in life and then helping them figure out ways to achieve those goals via concrete steps toward them.

ACT therapists will not just ask patients to choose one or two goals and work toward them. Instead, they will help patients to identify several goals and work on achieving them in the short term. For example, suppose a patient has identified several values (e.g., being wealthy and having good health). In that case, an ACT therapist may encourage them to take small steps toward achieving these goals each week or month (e.g., exercise more frequently or invest part of their income into mutual funds). This way, people can gradually move toward their ultimate values while not feeling overwhelmed by trying to achieve everything at once. ACT advocates an approach to therapy that includes getting people to develop a "coping life philosophy" in which they try to live up to their core values.

ACT does not aim only to get people to change how they think about themselves but also how they relate and behave with others. For example, ACT therapists will often ask patients with significant problems like autism or schizophrenia how they want other people in their life (e.g., family members and friends who tend to be critical) to act toward them. "For example, I may ask a patient, 'How can I start by being more accepting of my family's behavior toward me? What are some things you can do in your life that will help you to be more accepting of people?'" It is also true that ACT therapists will encourage some people with chronic illnesses or significant personal loss to work on acceptance.

In addition, someone trying to develop a core value like acceptance might decide to ask family and friends how they want them to behave toward them. In general, these gestures show patients how they might be able to make genuine changes in their patterns of behavior and communication with others. These changes might then help the patient to develop more meaningful relationships in their life. However, ACT therapists usually encourage patients to work on these issues one at a time rather than in bulk.

Psychologists often describe emotions as being "felt" with certain physiological sensations. For example, they may describe how anger is felt with a tightening in the chest area, while sadness is accompanied by a feeling of heaviness in the body. However, these associations are often not conscious, which means that people do not know why they feel that way; therefore, they have difficulty describing their feelings to others. Therefore, ACT therapists will often ask patients to be more specific about their feelings and why they feel them. This helps them be more aware of their feelings and communicate them better to others.

ACT therapists are interested in helping patients develop a clearer understanding of what they want from life, apart from the expectations of other people or cultural stereotypes. They will help patients get in touch with their values and find ways to achieve them.

How to clarify values and commit to valued-based actions

To clarify your values and commit to value-based actions, you must be willing to accept your thoughts and feelings without dictating how they should be. For example, if you are anxious about doing something because you fear rejection, instead of fighting the feeling or trying not to feel anxious, you must learn how to say "I am anxious" and "This makes me feel this way." It can help us learn acceptance skills if we label our emotions as they come up. Labeling your emotions when they first appear will help you understand what triggers a particular emotion or feeling.

Value clarification is not just about learning how to identify your values but, more importantly, how to hold value-based action simultaneously, and you are learning acceptance skills. Value clarification is a process that allows us to understand why we have goals, wants, and needs and what systems will help us meet them. We must clarify our values with other people for them to help us meet our valued goals.

For example, if you are involved in a group therapy group of people who want to stop drinking, then it may be helpful for you and your therapist to identify your values so that you know why it is important to stop drinking. Your therapist may also be able to offer you different techniques to stop drinking, such as Dr. Williburtons' model of continuing recovery.

Looking at your values will help you to clarify what goals and actions you want to accomplish to meet those valued motivations. However, it may also lead you to discover that your idealized self is buried in shame that has not been addressed. This discovery can be scary and hard to accept, but it will start a process for you where you begin the process of healing from the old wound or fears which have come up around conducting new behaviors and attaining your valued goals.

Moreover, commitment to value-based actions is the ability to do what is essential and meaningful to you, even when it is difficult. For example, if you are married and are trying to discuss essential relationship issues with your partner, your partner does not seem willing to listen or talk about it. Therefore, it may be helpful for you to commit to valued actions of expressing how you feel about the issue, even though that action may not be easy.

When we can hold our value-based actions and stay committed by saying things like "I know this is hard, and I am still going to do it" or " I am committed to, whatever happens, even if my spouse or significant other doesn't change," then these become action statements that help us move through a situation.

For example, if your therapist is trying to work with you to interpret your values and actions and focus on a specific goal, then it will improve the process if you state things like, "I know that this is hard for me to do, but I still want to do this." This type of commitment helps us hold our valued actions despite the difficulty.

Once we learn how to clarify our values and commit to value-based action statements, we can begin learning "how" we will hold and express these things. We must practice how we will operate in the world, for these new skillsets or beliefs systemically function better in our brains. How we relate to people and the world will change once we fully accept them, clarify our worldview and choose value-based actions.

Acceptance and commitment therapy is a process with many steps to complete the value clarification process. By learning to clarify your values, learn how you want to act based on those values, commit to valued action statements and practice these new behaviors, you can lead yourself out of old patterns of behavior that were not using your newly learned skillsets. Once you have completed this process, it will be possible for you or a client that you are working with or helping them complete Steps 2- 10 in this model.

Therefore, the following tips can guide on how to clarify values and commit to valued-based actions:

1. Clarity to confusion

This works by learning to accept the confusion around our values, worldviews, and actions. You will learn to allow yourself to see the picture in your head or observe your current unconscious behavior patterns.

2. Seeing ourselves as different

This works by learning that we are different people than we think and capable of doing new things than what was previously done in our life. Realizing that what has been done before is not who we are today will begin a healing process by seeing our old wounds in a new, more accepting way.

3. Being clear about your values

This works by learning to identify the essential things in your life and clarify your values. This can be challenging as we do not always know what is good for us or what we want for our lives, but this process is essential in uncovering our true feelings and needs.

4. Seeing through different eyes

This works by learning that you have essential lessons from life and other people, which will help you find new and better ways of relating with people and the world around you.

5. Being able to accept all points of view

This works by learning to be clear about what you feel is right, wrong, or indifferent without wanting to control anything or anyone else's behavior. Seeing both sides of the situation helps you accept that our worldviews will never be perfect, and it may be challenging to find the fine line between accepting and adjusting.

6. Learning how to identify what matters

This work by learning to focus and keep your mind on acting in a meaningful way and not being distracted by unimportant things, which will help you in your daily life.

7. Learning how to commit yourself

This work by learning how to commit to your values, even when it is hard, or something important comes up during the day.

8. Learning how to commit to valued-based actions

This work by learning how to say things like " I know this is hard, but I still want to do this" or "I am committed to whatever happens, even if my spouse or significant other doesn't change," which will create an action statement that helps you stay focused and continue your valued goals even if it is difficult.

9. Knowing what values you have

This work by learning the differences between different worldviews you have and being able to articulate what morals, values, beliefs, and principles are most important in your life so that you can make choices and decisions in a way that feels true.

10. Learning how to accept and express your values

This works by learning how to accept and express your values daily. You will learn how to create a meaningful and consistent life with who you are so that you can operate out of a sense of yourself, others, and the world around you.

Many people will have difficulty completing this process independently, as they may not know where to start or have support from other people. If this is true for someone you are working with, I would suggest they see a counselor or therapist who can guide them through the steps and ask questions if they need more help or insight into their life.

11. Learning how to define success

This work by learning how to clearly define and understand what is meaningful in your life and how you want it to be. By learning what is essential in your life, it will be easier for you to decide where you want to go and who you want to be. For example, maybe learning what is essential will help us know when we are wasting time on things that are not useful or helping us achieve our desired goals.

12. Learning how to live with failure

This work by learning how to learn from failure and change your beliefs, thinking and behavior in a way that will become more useful.

13. Learning how to express values

This work by learning what it means to be clear about what you want and need in life. We will learn new skills like expressing ourselves more clearly in everyday conversations, dreams, thoughts, and actions; this will help us become more explicit about our ideas and beliefs so that we can say them out loud without the fear of rejection or judgment from others.

14. Learning to listen to yourself

This works by learning to listen to what you need and want from people, events, and the world around you. This will help us become more effective in social situations and relationships, which can help us grow in our personal and professional lives.

15. Learning how to forgive others

This work by learning that everyone does not always mean well or even know the effect of what they do, so we will learn how to forgive people for their mistakes or areas where they are wrong. This will allow us to focus on what is 'real' or authentic about a person instead of letting our emotional sides get in the way of rational thinking.

16. Learning how to forgive yourself

This work by learning to accept who you are and your limitations around certain situations or people and not to blame yourself. This will help you accept your faults in different areas of your life so that you can move on and improve, rather than dwelling on things that happen in the past that we cannot change.

17. Learning how to acknowledge yourself

This work by learning how to express ourselves more clearly in everyday conversations, dreams, thoughts, and actions; can help us feel better about what we have done in our lives, thus showing appreciation for who we are today instead of wishing we were someone else or had a different life.

18. Learning how to be motivated to succeed

This work by learning how to create the beliefs, goals, and actions that will help us feel motivated in daily life so that we can take care of ourselves and make optimal choices. We will learn to develop self-confidence and higher motivation levels, which can positively affect our lives.

19. Learning how to stay motivated

This works by learning to maintain motivation internally with discipline, persistence, and consistency so that you can overcome your fears and doubts when starting something new or changing old habits. You will learn what does not work for you to commit more fully.

20. Learning how to make a vision for yourself

This works by learning to imagine, feel, and realize what you want and need to bring these visions into life through positive action. It will help you commit more fully to achieving your goals and dreams and break down any barriers or obstacles on the road.

21. Learning how to create a vision for others

This works by learning to project our values onto others constructively while not getting on their case all the time or trying to convert them. We will learn how to help others be more aware of their values so they can defend their ideas or stand up for themselves in a way that is consistent with who they are.

22. Learning how to dream

This works by learning how to create the beliefs and goals we have always wanted and how to convert our visions into life. This can help us know what we want from our goals and dreams and feel more connected to other people's dreams.

How to be present through mindfulness

ACCEPTANCE AND COMMITMENT THERAPY is a behavioral treatment for problems such as depression, addiction, and anxiety disorders. It was developed by Steven Hayes, Ph.D., and originated from the Buddhist practice of mindfulness.

The core principle of ACT is that it is not what happens to us in life that causes us to suffer emotionally but our thoughts about what occurs. Therefore, ACT teaches skills to help people engage with the present moment without judgment and with a quality of compassionate acceptance towards oneself and others.

ACT uses different metaphors that emphasize this idea, including "radical acceptance," "enlivening touch," and "what if it's a good thing.

The first step to taking control of your life and emotions is to be mindful. There are many different definitions of mindfulness, but what they all have in common is a focus on being present.

Mindfulness means being aware of the environment that you live in and the people that you interact with daily. This allows you to take your reality head-on and not judge it as good or bad, pleasant or unpleasant. It means seeing things for what they are, without preconceived notions or judgments of your own. It also means being aware of self, as well as other people.

Thoughts are just that: thoughts. They are not necessarily wrong or suitable for you, but they come from a place of emotion and affect your ability to think clearly throughout the day.

In mindfulness, a core belief is that all experiences are neutral as long as your mental state is clear. Most importantly, though, is the idea that our thoughts can be changed. When there is no judging involved in feelings and experiences, it will be easier to accept them. This will allow you to focus on the present moment with clarity of mind rather than on past hurt or traumatic events that might still affect your present behavior and emotions.

To be mindful, you must engage in a three-step process:

a. notice
b. acknowledge
c. accept to create a space between you and your emotions that allows you to live in the present moment instead of dwelling on the past or fearing the future.

ACT seeks out, accepts, and embraces negative thoughts, emotions, and physical sensations for what they are, without judgment. For this to work, three things must occur: 1) noticing what is happening around you; 2) accepting it without judgment; 3) committing yourself to positive action despite all these things that might be going wrong in your life.

The ACT model is based on acceptance and commitment therapy, initially developed for people with substance abuse problems. It treats various conditions, including depression, anxiety disorders, chronic pain syndromes (Somatic Experiencing), sexual addiction (Emotionally Focused Couples Therapy), and impulsive behavior. It also helps to prevent relapse in survivors of child abuse.

The last part of this process is the most important. When you can accept things, your mind is no longer clouded by judgments and self-judgment. You can then begin to notice the patterns that bring about negative thoughts and emotions. You can then remove yourself from situations that cause discomfort or stress and acknowledge that there are other paths to take. You can then change your environment or life to match your acceptance of yourself and others rather than being hard-pressed by a negative mindset or influenced by others who may use words or actions to keep you in a state of anxiety and despair.

ACCEPTANCE AND COMMITMENT THERAPY doesn't force you to deal with difficult situations in a state of mindfulness. Instead, it gives you the tools to walk away from negative situations to return to them later once you have regained control of your mind and emotions.

However, some say that ACT is a series of techniques used to manipulate people out of their comfort zone subtly. For example, that ACT manipulates the client into accepting what ACT Therapists say as truth without questioning. Critics also charge that this approach creates "a quasi-religious rather than therapeutic experience for many patients."

Therefore, the following tips can guide how to be present through mindfulness:

1.   Accepting the present moment has to be a priority

We are often taught acceptance in therapy, but it is a skill that we rarely practice. When you are busy planning your next move or worried about what will happen next, you can't notice the moment you are in. Moreover, criticism and self-judgment for being in the present moment cloud your mind and prevent you from accepting what is happening, which leads to suffering.

Consider eating, sitting, watching TV, taking a shower, or going to sleep as opportunities to practice acceptance. Linger over the sensation of chewing food or smelling a flower rather than cutting your meal short or walking past that flower. If you have trouble sleeping at night, focus on your breath and body rather than planning your day tomorrow.

2.   Be aware of what is happening in your environment

Mindfulness can be difficult when we are in situations where we feel like an outsider or when we are constantly bombarded with distractions. This can be difficult for people who are very narrow-minded about their world. However, something is always happening in our lives, so be present in those moments, too.

Imagine you are a child at a birthday party and you don't know anyone except one other child attending the party with his parents. You may feel awkward being at the party, but it's not strange because there is plenty to do that involves your imagination and creativity. Instead of having a wrong time at the party (this can include being bored), try to get into the moment and imagine what it would be like if everyone had fun together and you were able to interact with them during the party.

3.   Think about your reactions before you have them

When we get into unpleasant situations, we don't react in the best way possible. For example, if a classmate is rude to you during class, instead of reacting poorly by turning red and thinking that this person is terrible and everyone hates them, think about the situation from their perspective. What does this person see in you? Were they not included in the group for any reason? If so, why? Instead of jumping to conclusions about what's wrong with them, try to understand what's going on in her mind.

4.   Learning which events you can control and which you cannot

Sometimes, we might feel frustrated when we get into stressful or awkward situations. We might see our inability to control a situation as a fault; however, this is not necessarily the case. First, ask yourself whether you can change the situation at hand or if it's better to let it pass. Next, ask yourself why you want to change it in the first place. Finally, let it go and learn from your reactions if it's not a good reason. The more you learn about how your reactions affect your behavior and emotions, the easier things will be when they happen again.

5. Helping others

When you are in a situation, your attention will immediately be drawn toward others experiencing distress or discomfort. You will want to help that person, but you must be aware of your situation. Instead of comfort and care, sometimes people want to be left alone because they need to think through their feelings or overcome a fear or phobia. Moreover, you may react poorly if someone else is also trying to help you. You might feel like everyone is trying to change you instead of accepting who you are now.

If someone is trying to change your behavior or beliefs and make you uncomfortable, stop and think about the situation. If you know nothing is wrong with your actions, then let the person know how they are making you feel. If it doesn't stop, walk away and return when you have a clear head.

6. Changing your thoughts about yourself

When we are at our best, we are accepting of others and ourselves. To get to this point, it's vital to think differently about ourselves than we do when things go wrong in our lives. When someone makes a mistake and beats themselves up over it, look at the situation and determine whether it is worth beating yourself up over. Ask yourself whether it is possible to make a mistake without having something wrong with you. Think about what you should tell this person and consider their feelings.

If the answer is no, then make a conscious decision to think differently about yourself and others. For example, don't get angry or offended if someone calls you a negative name or accuses you of doing something that makes you look bad. Instead, try to understand why this person said that sentence and think about why they would say it in the first place. When we change our thoughts about ourselves, we can change how we view ourselves to be more accepting of who we are now and how we feel in the present moment.

7. If you are in a situation where you cannot control anything, accept this

Sometimes, we can't change a situation like last week's weather or a fight with someone. This doesn't mean that it's not possible to let go of the situation and be present in the moment. It might take practice, but it is possible to be still and accepting of difficult times. Think about how you feel when things aren't going your way and ask yourself whether letting go is actually what you want to do.

Asking questions like this can help us determine whether something is wrong with our thoughts. If we feel happy when things aren't going well and can still make decisions, there is nothing wrong with us. We might feel like something is wrong with us if we can't control our emotions, but this is not true. It's possible to find comfort in situations where we think it isn't possible.

8. Letting go of regrets

Sometimes we look back at something that happened in the past and regret things that didn't go the way they should have. For example, we might miss an opportunity because of a decision someone made or say something that hurt someone's feelings or break up with someone who, deep down, we know would be a great partner. If you think about the past, try to let go of your regrets.

As much as possible, think about why you made that decision and what you should have done to improve it. For example, if you broke up with someone because they did something that hurt your feelings, ask yourself what they were feeling at the time and if this was something meaningful or not. After all, it is possible to see situations from two different perspectives and come to two different conclusions about what happened.

9. Let go of your fears

Fear is always there, no matter what we do. Fear can be related to whether someone will like us, what kind of job we might get when we graduate and which people will like us. However, most of the time, fear is not a good thing that our minds should control. Every time you find yourself experiencing fear, ask yourself whether it's worth it to let it control you or if you could do something to overcome it instead. The more you look at fear as a positive feeling and investigate the reason behind your fear, the more control you will have over it.

The only way to overcome fear is to keep trying. There are numerous things we can do to control our fears, but the best way is not just to try to control them but also to find a way to accept them as they are. Consider the situation and figure out whether you could be afraid of something that isn't that bad in the first place. You might also ask others who know what you're feeling if they think there's a reason for your fear or if it isn't worth worrying about.

How to help clients commit to act by setting goals

Acceptance and Commitment Therapy (ACT) is a form of cognitive behavioral therapy that is particularly effective for individuals with a high degree of avoidance. Individuals who commit to their goals are more likely to reach their desired end or ultimate goal. Thus, setting the appropriate goals before taking any action has led many people in those cases where avoidance may be a factor in success (or lack thereof) in committing. The ACT contains an extensive array of specific strategies. Still, the most well-established ones include identifying and clarifying one's values and looking at aspects of the self that may be holding back change or success. This is done by using "the worksheet," a form in which goals are generated and then revised over time to help people reach the goals that they set themselves.

The worksheet can be used in different ways to approach goal setting, such as:

a. Identifying Desired Characteristics and then Experiencing Them
b. Asking About the Future and then Evaluating Actions/Behaviors.

It has been said that ACT is more than just an effective way of helping someone commit to change, but a "way of life" taught to help people live better lives. ACT recognizes that many people are not the way they would like. Therefore, rather than the negatives, it focuses on the positives and how one can get there through setting goals and observing their progress.

ACT uses a variety of different exercises to help individuals reach their goals by following a series of steps, such as:

a. Identifying Goals
b. Setting these Goals
c. Focusing on the Values/Beliefs that are Important to the Person
d. Estimating How One Would Feel if They Reaching Those Goals.
b. Experiencing Those Desired Feelings by Using Helpful Methods
c. Instilling a Sense of Direction
d. Applying Exercises from Session to Daily Life, e. Learning how to Accept and Commit

Clients who struggle with setting goals may find it helpful to identify their values to help them determine what they want out of life. Removing the word "should" from clients' vocabulary can also help them to change their outlook on the future and their goals, as well as help them anticipate what they would feel like if they managed to reach that goal.

Studies have shown that values help individuals identify specific goals worth setting and are likely to be valued by them and not just by others. In addition, it has been found that individuals who believe in their values are more likely to follow through with a goal when there is no outside pressure involved in the process.

When looking at the process of setting goals and having a sense of direction towards them, it is helpful for the client to have a journal. Having a journal allows the client to keep track of their experiences and feelings that may arise for them to develop more in-depth self-awareness. Through journaling, it is often recommended that clients practice their "negative visualization" to help them identify what they do not want while recognizing what they do want. This specific exercise helps the individual by helping them to see the adverse outcomes of not reaching those goals.

Therefore, these tips can guide how to help clients commit to act by setting goals:

1. Identify the client's distressing thoughts or problem

Distress identity refers to the identity one has for themselves, their "who I am." The term is used to show how even though that person may experience other people's verbal or physical abuse, they do not feel they belong to that group. In addition, this identity can help identify what the client does not want to be identified with, for example: "I am a very accepting person" and "I do not like being judged."

2. Identify the client's distressing feelings

Distress feelings refer to the emotions and sensations from experiencing distressing thoughts or problems. When considering distressing feelings, they often have a solid emotional connection attached. For example, "I am worried about the future" versus "I am worried about being a burden."

3. Identify the underlying desire that is being thwarted by the thought or problem

The underlying desire is most likely the opposite of the distressing feeling that the client has, such as "worrying." This term refers to how clients view themselves concerning other people. The underlying desire may be "I am a good person."

4. Help the client identify a specific workable goal

The goal must be within the client's life and be significant enough so that it will matter to them daily. When there is no specific goal, distressing thoughts continue to haunt the individual or cause further disturbances in mind. "Other people will always judge me" can become "I am a good person," which leads to more positive feelings.

5. Have the client estimate how they would feel if they reached their goal

There must be an emotional attachment to something deemed necessary to reach, such as a goal that may be money-related. For example, "I will feel confident" versus "I will be a good person" allows for more positive feelings.

6. Help the client experience the desired feelings by using helpful methods

Once the client states the goal and estimates how they would feel if they reached it, ways of reaching that goal should be outlined. Clients must then write about their goals daily to encourage them to take action (specificity). The client can set daily reminders such as alarms or call friends and family to remind them of their goals. Also, setting goals helps individuals become more aware of what they do not want rather than what they do want because it is essential to recognize how one feels when they are unsuccessful.

7. Encourage the client to participate in an ongoing process of self-awareness

The final step is to help the individual become more aware of how they are progressing and what they are doing to make progress. Once this awareness is reached, the individual can be confident that they are not getting back on track and can accept themselves for who they are now.

8. Help the client identify a means to improve and adjust their long-term goals

The goal should not be something that one thinks they will "do" or "be," but it should be something that one believes they can choose to do or be, such as "to earn an advanced degree in a certain area."

9. Have the client apply these techniques to their daily life

The suggestions in this book can be helpful for anyone struggling with setting significant goals and motivating them to take action. This book will teach readers how to help clients identify distressing thoughts and problems and how distress is experienced using helpful methods. This book will focus on teaching them how to reach their goals and apply them to daily life so that they do not get distracted once they have made progress. This book suggests that having a journal will be helpful for clients and identifying one's values, which are personally significant enough to create a positive change in the individual's life. Therefore, the book can be helpful to those who are interested in helping others set their goals and reach them.

10. Provide encouragement and support in reaching that goal

Having a support system can help someone who struggles with setting goals. By allowing them to address issues and concerns in a safe place, clients will be able to feel more comfortable and confident about reaching their goals.

11. Help the client identify a relapse warning sign

Sometimes when one reaches one goal, other issues are difficult to recognize and address. Therefore, it is essential to identify if there are any warning signs that the client may observe themselves experiencing. When one is aware of these warning signs, action can be taken immediately before they have a chance to fall back into old habits again.

12. Help the client identify a method of preventing a relapse

When individuals reach one goal, they may feel satisfied and as if they do not need to work towards anything else in the future. Therefore, it is important to identify methods that will encourage them to continue putting in effort towards their goals. These methods can be different for each individual and should be considered accordingly.

13. Encourage the client to ask for help when needed

Setting goals can be challenging, especially if the individual is experiencing difficulties or is distracted by other outside factors, such as other people's negative comments or behaviors. When one is exhibiting these warning signs and starts to experience symptoms of relapse, it is best to seek help because they are experiencing a significant problem and cannot handle it independently.

14. Have the client recognize their strengths

The strength of someone is an essential factor in setting significant goals. When one has these strengths, one can commit to a goal and stay committed.

15. Have the client identify their challenges

To reach an important goal, it is essential to identify the challenges in one's life. One may face these challenges and be unwilling or unable to change their current condition because they believe it is who they are or will continue being this way forever. It is best when they think that there is no alternative or that there is no other solution besides their current situation—it will not change.

16. Help the client identify past and current challenges

When facing challenges, examining past and current problems can be helpful. Past problems may be attributed to previous adverse events. Examining these issues allows individuals to recognize their failures and develop new coping strategies. Current problems can relate to obstacles unique to the individual's daily life, such as relationship issues or work stress. This allows them to recognize difficulties and work on improving their situation while still having a choice.

17. Have the client identify their goals for themselves personally

One can think about their strengths and identify those that are personally significant, whereas one can think about their challenges and allow them to have personal significance. One may have difficulties with one of these two factors but no problem with the other. As a result, they can better identify how they can progress towards significant goals because they do not have a problem with one area, making it challenging to work on the other aspect.

18. Help the client identify ways to influence others

When one is trying to influence other people, they experience trauma. Therefore, it is essential to have a plan before taking action. When one gets upset or frustrated while trying to help others, they may experience difficulties and frustration. Therefore, it is best to have a concrete plan before taking action and prepare them beforehand with different ways that they can inspire and encourage them through their actions. This will prevent either side from getting frustrated quickly and allow the individual to work on their personal goals while they can use the previous methods on others once more.

How to stop intrusive and obsessive thoughts

One of the most common challenges people face with anxiety is intrusive and obsessive thoughts. These thoughts may take many forms but are often unpleasant, repetitive, and distressing.

Expert opinion is that these are a form of mental activity called worry or rumination, and they can be closely linked to an individual's feelings of worry or self-doubt. Indeed, research has shown that people with OCD often have above-average levels of worrying about everyday issues in their lives.

To overcome intrusive and obsessive thoughts, we need to break the link between worrying or rumination in the case of OCD and these thoughts. This is the first step in developing new, more helpful ways to tackle unwanted thoughts.

Step 1: Decide what makes you worry a lot.

What does it mean for someone with persistent intrusive thoughts to 'worry a lot? To answer this, it is necessary to understand what it means for you. For many people with anxiety, worrying a lot means spending some time thinking about something before they go to sleep at night. It may mean being unable to settle on one topic in conversation with another person or having repetitive images run through their head during the day.

Often we do not like thinking about ourselves and how we feel. As a result, we may avoid thinking about what is bothering us, which often leads to anxiety or worry. If you find it difficult to think about yourself positively or take the time to evaluate what is worrying you, then it might be because you care too much or are simply unwilling to think about how you feel.

If this is the case, it may be useful to consider whether sometimes worrying a lot is healthy and, as they say in Eastern culture, "When in doubt - leave it out." While sometimes worrying can be helpful (for example, when facing a tricky medical appointment), a more serious issue might occur with persistent intrusive thoughts. It might help to try and see if there is a way you can stop thinking or worrying about certain issues.

Step 2: Try not to focus on the content of your intrusive thoughts.

It is often useful to think about a time when you had the same intrusive thoughts you are having now, but instead of dwelling on them (which tends to make things worse), try to change your relationship with them. For example, if you have an intrusive thought that keeps coming back to your mind, it might be useful to see whether you can find a different way of dealing with it. Also, do not focus on its content if you dwell on why this thought came into your mind. Instead, focus on other issues, such as whether the thought makes you feel more anxious or less anxious or whether it is helpful to think about the content of your thoughts. It might also be useful to ask yourself if there is any benefit in repeatedly thinking about your intrusive thoughts. If there is, then what is that benefit?

In many cases, people with OCD notice that focusing on the content of their intrusive thoughts or trying to change how they think about them can worsen things. This is because as soon as an individual tries to stop having a particular thought, it becomes more difficult for them not to think about it again. After all, when we try and control our minds, we cannot do so without effort.

Step 3: Work out if you can find a way of trying to stop having your thoughts

This is similar to Step 1 but focuses more on the process of trying not to think about something than simply looking for a change in relationship with your thoughts. For example, if you try not to think about your intrusive thoughts (or find ways of trying to stop them) without changing the meaning behind your thoughts, they are likely to come back again. It may be useful at this point, however, not just to ask yourself whether you can think of ways of stopping certain thoughts from entering your mind but also whether there is any benefit in continuing to have certain types of thoughts. If there is, then what is that benefit? For example, if you believe it will help you to think about your intrusive thoughts, then ask yourself whether this belief makes any sense and, if so, why.

Step 4: Try to accept unpleasant thoughts without judging them.

Sometimes when we have intrusive thoughts, we tell ourselves that they are wrong or upsetting, making them more likely to come back in the future. However, one of the core principles of ACT is that anxious thoughts do not necessarily mean anything negative about a person. It may be useful, therefore, not to accept these thoughts without first questioning whether they have a purpose in our lives.

A useful way to try and work out the purpose of your thoughts is to see whether you can find any evidence for them. It may be helpful, for example, to ask yourself if there is any reason why you have these intrusive thoughts. Examining this question can prove helpful because we often only consider ourselves guilty of something when we have guilty feelings, which are often painful and distressing. If the thoughts do not seem to make sense or lead us anywhere, then it might help to consider whether you could benefit from letting go of them altogether. If there is any benefit in continuing to have these types of thoughts, what is that benefit?

Step 5: Make a plan to get rid of your thoughts.

This step examines whether it would be helpful to take practical steps using a three-column worksheet to eliminate or reduce the impact of unwelcome intrusive thoughts. The worksheet has three columns on the left: Yes/No and Agree/Disagree. The first column is for rating the extent to which a certain thought is true (from 0% meaning not true at all to 100% meaning true). The second is rating the extent to which a certain thought is helpful (from −100% meaning completely unhelpful to +100% meaning completely helpful). Finally, the third column is for rating the extent to which a certain thought is unwanted (from 0% meaning not wanted at all to 100% meaning wanted).

When completing these columns, it may be useful, in some cases, to consider what you are doing when you think about your intrusive thoughts. For example, you may ruminate on them or engage in other behaviors that will cause you distress. If this is the case, it might be useful to ask yourself whether there is a more helpful way of dealing with these thoughts.

In addition, it may be helpful to focus on your willingness to carry out certain assignments to reduce the impact of intrusive thoughts. A key question in this step will be whether you are willing to complete assignments related to trying not to think about your intrusive thoughts or thinking about them differently. You can check how willing you might be by asking yourself whether you would agree or disagree with statements such as "I'd like to get rid of my unwanted thoughts. I am willing to do this". If you wish to challenge many of your intrusive thoughts, then it would be a good idea to download the following worksheet.

Step 6: Confront your thoughts and change the meaning of them

This is not an individualized process because it can be useful for people with OCD to access external help and support at this stage. However, several tools may be helpful for people with OCD when they are ready to confront their thoughts and change the meaning behind them.

The first is an "unwanted thought diary," which helps people to record the number of unwanted intrusive thoughts they have each day. In addition, the diary can monitor how a person's vulnerability or risk of experiencing unwanted intrusive thoughts increases or decreases when they change their behavior in certain ways.

Second, it can be useful for people with OCD to make action plans to prepare themselves for situations that are likely to increase their risk of experiencing intrusive thoughts. Action plans may also help individuals to carry out other assignments more easily, such as confronting the meaning behind their intrusive thoughts, eliminating them from their minds, or looking out for alternative ways of living with these types of thoughts without letting them get in the way of their lives.

Third, people with OCD need to engage in behavioral experiments because they may need to determine whether their thoughts are true. For example, they may wish to challenge the thought, "I will not be able to stop myself from carrying out this type of behavior." But, of course, it is impossible to show that one cannot do something, so a more reasonable question would be, "Am I able to stop myself from doing this behavior?" This question can then be answered by carrying out different behavioral experiments.

A final point about confronting your thoughts is that it might help considerably if you have someone else who can provide external support as you carry out these experiments.

Step 7: Carry out assignments and practice new skills.

Here there are several exercises that you might consider. For example, the "unwanted thought diary" can monitor how a person's vulnerability or risk of experiencing unwanted intrusive thoughts increases or decreases when they change their behavior in certain ways. Often people with OCD find they can eliminate intrusive thoughts by carrying out behavioral experiments, particularly if they are performed in combination with other assignments. Moreover, many people with OCD have found it useful to keep a journal of their progress using the following worksheet.

Finally, as already mentioned, it is important to change the meaning behind unwanted thoughts, which can be done in several ways. One way is to employ thought-stopping. Another way is to participate in slow-wave therapy (SWT), based on research showing that people with OCD have hyperactive brains responsible for their intrusive thoughts. SWT tries to slow down a person's brain activity using visual or auditory stimulation. The visual stimulus involves having light in the person's eyes while inside an MRI machine (a safe type of magnetic resonance imaging scanner). The auditory stimulus involves listening to specific sounds while they are inside the scanner. SWT has been shown to reduce the impact of intrusive thoughts and is associated with improvements in cognitive function.

It is also important to carry out the suggested assignments because they may help you to challenge your thoughts and tell yourself that they are not true. This can be difficult when you have a genuine experience of anxiety, but it is important for you not to feel that you are doing a worthless thing, as this can make intrusive thoughts seem more powerful. In summary, your assignment might be to think about how much your thought bothers you, whether you could think about this without being anxious (or at least without being bothered) and whether there is any better way of coping with it.

Step 8: Use exposure and response prevention (ERP) to change your behavior

It is important to note that ERP is ineffective if it is not carried out consistently and regularly. Therefore, whenever you carry out assignments, you should try to do so as thoroughly as possible and with a high degree of commitment. For example, you should make sure that when carrying out exposure tasks concerning confronting your thoughts, you ensure that you are in the same environment each time (e.g., at home), so it might be helpful to try to carry these out at the same time each day.

ERP involves trying to think about your unwanted thoughts without being anxious. It involves consciously stopping yourself from carrying out the type of behavior you have been anxious about. These assignments aim not to get rid of intrusive thoughts but to practice not thinking about them for a short period. To do this, carry out at least one exposure task and one response prevention task each day to challenge your intrusive thoughts.

It may be helpful if you find it difficult to change your behavior by yourself, for example, if you are very anxious about not carrying out your assignments. You should seek help from a therapist or another person who can support you in your attempts to manage your intrusive thoughts and help you with other aspects of OCD.

A therapist or other professional must help with exposure tasks and response prevention, as you may need regular feedback on how well these are going. Still, it can also be helpful if the task is done in a supportive way.

How to overcome addiction and substance abuse

Rehab. It's something a lot of people have to go through, but it's not always easy. When you're coming from an addictive lifestyle, it might seem like you'll never be able to fully recover from the drugs or alcohol that have been controlling your life for so long. You might feel hopeless and like rehab is just a waste of time. But here are some important things to know before making this decision:

The first step in overcoming addiction is understanding that there is no "just one drink."

This is a common tactic used by people in denial – they will rationalize their way around their addiction and attempt to convince themselves that this one drink isn't a big deal. But it is a big deal because no matter how much you want to be sober, you cannot trust yourself around alcohol. You would not be reading this book or considering addiction treatment if you weren't already convinced it was okay to give up alcohol entirely.

You may have been using alcohol daily for a long time, so your decision to enter treatment is a lot riding on. If you decide not to go through with it, you will have the rest of your life to regret it.

Take some time to consider if you want to do this. You might be wondering what's so scary about getting clean and sober – even considering that the only thing worse than an addict could is an addict who doesn't ever get clean. The truth is that addiction takes hold of you in ways that can be very hard to control once it gets a hold of you and keeps you trapped in its grasp forever. You will be much happier and healthier if you get sober now.

Stay clean and sober if you are deathly afraid of being an addict for the rest of your life. It's much better to be a recovering alcoholic than it is not to be an alcoholic at all. If you're not ready yet, don't feel bad about that – after all, what kind of self-respecting addict would even consider entering rehab if they weren't at least a little bit concerned about their future? But once you've decided, do not doubt that doing so is right for you.

If you've already tried rehab, or if you're not sure whether or not you're ready to get sober, go into recovery by yourself.

This is one of the smartest things that can be done to deal with a problem as serious as addiction. While it might look like you're going in alone, some people have gone through similar experiences in the past and are more than willing to help any newcomer out. That person could be a family member; a friend; or an acquaintance who has done it before and can tell you how the process works. It could even be someone at the treatment center getting ready for their trip through rehab.

You will feel alone at first in this situation. Even if you're going through detox and feel that it's not as bad as you thought it would be, there are still many difficult things to get through on your own. That makes every day in recovery feel like a new beginning to all the old feelings and behaviors you have been accustomed to. At this point, the best thing to do is to go with the flow and try not to stress over your recovery too much. The fact is that getting clean, sober, and staying that way is hard work on its own. But when people show love and support during this time of transition, they can help keep you on track in your journey towards long-term sobriety.

Many drug and alcohol rehab centers can help you if you don't know where to start. They have licensed professionals who can guide you through all of the steps involved in getting clean. In addition, they have all the facilities and resources needed to ensure that you don't just go through detox but also go through detox and treatment in a way that is safe for your physical health, mental health, and entire lifestyle as a whole.

When entering any drug or alcohol treatment, it's important to remember that recovery takes time and to understand the expected results of different programs.

Therefore, these tips can help you overcome addiction and substance abuse:

1.   Commit to Developing and Following a Personal Recovery Plan.

A personal recovery plan is a powerful tool that helps people learn what they need to do to overcome addiction and substance abuse. A personal recovery plan is a document that lays out all the steps involved in getting clean and sober. It centers on what must be done, how it must be done, and when it must be done.

A personal recovery plan is designed for people who are still in the process of trying to understand addiction and substance abuse. A personal recovery plan guarantees that people will understand the problem and know what needs to be done about it.

A personal recovery plan provides a sense of responsibility for oneself, family, friends, and loved ones who might experience adverse drug or alcohol abuse effects. A personal recovery plan is an effective tool that can be used by people of all ages, genders, nationalities, and religious affiliations. A personal recovery plan is the cornerstone of managing addiction and substance abuse.

A personal recovery plan ensures people have a sense of ownership over their lives and well-being.

2.   Learn Effective Coping Skills and Life Skills During Addiction Treatment.

Life skills are essential to help people understand how to control their life instead of letting alcohol or drugs control them. Life skills also help people manage their everyday stress positively, so they won't be tempted to resort to drug or alcohol consumption just because things aren't going right with their lives.

Effective coping skills can also help people manage their emotions and lower the stress in their lives. For example, one successful approach would be learning a new skill, such as how to fold laundry or make a nutritious meal for dinner. In addition, people who go through addiction treatment and recovery can use these coping skills to keep themselves out of trouble and on the right path.

The more effective coping skills people use, the less likely they will resort to alcohol or drugs because of stress. Effective coping skills combined with other techniques, such as learning effective life management techniques, have been proven to help people quickly overcome addiction issues by preventing relapse.

3.   Do Not Fret About Relapse During Addiction Treatment.

Relapse is a natural part of recovery, and it's something that all people will experience during addiction treatment. However, relapse does not mean failure. Instead, relapse happens because it is a part of the recovery process. Addiction treatment approaches and techniques can help people mitigate this challenge through relapse prevention techniques and therapies.

There are many approaches to help prevent relapses in different stages of recovery. Therapies that prevent relapse are very effective as they can be offered to anyone thinking about relapsing or someone who has been identified as having a higher risk for relapse. In addition, effective therapy can be done in a short period, providing long-term benefits to the person undergoing treatment.

4.   Find a Mentor in an Effective Addiction Treatment Program.

When people go through addiction treatment, they have to engage in an interactive experience that involves more than just attending lectures and watching videos. The experience should involve people learning from other human being who has been through what they are going through right now during their recovery process. This person doesn't have to be a professional counselor. One of the best mentors is another individual who has successfully overcome addiction issues and is living a clean and sober lifestyle today.

Mentors can show people the steps needed in their journey to help them overcome addiction and substance abuse issues. They can help people understand what works for them, as well as what doesn't work for them.

Mentors can be a driving force in helping people succeed in their recovery endeavors. They can act as mentors, teachers, and role models during the treatment process. In addition, mentors are often important to keep people connected during this transition, so they can continue performing on a positive note after they are released from rehab.

5. Learn About the Recovery Process.

People entering addiction treatment should be prepared for what will be expected of them during the recovery process. They should be prepared to follow a good approach to achieve a successful and sustainable recovery. This can help them successfully learn how to overcome addiction and substance abuse issues in the long run.

The good news is that there are many effective ways of getting clean and sober, and people who want to get sober can learn about these ways in addiction treatment programs. There are many types of programs like residential treatment, outpatient treatment, intensive outpatient treatment, day programs, and more. These programs are tailored according to an individual's needs and their commitment to recovering from this life-shattering disease called addiction or substance abuse.

There are also many addiction treatment approaches like 12-step programs, non-12-step programs, holistic approaches, and more. These different approaches work in different ways to provide effective addiction treatment.

By learning how these different approaches work toward helping people get sober and stay sober in the long run, people will be able to make better choices in their recovery process. In addition, people can make more right decisions without relying on others during their recovery process.

Addiction Treatment Can Help People Get Clean After Neglecting It For So Long

There are many reasons why people end up neglecting addiction treatment and recovery for such a long period. The good news is that no matter why people neglect addiction treatment, it's never too late to get some help and create a new and better life for themselves. The earlier they get treatment, the easier it will be for people to overcome addiction issues throughout their life.

Addiction treatment can positively change lives so that people who have neglected to get help in the past can be more confident in their future. People struggling with an addiction issue right now should take advantage of available resources by attending effective drug rehab. It's never too late to get sober, so there is no need for addicts to wait when help is readily available at their doorstep.

Recovery is a process that requires accountability and commitment. Recovery is not just about what an individual does but how the individual behaves after participating in the recovery. People who truly want to recover from substance abuse problems and addiction must ensure they get the most out of their recovery. The sooner people get treatment, the easier it will be for them to overcome addiction problems.

Many different types of programs are available today, so there is no reason not to be willing to get help if you have denied yourself this type of support system before. The more time passes without attending an addiction treatment program, and the more difficult recovery will become. Don't let your fear of recovery stop you from getting help by attending a good addiction treatment program.

Many decisions can be made in life, and people often find themselves paralyzed by the choices in front of them. People who want to recover from an addiction or substance abuse problem must commit to getting the help they need. When people get treatment, they can address their addiction issues head-on effectively, improving their long-term chances of recovery.

People who avoid getting help only make it difficult for themselves and their loved ones to address addiction problems as they progress further into their addictions.

How to understand yourself through ACT

Acceptance and Commitment Therapy (or ACT) is a 4 – step psychological process that can help greatly in improving one's life. The first step of ACT, as stated by its founder -- Steven Hayes, Ph.D. -- is to "take an accurate inventory" of oneself. This means objectively assessing how the person views themselves and their current situation.

In the second step of ACT, one must analyze whether the thoughts and feelings they have about themselves are based on reality or if they are instead based on unrealistic expectations that are not being fulfilled. The person is encouraged to accept if they are not based on reality. The third step of the ACT discusses how one's feelings and thoughts influence behavior. The third step helps one understand how they act and how this compels them to continue to act in certain ways.

In the fourth step, the person is encouraged to commit to change. This involves making an active choice to stop doing things they are now doing and start doing something different.

Steps 1-3 can be difficult for some people because it means accepting flaws, imperfections, or setbacks that have affected their lives in the past. It means facing emotions from the past. It also means looking clearly at the present situation because that is where one's behaviors are most likely to be repeated.

ACT is not a quick fix. Most people who use the methods of ACT for self-improvement will report that it takes time to accomplish their goals. The first step alone can take months or years because it involves an honest self-assessment and some difficult emotions.

Step 2, where one looks at the relationship between thoughts, feelings, and behavior, also involves facing both old experiences from the past and painful emotions from those experiences. This can also take time to work through because most people don't know how to go through this process. It requires gaining knowledge about one's personal history and understanding how they learned their behaviors as they grew up.

Every person says they want to improve themselves in some way. Unfortunately, many try to do this based on advice from other people and not by using the actual processes available through ACT. As a result, they may waste time and get frustrated and discouraged. However, people who have been helped by ACT can report that the methods have made a profound difference in their lives, leading them to higher levels of self-esteem, better relationships with others, and greater happiness. Instead of being constrained by the past, they can say they have learned to live in the present and plan for a bright future.

These tips can help in understanding yourself through ACT

1. Acceptance:

Acceptance is the first step in the ACT. Accepting is accepting that you are imperfect, flawed, or incomplete. You can't change what you don't acknowledge first. For example, frequently resentful or unforgiving people cannot accept themselves because of their inability to accept others as they are. Accepting others helps us to accept ourselves, too, because we realize there is nothing wrong with us and that we need not be so hard on ourselves.

2. Commitment:

Commitment is the second step of ACT and involves making a genuine choice in favor of your growth objectives (our goals). We commit to improving our life by making an active choice to stop doing something that is not working and start doing something else that will work better for us. Commitment means putting forth a higher effort and doing what is required to reach our goals.

3. Values:

A value is something that you think is important and meaningful in your life. It may be a goal, ideal, belief, quality, or experience you want to increase in your life. There are two types of values: terminal values and instrumental values. A terminal value is an ultimate aim or the highest goal you hope to achieve in your life, while an instrumental value refers to the steps needed to reach a terminal value. If our behavior conflicts with our values, we experience cognitive dissonance, which refers to psychological stress experienced when two attitudes or beliefs are inconsistent.

4. Life Compass:

The life compass is an easy way to remember the steps of the ACT. The steps are A-Acceptance, C-Commitment, and T-Values. This is a simple way to remember these terms and the order of the process (A-C-T). Remember that this process cannot be rushed; it takes time, patience, and growth on your part, but it can make all the difference in your life.

5. List Activities:

It is important to know what activities you perform daily and then identify the ones that work and those that don't. You want to identify the activities that keep you doing what you are doing when you are not working on improving yourself. Once you have identified these activities, one of the best ways to change them is by identifying those that lead to a healthy life. If most of your daily life has been filled with unhealthy habits, it will be much easier for you to change them.

6. Observe Your Thoughts:

People who have friends or family members who think they are depressed but aren't are often unaware of their thoughts. However, this may indicate that they are depressed because they have been close to them for so long. This can also make it seem like the depression is less intense when it may be more severe. Listening to your thoughts can help you better identify the reasons for your depression and what makes you feel good about yourself.

7. Positive Affirmation:

A positive affirmation is a statement that reflects or describes a positive truth about yourself. This helps you recognize your positive traits, acknowledge them, and appreciate how they make you feel good about yourself.

8. Mindfulness:

Mindfulness is the ability to be fully aware of and attentive to what is happening in the present moment. It means being aware of your thoughts and feelings without judging or getting caught up in them.

9. Self-forgiveness:

This is when you accept yourself for who you are, forgive yourself for the mistakes you make, and move forward with your life. Self-forgiveness means releasing regrets from the past, forgiving others to free yourself from guilt, and finding a new way to live that is full of love and joy once again.

10. Mindfulness Meditation:

Mindfulness meditation teaches you how to sit quietly and focus on your breathing as you pass judgment on any other thoughts that interfere with your concentration. This allows you to be more aware of your thoughts, feelings, and emotions without being attached.

Mindfulness meditation is a simple way to learn how to achieve a state of mind that is more connected to oneself, others, and the world around them.

11. Acceptance and commitment therapy online:

There are many online courses that you can use to learn about acceptance and commitment therapy. This will greatly increase your understanding of ACT (Acceptance and Commitment Therapy) which can help you achieve a better balance in your life through these processes. Moreover, reading self-help books is also a great way to learn more about ACT.

12. Change:

Change is inevitable, and it is important to embrace it to improve your life. Change can be hard at first, but once you can accept change, you will find new ways of reaching your goals and improving yourself as a person. If you do not want change, you are likely doing something that is not working for you and will add stress to your life, leading to depression.

13. Self Regulation and Values:

Self-regulation is the ability to control your emotions and thoughts to achieve your goals. This is a crucial part of ACT because it helps you deal with any obstacles that prevent you from reaching your valued goals.

14. Relationship:

It has been said that we are never more than 6 degrees away from one another. In other words, everyone is connected in some way or another. Therefore, healthy relationships with others can help improve our feelings about ourselves, our environment, and the world around us. In contrast, unhealthy relationships can cause stress and anxiety, interfering with our ability to learn, grow and improve.

15. Explore:

Sometimes it is good to explore new things that can help improve your life and learn new skills you never thought you would have. Remember that if you don't try, you will never know what could have happened, and exploring new things can also help prevent depression because this gives you something positive to focus on in your life.

16. Act:

Yes, action is one of the steps in ACT, and it is important to take action by following the step before it (that is, the pre-conditions). You are making changes and improving yourself by taking action, which means that those thoughts and feelings will no longer burden your mind.

17. Routine:

Having a routine can help you improve your life by teaching you discipline and giving you a better sense of structure in your daily life. In addition, when you follow a routine, you are more likely to accomplish your goals, feel happier and be more successful. But remember that having a routine does not mean that your life will be dull; the key lies in finding a balance between the excitement of your daily life, spontaneity, and adding new things into your routine.

18. Tell Others:

Telling others is a powerful way to address any problems, issues, or concerns we may have as individuals. It is important to remember that while others may not understand you at first, they can be great support mechanisms and provide the guidance, comfort, and feedback that we need.

19. Problem Solving:

Problem-solving is one of the most important steps in the ACT because this step helps you deal with your emotions and thoughts by finding a solution to them instead of letting them control you. This step often works hand-in-hand with acceptance because it allows us to learn from our experiences, deal with emotional pain and find meaning in our actions.

20. Find Help:

If you feel that you cannot make progress in your life, if you cannot solve problems or find meaning in your life, then it is best to seek help from a professional psychologist or counselor. It can improve your life if you learn about the things that are affecting it, such as your thoughts and feelings, and understand what needs to change to achieve balance in your life. ACT has been proven effective in treating many psychological issues such as depression and anxiety; learning more about this process will help you heal yourself more effectively

Application and benefits of ACT in everyday life

ACT is a therapeutic process that helps individuals and groups to accept who they are, work on unmet goals, and commit to positive change. The following book explores the possibilities of ACT in everyday life.

ACT is founded on the work of two models. The first, ACT, was developed by Jim Reinecke and first published in 1985 in his dissertation. The second model, called "The Interpersonal Theory of Conflict" (ITCC), was developed and published by David Shapiro and his colleagues Sheila Kitzinger and Stephen Hayes in 1983. While many therapists use elements from both approaches, some important differences are worth noting.

ACT promotes a goal-oriented clinical approach to working with clients. A therapeutic relationship is viewed as embracing at least one client together throughout an agreed-upon period. The therapist encourages a commitment to the therapeutic task and informs the client that changes may occur in how they define themselves and their world. The goal is not to set up a relationship that can be maintained indefinitely but can be used effectively in the here-and-now. ACT assumes that therapy is a change process to increase healthy behaviors and decrease dysfunctional ones rather than a process of understanding or insight. Ideas about this approach are drawn from both cognitive-behavioral and other related therapies.

ITCC seeks to understand how individuals relate to others as it relates to dysfunctional interpersonal behaviors. It is based on the assumption that there exist "conflictual cycles" in which persons engage in unfair treatment of others, resulting in a similar cycle of abusive and abusive responses by other persons toward the individual. The therapist's role involves fostering an ability to recognize these cycles and become aware of their existence. Thus, ITCC therapists aim for collaborative relationships with their clients with the view that such a relationship is the basis for change.

ACT and ITCC offer clinicians different ways of approaching their therapeutic tasks. While the emphasis is on collaborative relationships, the underlying belief systems differ. For example, ACT assumes that change relates to people's beliefs about themselves and the world. On the other hand, ITCC assumes that change involves learning to recognize and deal with conflictual behavior patterns rather than trying to effect personality change.

Therapists use either a behavioral or a cognitive approach in working with clients. A behavioral approach focuses on behavior as the vehicle for change; it is based on a belief that better behaviors are likely to occur when clients are aware of them (e.g., self-monitoring of client) and able to make and follow up on plans for achieving them. A cognitive approach focuses instead on the nature of thoughts, feelings, and perceptions concerning behavior. It emphasizes interpersonal processes in which clients consider how they think about themselves and others, how they feel about them, their relationships, their interactions with others, and so on.

The focus in therapy with ACT clients tends to be on what is happening in "here-and-now" situations as opposed to theory or conceptualization. The therapist uses the "experiential avoidance" framework to clarify with clients the unnecessary costs of attempting to control their subjective experiences. The idea is that therapy involves learning to "pay attention" rather than hiding from or trying to avoid internal experiences and feelings. The emphasis is on helping clients commit themselves to a course of action in which they will see consistent positive results rather than a course of action that may result in failure or negative consequences.

Therefore, these tips can guide the application of ACT in everyday life:

a. Identify the "here and now" situations in which you are currently trying to manage your life by avoiding unacceptable feelings/subjective experiences.
b. Identify the "abusive strategies" you've used to manage these situations and consider how these strategies have affected you in terms of interpersonal relationships with others, self-esteem, and health.
c. Make a concrete plan to begin using more healthy strategies for overcoming your negative patterns with the hope that this will bring about positive change in "here-and-now" situations regardless of what has happened previously in your life or what might happen on a theoretical level of planning, etc.
d. Commit yourself to making this plan work by practicing it before committing.
e. If you are experienced with ACT and ITCC, you may consider using a behavioral or cognitive approach in everyday life. If you are interested in learning more about behavioral approaches, please refer to the following book:

As we go through our everyday lives, we try to manage what happens using certain strategies. But not everything works well. Some strategies can be hurtful and harm others as well as ourselves. ACT therapists help individuals make the necessary changes in their lives by first gaining awareness of what they are doing now that gets them into trouble with others while hurting themselves.

Some things to watch out for are:

a. Trying to force other people or situations to do things your way. This can backfire and make the situation worse.
b. Not being truly present in any one moment of your day. For example, suppose you are in a meeting or interacting with another person. In that case, you may step away from that interaction just as it is getting interesting or exciting, and then when others try to bring you back in, it will be too late for them to continue what they need to say to you at the time it needs to be said.
c. Mind reading about the feelings of others is more accurate than their feelings (i.e., when you say to a friend, "I just know that you are angry with me because..."). This hurts the other person and can make them feel misunderstood.
d. Using the words "should" or "must" or attempting to be perfect at everything all the time. If you use these words, it will only bring about more unwanted pressure on yourself and others (i.e., saying to your spouse, "You should know by now that I 'must' be home from work no later than 6:30. It is 'should' be obvious to you that I need those 15 minutes to decompress before seeing the kids, etc.").
e. Attempting to control the outcome of events. In some circumstances, the outcome of an event is not possible to control, but in others, it is. (i.e., "If I am late for work again, I 'should' feel guilty about that and then should try harder to make my presence at work more predictable by taking my car in for an oil change, etc.")
f. Trying to control your feelings or what you feel or not feeling. It is helpful to know when you have used such a strategy and let it go now (i.e., "The other day I felt really angry when.").

Moreover, these are the benefits of ACT in everyday life:

a. Increased ability to tolerate or accept thoughts and feelings present at any moment.
b. More willingness to experience feelings as they are without trying to change them. This is an important component of being more fully human and staying connected to others (e.g., "I am not proud of myself for feeling 'this' way, but I can be proud of my willingness to step up and feel 'this' way.").
c. Breaks old patterns of avoiding and managing negative feelings, thoughts, and experiences.
d. Increased ability to be yourself in any given situation (except when controlling the outcome of events is desired).
e. Increased self-acceptance and a general feeling that life is more predictable and controllable (in general).
f. Decompression from chronic feelings of being overwhelmed by feelings or emotions, thoughts or actions that are upsetting to you.
g. A feeling of courage to follow through on an action plan you have made after carefully considering all the aspects of a situation.
h. Increased personal power over your immediate choices in spaces where there are few options available to you (i.e., when you are in a meeting, and the main speaker does not allow for input from others, you may say to yourself, "I can choose to 'stay' at this meeting or choose to 'leave' this meeting. Either way, I will survive it, and there are things I can learn from my experience here.")
i. The ability to take risks rather than being opposed to them (i.e., taking chances, making mistakes, and failing; these do not equal 'badness' or 'evil').
j. Feeling more confident in your abilities to handle situations that may arise from taking chances and making mistakes.
k. Increased ability to stand up and say "no" if necessary.
l. Increased feelings of self-compassion, love, and respect for self and others.

m.   The ability to step away from any thought or feeling that is upsetting to you when you are with others (i.e., if someone says something that triggers an angry response in you, you can say to yourself, "That's just the way they are talking right now" so that you can step back from your angry response).

n.   Greater access to what matters in your life and less time spent on things that don't matter (i.e., things like getting ready for work in the morning).

o.   Increased ability to "let go and be" in all of your experiences (i.e., in any situation, you can decide to "just let it be what it is" and "not try to shape or control events").

However, those new to ACT will sometimes initially feel overwhelmed by their thoughts, feelings, and behavior. This is normal and should not force you to decide on your life, but just an indication that you need some time to get comfortable with the new ideas. So do not worry if you feel disappointed, confused, or lost after hearing the above explanations for why you are doing what you are doing.

Therefore, it is very important to accept each new idea in the ACT and give yourself time to see if the idea works for you and fits your life. Some ideas might be useful soon, while others might take some time to work through your system.

When you first begin using ACT, it can be helpful to set aside a specific time every day for 10–15 minutes or so when you can read through the above explanations in one of the ACT books or listen to one of the tapes multiple times, until you understand the idea enough that it becomes a part of your life.

It is also a good idea to practice applying ACT to your life in real-time whenever possible to see how well it works for you.

Although you can take the above ideas from ACT and apply them to your life in any way that seems useful to you, you need to remember one thing:

ACT does not aim to change you or your behavior in any way. It aims to help you accept how things are, make sense of what is happening and then step up so that you can act in your own life instead of being stuck in old, harmful patterns. ACT will never ask you to stop caring for yourself or be perfect at everything. That would be another way to control others, feelings, or events (which would create more unwanted pressure on yourself).

ACT is about seeing the big picture of your life and figuring out what works for you, not just in your mind but in the real world. So be sure to only take the parts of ACT that fit you and your life while leaving all the rest behind.

Therefore, getting a feel for what will work well for you and what won't. Then, experiment with ACT to see if it helps you live a better life (rather than just letting new ideas overwhelm you). And no matter how well or poorly things go at first, do not give up too soon. Be prepared to try again and see if something eventually sticks with you or not (and then throw away whatever doesn't work).

How ACT can help you overcome rethinking holiday stress

According to the Anxiety and Depression Association of America, anxiety disorders affect 40 million adults (18.1%) in the United States aged 18 and older. If we look at just general anxiety disorder alone, that number jumps to 8.7% of young adults (ages 18-29) in this country.

It's easy to feel helpless when combating common anxieties such as the fear of public speaking or a fear of heights, but acceptance and commitment therapy is an evidence-based practice that can help you find peace with these fears by teaching you how to commit yourself fully to your desired goal despite any discomfort or negative feelings accompanying them on your path towards success.

The basic premise of acceptance and commitment therapy, or ACT for short, is that when we hold on to negative feelings about a situation – in other words, we continue to fear the future and thereby prevent it from happening – the only way to truly overcome the consequences of our developing anxieties is by admitting that those fears are a part of us.

To understand how ACT works, first, it's important that you understand what causes anxiety disorders. Dr. David Barlow offers this explanation in a New York Times book:

Anxiety disorders often begin in early childhood and are often linked to difficult experiences as children or teens. As children, we learn the rules of our culture and are forced to make decisions and take actions we don't want to do. We may feel ashamed or fail at those tasks, and when we're scared, we are also caught in a society that demands perfection.

As adults with anxiety disorders, we struggle with these same issues. We are often encouraged by our families, peers, and other people around us to be perfect; they want us to succeed in our careers and ambitions. However, when we experience an anxiety attack because of our fears about failure or imperfection, it can become very difficult for us because it's natural for us to be threatened by failure even if no one is trying to hurt us.

ACT teaches us that our anxiety disorders don't stem from the present; they stem from our past; each of us has learned to fear and react nervously towards certain situations. ACT helps individuals with their anxieties by teaching them how to identify and accept the feelings of their anxiety as a part of themselves, rather than trying to suppress them or run away from them.

It's important for you to understand that accepting your own anxieties doesn't mean that you approve of your anxiety disorders; it simply means that you are willing to fully experience the emotions that come with them. This is the first step towards being able to overcome your anxiety, but it's a step that's easier said than done. To illustrate this point, let's take a look at some of the common symptoms of anxiety disorders as defined by the Anxiety and Depression Association of America:

Therefore, ACT can help you overcome rethinking holiday stress through:

a.   Recognizing the triggers and triggers of others

This is important since many anxiety disorders are brought on by common triggers. For example, the fear of public speaking is brought on by social pressure and the fear of failure. If we're able to learn more about the situations that arise during our holidays (for example, large crowds, uncomfortable social interactions, and holiday pressure), we can better manage our anxieties.

b.   Learning to accept our own feelings

For us to accept our feelings and therefore overcome our anxieties, we must first acknowledge them as real parts of ourselves. It's important to understand that everyone experiences anxiety at some point in their lives; it's merely a matter of how much we allow these feelings to control our lives. ACT will teach you how to identify and fully experience your feelings without needing to change them.

c.   Practicing mindfulness

Mindfulness is a basic principle of ACT that teaches us how to be fully aware of the present moment – the good, the bad, and the ugly. It helps us take an analytical look at our emotions and understand that sometimes our anxiety disorders can rise out of fear, but they can also lead to positive outcomes if we are willing to embrace them.

For example, let's say that you're afraid of talking in front of a large group because you're worried about making mistakes or being humiliated in front of others. If you practice mindfulness, you will become more aware of the anxiety and the need for action that's incorporated with it. Mindfulness teaches us to:

1. Notice when we feel or think about our anxieties – for example when we're waiting in line at a crowded store
2. Accept and fully experience our feelings – for example, let's say that you have a fear of public speaking because your shyness makes it hard to speak up at work or in social situations
3. Remain present in these moments – even if they seem like embarrassing moments, you must remain mindful and do your best to keep cool and be attentive
4. Act with deliberate awareness – in other words, you must make a conscious effort to work with those feelings of anxiety instead of attempting to run away from them.

d. Remind ourselves that we're not alone

Even if you're the only person in your family who struggles with anxiety, it doesn't mean you must suffer silently. By being aware and accepting of your own feelings, you can lean on the support of others around you and ask for help when attending big holiday gatherings or traveling.

e. Finding personal rituals

It's important for us to have our own personal rituals that remind us that we are in control, not our anxieties. For example, if you're afraid of flying, you might want to write a list of things that make you happy and remind you of your loved ones. If your anxiety makes it hard for you to be alone, then try creating a playlist with songs that calm you down. And if you have the holiday blues, it may be helpful to listen to music that reminds us of the joys of the season.

f. Understanding the uncomfortable feelings

This is one of the most important parts of ACT since we must learn how to accept our feelings instead of bodily or emotionally pushing them away. The more we resist uncomfortable feelings or try to run away from them, the more they control us. If you feel that the holidays are a time in which you struggle the most with your anxiety, then it's recommended that you try to accept these feelings and find ways to be mindful of them.

ACT is an active treatment that teaches us how to be aware of our own feelings and thoughts instead of ignoring them or trying to run away from them. By implementing the five steps discussed above, we can overcome our anxiety over the holidays and eliminate many negative emotions and situations that arise during this stressful time of year.

g. Being willing to accept your own feelings

This is the most important part since it teaches us to take a step back from our emotions instead of trying to escape them. The more we try to avoid unpleasant situations or feelings, the more out of control we feel and the more anxious we become. It's important for you to understand that accepting your feelings doesn't mean that you approve of them. You must be willing to put yourself into uncomfortable situations for you to overcome your anxiety disorders.

ACT has helped many people with anxiety disorders, whether it's a fear of public speaking, performance anxiety, or even the holiday blues. There are a variety of techniques that can be used to help you overcome your fears, but one of the best ways to get started is by attending an anxiety treatment group where other people with similar disorders can offer their support and advice.

Since an increasing number of people suffer from anxiety and depression during the holidays, it's important for all of us to take action to help those who struggle with these difficulties. We can do this through practices such as mindfulness meditation and cognitive behavioral therapy (CBT), which have been proven effective in treating anxiety disorders.

h.   Don't fight your emotions

Our anxiety is often caused by our attempts to fight or avoid negative feelings and emotions. Instead, try practicing acceptance of these feelings and attempt to make sense of them. This means that you must stop trying to push away your worries and accept them as a natural part of life. By making space for uncomfortable emotions, you free yourself to live more fully in the present moment.

ACT teaches us that some of our most challenging emotions can be faced directly with mindfulness practices and acceptance exercises. These steps help us become more aware of our own thoughts, feelings, and sensations – even the painful ones – so we can reframe them and make sense of them instead of running from them or trying to change them.

i.   Finding meaning in our emotions

This means we must find a way to make sense of our feelings and thoughts. This never happens overnight, but by identifying what causes our anxiety and finding ways to explore and understand them, we can begin to unravel the thoughts that lead us down a path of confusion and depression.

To help ourselves with anxiety disorders, we must accept that these feelings are part of life. By learning how to work with them instead of fighting or avoiding them, we can begin building awareness and acceptance in our lives. By practicing acceptance, we become more mindful of the present moment instead of worrying about the past or future and how our anxiety will affect us.

j.   Acceptance is a process

If you struggle with anxiety, then you must understand that it's a disorder that will take time to overcome. You cannot fix these feelings with a magic pill or short-term solution. Instead, you must accept these feelings as part of your everyday life and work towards living a more fulfilling life. It's important for all of us to learn how to live with our problems instead of hoping that they will magically disappear. And once accepted, it's important to find a way to bring the anxiety into our daily life and learn to accept that these feelings will always be part of us.

ACT teaches us that we must accept our feelings, thoughts, and emotions as they come and that they are not necessarily bad or wrong. Our emotions are often a sign of things we need to work on or problems we need to solve to live fuller lives, which is why we should make a habit of accepting them.

k.   Our feelings are a part of us

ACT teaches us that our feelings are not necessarily good or bad, but they show us things we need to work on. By learning how to control our thoughts instead of our emotions, we learn how to move on with our lives and overcome issues that previously held us back. Since anxiety is a disorder in which negative thoughts cause anxiety and depression, it's important for us to understand the difference between feeling anxious and thinking the thought "I feel anxious".

Mindfulness with ACT

Mindfulness with ACT has helped me more than any other therapy I've tried. It has given me a greater sense of self-awareness, and my mind has also been infinitely calmer and happier. It's the most amazing thing that's happened to me so far in my life, and I would encourage anyone to try it out if they're interested in changing their lives for the better.

It's made such an impact on how I view myself and what I can do that I've taken part in a recent study conducted by MIND UK/NHS on its effectiveness: 'The Effect of Mindfulness-Based Therapy with Acceptance and Commitment Technique Compared to Behavioural Activation Treatment for Depression, which is published online today.

It's a groundbreaking study, one of the first of its kind to compare mindfulness to CBT for depression. It has raised many questions among awareness groups that I'd like to address here. Mindfulness with ACT (MwACT) is used for many conditions, including depression, anxiety, and addiction. Clients who have benefited from this approach report a reduction in their symptoms: an increased ability to feel better; fewer negative thoughts; and an overall sense that they have more control over their lives. As someone struggling with depression for some time, I'd like to share my personal experience with you and explain how it changed my life.

The arguments for the effectiveness of MwACT are simple. First, ACT is a therapeutic approach designed to help people understand how they think and feel and how those feelings affect their lives. It does this by training people to become more aware of their thoughts (cognitive) and feelings (affective) – not necessarily to change them, but so that we can be more effective at choosing our actions and how to best deal with them. This is an important skill that is often lacking in the lives of many people suffering from anxiety and stress, especially those who have ongoing problems with depression.

The use of mindfulness in treating depression is not new. Still, the excellent research on this topic led by Professor Mark Williams and colleagues at Cardiff University has made it clear that mindfulness can help people suffering from this condition. This explains why MwACT – i.e., mindfulness with ACT – has become popular among therapists who treat mental health conditions and sufferers.

Mindfulness is used within ACT to help us become more aware of the thoughts that typically upset us and lead us down into a battle with ourselves regularly, or 'fear-rages' as I call them (see here for more information). ACT helps us to become more able to observe these thoughts and their effects on our emotions and stop avoiding them by arguing with them or trying to 'fix' them. The resulting quietness is subsequently followed by a sense of greater freedom, perspective, and connection with ourselves, which leads to improved well-being.

With all this in mind, I want to give you my experience using mindfulness with ACT. I've been working with a therapist called Mark Jenkinson since May 2013 – and started doing the mindfulness element within my therapy shortly after that – so I'd like to share some of what I've learned over the last four months.

ACT therapists work with their clients directly. First, they ask you to set goals and targets for yourself, then work with you to identify the thoughts (cognitive) and feelings (affective) relevant to your situation. Once these are identified, they work together with you to encourage relaxation through breathing exercises to calm your mind and allow these thoughts and feelings to surface.

This means identifying the thoughts and feelings that are causing me distress (there are several ways to do this, including writing some down in a journal) and encouraging the body to relax to allow them to surface. Once I've settled down, I ask myself questions to identify what is happening (i.e., what am I thinking/feeling?). This usually involves asking myself if this thought or feeling is true or not – for instance, am I angry at someone? If the answer is yes, I would like it to be less likely that this will happen again – so instead of getting angry all the time, perhaps act milder next time. If the answer is no, I would like to eliminate it (i.e., not be angry at someone or anything).

Mindfulness with ACT can only really be understood by trying it out for yourself, and you can do this in many ways: try engaging in a simple mindfulness exercise, such as the one described here. Alternatively, you could do some research into the work of Jon Kabat-Zinn and his program Mindfulness-based Stress Reduction (MBSR), one of the best-known approaches to mindfulness today.

The results for MwACT are very positive. Essentially, it's about helping you to become more aware of your thoughts and feelings and allowing you to observe those thoughts in action. ACT helps you to do this by training you to become more aware of the present moment – that is, the reality around you – while simultaneously not trying too hard to change anything.

I believe that this approach is helpful for many different conditions, not just depression. I would point out that the research on the use of mindfulness with ACT is comparatively low, but this is changing with more and more studies being done every year. What's clear so far, however, is that it offers a very positive approach to dealing with the thoughts and feelings causing distress.

Mindfulness with ACT can help people overcome difficult thoughts by helping them become more aware of their everyday experiences and where they're thinking from within their own experiences. It helps them become more aware of their thoughts – although perhaps less so than traditional CBT – to let them go (i.e., let them exist rather than judge them). In this way, mindfulness with ACT leads to a state of awareness that helps to remove distress and improve well-being.

This leads to a much greater sense of calmness and control over your life, which I'm grateful for as it helps with my current depression. This is something that everyone can benefit from through mindfulness with ACT, including people who struggle with anxiety or stress.

Benefits of mindfulness with ACT include:

a. Greater self-control: as well as helping to remove the thoughts and feelings causing distress, ACT helps to identify your thoughts and feelings to understand them. It then helps you develop greater control over those thoughts rather than feeling powerless against them.
b. Self-knowledge: through mindfulness with ACT, you can gain greater awareness of yourself, including your values and what's important to you.
c. Greater self-acceptance: mindfulness with ACT helps you to accept yourself by allowing you more time to be by yourself without feeling judged or needing to change anything in particular.
d. Greater motivation: mindfulness with ACT helps you remain motivated to do things important to you (e.g., making art or music, etc.) and allows you to focus more on your values.
e. Greater connectedness: mindfulness with ACT leads to greater connectedness with yourself, others, and the world around you. This is because it helps you become more aware of your thoughts and feelings, rather than struggling against them or avoiding them by turning away (which often leads back into a battle).
f. Greater freedom: mindfulness with ACT helps you become freer from the thoughts and feelings causing distress. Again, this can be in terms of being less compelled to act in ways that lead to unhappiness or suffering (e.g., needing to control others – e.g., by finding a new partner, changing jobs, etc.).
g. Greater happiness: mindfulness with ACT leads to greater happiness because it helps you to become more aware of yourself and what's happening within your life, which helps you to be more at peace and content.

h. Greater satisfaction: mindfulness with ACT allows you to experience your thoughts and feelings as they are, without needing to change or avoid them. This leads to greater satisfaction (we can only be this way within ourselves).

i. Greater courage: mindfulness with ACT provides the space and trust required for you to do things that aren't normal or right but are important for you (e.g., get a new job, leave a current job, change course at university, etc.).

j. Greater optimism: mindfulness with ACT helps you to be more optimistic by helping you learn how to cope better when faced with stressful events and difficult situations.

k. Greater empathy: mindfulness with ACT helps you to develop a more compassionate attitude towards yourself and others (e.g., if you're sad, you don't feel the need to blame yourself or others for this).

l. Greater compassion: mindfulness with ACT helps you to develop a more compassionate attitude towards yourself and others. It helps you to stop judging yourself and others and allows you to become more humane.

m. Greater awareness: mindfulness with ACT helps you to become more aware of what's happening within your life, not just your ideas about things or the meaning that they have for you (e.g., failing to achieve something important, losing someone important in life).

n. Greater openness: mindfulness with ACT allows you greater openness towards life by helping reduce internal barriers that might be stopping you from being or feeling open (e.g., holding onto beliefs about how things should be, but it's different from reality).

o. Greater trust: mindfulness with ACT helps you gain greater confidence in yourself, including your self-efficacy (e.g., how capable you manage difficult thoughts and feelings).

p. Greater willpower: mindfulness with ACT helps you to have better willpower (e.g., to resist unhealthy food or habits, etc.).

q. Greater creativity: mindfulness with ACT leads to greater creativity in various ways, including music, painting, writing, and many more. This includes a greater sense of freedom and choice (e.g., being able to decide that it's okay not to do something).

r. Greater success: mindfulness with ACT leads to greater success in various areas, including personal and professional (e.g., moving forward at work to create something that you're passionate about or finding new friends who are supportive of your efforts).

s. Greater happiness and well-being: mindfulness with ACT helps you live a fuller life by lessening the stress and unhappiness you experience.

t. Greater contentment: mindfulness with ACT helps you to gain greater contentment by reducing the negative thoughts and feelings (e.g., self-criticism) that get in the way of feeling happy and satisfied with life.

u. Psychological flexibility (including flexibility of your mind), which leads to greater happiness and well-being: as mentioned above, psychological flexibility leads to a greater sense of happiness and well-being because it helps you to see things for what they are, rather than through them being colored by your thoughts or feelings about them. This includes accepting your thoughts and feelings, even those that might be causing you distress or making life difficult for you in some way (e.g., anxiety).

v. Psychological resilience (including resilience of emotions): this refers to higher levels of emotional and physical resilience, including more resilience of your emotions and other aspects of your life. This means that you are less easily stressed out about life's difficulties and less likely to suffer from depression and other mental health problems caused by stress.

How to introduce patients to mindfulness.

Acceptance and Commitment Therapy is trauma-informed, client-centered psychotherapy that was first introduced in the late 1990s. It can be applied to any issue — including to patients who suffer from PTSD or addiction.

It's based on the idea that we all have three important aspects of ourselves: our thoughts, our feelings, and our behaviors. ACoT aims to help patients become more aware of their thoughts, their emotions, and how they act to live more fulfilling lives by either changing or accepting their behaviors.

Acceptance is important to this foundation because it helps patients learn to accept their thoughts, feelings, and behaviors. A big reason we act in negative ways is because of the shame we give ourselves for being unable to change. To change mental health behaviors, we have to be able to accept what is happening.

Acceptance doesn't mean that problems go away; it just means that you don't fight them because you decide it's better to accept your situation and move forward differently.

Acceptance is a complicated and important concept that can be difficult to learn. However, with mindfulness training and therapy, you can start to develop acceptance toward yourself. Mindfulness involves maintaining a nonjudgmental awareness, or curiosity, of your thoughts, feelings, and body sensations.

To do this, you're challenged throughout your therapy sessions to observe these thoughts and feelings as if you were watching a movie rather than living it yourself.

This process helps you understand the root of your negative behaviors and thoughts to stop judging yourself for who you are or what has happened in the past. It also provides insight into changing your unhealthy behaviors into something more productive.

Mindfulness practices can help you accept your feelings, which is a vital step in therapy and recovery. Through mindfulness, you can understand what your feelings are telling you and how to respond more appropriately.

This practice is also important because it helps you understand the connection between thoughts and feelings. For example, when we get into certain situations that make us feel a certain way, we often think about our past experiences or worry about things going wrong in the future.

Mindfulness helps remove these thought processes from the equation so that we can focus on the present moment — which helps us understand what's causing our emotions to surface in the first place.

Finally, mindfulness can help you establish acceptance toward others by reminding you that there's a good chance that they're experiencing similar challenges. This outlook helps you focus on the present — your relationship with them, what's happening right now — as opposed to dwelling on how they may have hurt or wronged you in the past.

Another important practice is monitoring what you say to yourself and others. This practice is done through self-talk. Self-talk is a type of dialogue that takes place inside your head, and it usually involves words and phrases like "I should," "I must," or "I have to."

We don't usually realize we're repeating these things to ourselves so that we can become more aware of how our negative thoughts affect how we act. As a result, we can begin to reframe these kinds of statements and change how they affect us.

Examples of self-talk include: "I shouldn't be here, I should have brought a book to read," or "I can't stand this pain. I need a drink and a cigarette." During sessions, you can practice mindfulness exercises like observing your thoughts as if watching a movie rather than living it as you talk about your past experiences or worry about what may happen in the future.

The following tips can help you learn how to introduce patients to mindfulness:

a. Find a comfortable space

Mindfulness is all about being present in the moment. So, finding a space where you can comfortably sit and focus on your breath without distraction is important. It's best to find a space that doesn't have any distractions like television or cell phones.

b. Start with one minute at a time

When introducing your patients to mindfulness practices, start with one minute of concentrated breathing.

Start by focusing on your breath and counting each time you exhale for 30 seconds. After 30 seconds, take 1-2 deep breaths and then return to concentration.

Once this becomes easier, increase the time you spend on concentration from 30 seconds to 60 seconds. Once you feel comfortable with this, increase the time to one minute, the recommended length of a mindfulness exercise.

c. Start with your breath and then move on to your body

So many of us are so distracted by our thoughts that we lose touch with our bodies. Start by focusing on your breathing and then slowly move to include other body parts that you may normally shut out, like the pain in your back or feet.

d. Practice what you've learned regularly

The more you practice mindfulness, the easier it will be to apply it to daily life. Practicing mindfulness is the same as any other skill; it takes time and practice to become comfortable with the new way of thinking.

e. Start by merely observing your thoughts

You can learn more about yourself and others by observing your thoughts and feelings without judgment. Try not to judge or react strongly when negative thoughts enter your mind during this exploration. Instead, focus on being present in the moment as if you were watching a movie — which means no reacting or saying anything because that would be like being in the movie too!

f. Let this be the beginning of a new behavior

Mindfulness has many benefits, including the ability to focus on your breathing while having a conversation with another person. But mindfulness can also help you make more positive choices in your life that can benefit you and others.

g. Keep it simple

Simplicity is important to understanding mindfulness, so try focusing on one part of self-talk or movement at a time. Also, when using guided imagery, this should happen very quickly so that it's easy for patients to follow along without being distracted by too much detail.

h. Don't force the process

Not everyone is interested in mindfulness or what it can do for them. Take things slow and make sure that your patients are receptive to mindfulness before trying to make it a more regular activity in your sessions together.

i. Have your patient practice with a partner or therapist

Partners, friends, and family members can also be good candidates for practicing mindfulness exercises with patients. Practicing mindfulness with another person provides an added benefit because it creates a bond between people. Also, it's easier for patients to practice with someone who may have similar problems and can relate to their struggles rather than someone who will judge them for having similar feelings or thoughts.

j. Don't forget to ask your patient about the benefits they have noticed

Whether your patient is having trouble sleeping, staying focused on a task, or thinking positively, ask your patient if they notice a benefit from practicing mindfulness. If so, encourage patients to continue practicing on their outside of sessions.

k. Be prepared for setbacks

Patients often have strong beliefs about what will help them in life — be it alcohol or drugs, working long hours, and not taking time for themselves or even relationships with other people. These beliefs may surface before the benefits of mindfulness can be realized, and they can create temptations that make it difficult to stay on track with mindfulness practice.

Once patients feel like mindfulness is a beneficial lifestyle change, encouraging them to practice mindfulness on their own at home can help them maintain the benefits.

l. Keep yourself grounded

It's important to note that self-doubt can be just as much of a problem as an addiction for patients.

As an addiction treatment center counselor, it can be easy to get caught up in the success of your patients. But you mustn't lose yourself in their experiences and remain grounded in what your own experiences have taught you about mindfulness and recovery from addiction.

m. Don't overdo it and burn out

Sometimes less is more when introducing people to mindfulness because they will automatically incorporate mindfulness into their lives without trying too hard once they understand the concept.

But it's important to remember that mindfulness is not an on-off activity — it's a way of being present in the moment and living.

n. Make mindfulness available at your addiction treatment center

Being available to patients interested in learning more about mindfulness will help you get through practicing mindfulness at home more quickly.

o. Be willing to make changes as you learn more about your patients and their needs

It can be hard for counselors and addiction specialists to change their practices as they discover new ways to help people move forward in recovery from addiction or other mental health conditions. However, being open to new techniques will allow you to better serve your patients and see the best results.

p.   Use mindfulness in other ways at your treatment center

Like how you incorporate mindfulness into individual treatment sessions, you can include mindfulness in group counseling and other activities at your addiction treatment center. Mindfulness can benefit active addiction care programs, relapse prevention programs, and inpatient sub-acute mental health addiction treatment programs.

q.   Observe how people respond to different exercises or practices

Like anything else, some patients will respond better to one type of exercise than another. This varies from person to person, so experiment with different exercises or practices to find out what works best for your patients.

r.   Ask your patient to create their mindfulness exercise

Patients need to do their mindfulness exercises at home because this provides a sense of ownership over the practice. This allows them to set goals for themselves and take ownership of the results they are getting from practicing mindfulness on their own.

s.   Provide ideas or resources that will help your patient learn more about mindfulness

You can help your patients find resources related to what they have learned in therapy if they are interested in learning more about different types of exercise that may be helpful with their recovery process.

t.   Refer your patient to other resources if they are interested

There are several techniques, practices, and ideas that you can use when introducing mindfulness exercises to patients. If they are interested in learning more about other techniques, take the time to learn more about mindfulness and share what you have learned.

u.   Encourage your patient to share their successes with others

If your patient is practicing mindfulness exercises at home, ask them how they feel about the results and if they want to continue following through with the practices after treatment.

Mindfulness is a therapy to treat depression, anxiety, stress, and sleep disorders. Mindfulness-based therapies such as mindfulness meditation are regularly used to treat pathological levels of thought patterns and negative emotional states in treating children with ADHD. When used with children, mindfulness-based therapies have been shown to reduce hyperactivity and academic challenges, improve concentration and reduce depression and social anxiety symptoms in children. It has also been shown to help treat physical ailments such as pain and blood pressure.

Stress management through mindfulness

Stress management through mindfulness is becoming increasingly popular. As a result, more and more people are trying to find ways to reduce their levels of anxiety by enrolling in acceptance and commitment therapy (ACT). ACT is a cognitive-behavioral therapy designed for people suffering from psychological issues such as depression or anxiety. It is based on the idea that our lives have three systems: automatic thoughts, values, and action tendencies. Automatic thoughts can be beliefs about ourselves or others that seem true but do not match reality; values are things we care about; action tendencies are the patterns of behavior we have associated with our goals at any given time. A therapist will help an individual address stressful thoughts with evidence-based strategies. The client will then develop a written acceptance plan, or effortful commitment plan (ECP), that looks at values, action tendencies, and automatic thoughts associated with their goals in life. An ECP will help the individual identify how they can reduce their anxiety and negative affect levels by taking specific actions towards their goals in life. An ECP is often used because it is quick and easy to fill out and a very effective method of managing stress. Individuals can refer to their ECP whenever they need a reminder of what they should do to meet their goals.

Despite the positive results that ACT has shown, many therapists report that adherence is still a problem in their practice. This is because people often struggle with understanding the concepts of mindfulness, automatic thoughts, and values. It can be difficult for an individual to understand the connection between mindsets and automatic thoughts. Understanding the difference between mindfulness and values can also be confusing and overwhelming.

The key reason adherence has been so difficult for many therapists is that there are many different ways to achieve mindfulness. For example, in ACT, many different mindfulness strategies can be used. They include mindful awareness, compassionate acceptance, and non-judgmental observation. Each strategy has a unique purpose and is designed for a different goal. For example, attentive awareness is often used to curb negative thoughts and damaging beliefs about oneself or others.

In contrast, non-judgmental observation can be used to develop more positive feelings about oneself and others by practicing thought sampling. The idea behind sympathetic resonance is that clients will start feeling better because they will recognize when they hear their inner voice (automatic thoughts) instead of engaging in repetitive cycles of negativity towards themselves and others. Thus, this is a very specific and targeted technique that focuses on the individual's goals in life.

For therapists, it can be difficult to understand how mindfulness can help individuals manage stressful thoughts. This is because it is a very complex concept that concerns the mind and body. As a result, ACT therapists often ask their clients to practice mindfulness meditation. This meditation technique involves concentrating on a single point of focus for as long as possible, which can look like following one's breath or focusing on one's body weight in a certain way. However, although therapists sometimes recommend mindfulness meditation, it has often been shown to have little effect on a person's situation. This is because the different forms of mindfulness are not all intended for the same purpose. Therefore, it can be difficult for an individual to practice one form of mindfulness alone without practicing the other forms that ACT suggests. In addition, those who practice meditation for a long period may suffer from various health problems such as back pain or insomnia.

Mindfulness is effective in reducing stress and anxiety in both adults and children above the age of 8 years old. However, research shows that this can only be achieved when there is a safe environment where people can practice mindfulness. Mindfulness is not only about the practice of attending to full awareness of one's experiences and inner thoughts, but it also involves the reduction of harmful thoughts and stressful experiences. Because it can be very difficult for people to learn how to deal with their stress and anxiety on their own, many therapists will recommend that their clients attend group therapy to practice mindfulness and learn new skills. For example, a therapist may ask one of their clients to go over goals with a partner they both know to stimulate conversations about what they are doing in life and how they plan to achieve them.

Therefore, these tips can guide stress management through mindfulness:

a. Practice mindfulness meditation daily by focusing on one single point of focus, such as following one's breath or focusing on one's body weight while standing up. If a person is already practicing mindfulness, they should practice paying attention to the moment rather than concentrating on a particular thought or feeling. For example, if a person feels anxious, they should instead notice their breath coming in and going out rather than thinking about how anxious their feelings are. This will help them reduce their anxiety levels and improve their states of mind.

b. Practice mindful awareness daily by using compassionate acceptance as a different way to perform mindful awareness. For example, in compassionate acceptance, a person should not try to control their thoughts but rather try to notice thoughts connected to their goals.

c. Practice sympathetic resonance every day by trying to listen without judging the inner voice of oneself or others. This means that you will start to recognize when your automatic thoughts are repeating themselves and can change how you respond to them. You will also be able to acknowledge and value your feelings, even though these feelings may sometimes differ from those of others around you who share similar goals in life.

d. Practice mindful awareness by identifying and then working through any harmful automatic thoughts that may be causing problems for an individual's goals in life. For example, suppose a person notices that they have fallen back into their old ways of thinking and responding to stressful experiences. In that case, they should try to identify these harmful thoughts as quickly as possible to return to their goals. For example, if an individual feels sad or angry toward their partner, they should try to pay attention to the situation to identify what is causing this emotion.

e. Practice mindful awareness by maintaining proper posture when standing and sitting. For example, an individual should sit with good posture and ensure they are not slouching while exercising or feeling stressed. This will help them feel better physically while helping with their anxiety and stress levels in the long run.

f. Practice sympathetic resonance by listening to the internal voice of oneself or others without judging it. This way, you can avoid getting into a negative cycle of repetitive harmful thoughts and feel better about yourself and your life goals.

g. Practice mindful awareness by focusing on personal values rather than getting caught up in harmful thoughts about an individual's close relationships. For example, people should concentrate on their relationships rather than comparing themselves to those around them who may be more successful or have achieved more overall goals in life thus far.

h. Practice mindful awareness by using positive self-talk instead of talking negatively to oneself or others throughout a stressful experience. Research shows that this can increase a person's self-esteem, decrease their anxiety and stress levels and improve their overall outlook on life.

i. Practice sympathetic resonance by listening to the internal voice of oneself or others without judging it. This way, you can avoid getting into a negative cycle of repetitive harmful thoughts and feel better about yourself and your life goals.

j. Practice mindful awareness by focusing on personal values rather than getting caught up in harmful thoughts about an individual's close relationships. For example, people should concentrate on their relationships rather than comparing themselves to those around them who may be more successful or have achieved more overall goals in life thus far.

k. Practice mindful awareness by using positive self-talk instead of talking negatively to oneself or others throughout a stressful experience. Research shows that this can increase a person's self-esteem, decrease their anxiety and stress levels and improve their overall outlook on life.

l. Practice compassionate acceptance by understanding that children may not be able to follow in their parent's footsteps. Instead, parents should try to nurture their children's talents and strengths and help them to overcome some of their weaknesses. This will encourage children to feel better about themselves more consistently and more confident in pursuing goals in life.

Mindfulness can be applied as a therapeutic intervention in any field of medicine but is particularly beneficial and highly recommended as a coping mechanism for chronic illness management. As a result, the medical community has suggested that mindfulness training should be incorporated into many treatment plans for various health problems. Mindfulness can be beneficial for improving coping with chronic pain, stress, anxiety, and depression. For example, in one study, patients who practiced mindfulness meditation for eight weeks reported significantly less pain and psychological distress than patients who did not practice. Similarly, patients participating in a 12-week mindfulness program could also decrease their stress levels, depression, and negative outlook on life. In addition to these improvements in psychological health, many participants also experienced an improvement in their chronic health problems (for example, a reduction in pain), indicating that mindfulness may be especially beneficial to people with chronic illness management.

Mindfulness has been defined differently, but a few common components are found in these definitions. One definition is "a moment-to-moment awareness of thoughts, feelings, and bodily sensations." This means that mindfulness is not only about the practice of attending to full awareness of one's experiences and inner thoughts, but it also involves the reduction of harmful thoughts and stressful experiences. Mindfulness also involves being aware of and accepting emotions like pain while decreasing suffering, which is beneficial in managing chronic pain. Another definition of mindfulness is "the awareness that emerges through paying attention on purpose, in the present moment, and nonjudgmentally to the unfolding of experience moment-by-moment." This definition stresses the importance for practitioners to observe when a client's mind wanders onto a negative thought that may perpetuate thoughts in an ongoing cycle that causes harm. Mindfulness can be applied as a therapeutic intervention in any field of medicine but is particularly beneficial and highly recommended as a coping mechanism for chronic illness management.

The next chapter will discuss Highly Sensitive Empath. This is when people are highly sensitive to pain, emotions, and their surroundings. Their nervous system is hyperactive and can be overwhelmed by many stimuli. As a result, they often have high anxiety and depression but can also be high functioning on many levels because of the challenges they face in the world.

This brings us to the second kind of Sensitivity. Highly sensitive people are very aware and reactive to all things happening around them, especially related to pain and emotions. These individuals' nervous system is hyperactive and can be overwhelmed by too many blissful stimuli like music, smells, sensations, tastes, etc. They often have high anxiety and depression but can also be high functioning on many levels because of the challenges they face in the world. They are more often introverted than other groups of people. Highly sensitive people have greater empathic abilities and are more intuitive. Unfortunately, highly sensitive people can suffer from underemployment; they lack the resources to manage their higher awareness and sensitivity (possibly because they do not know how).

HIGHLY SENSITIVE EMPATH

CHARACTERISTICS OF A HIGHLY SENSITIVE PERSON

Highly Sensitive Empaths are people who automatically feel others' emotions and the world around them, just as other people feel the good or bad colors in their immediate surroundings. They might constantly be moved by different sights, like a church mural, which is why they may appear distracted or in tears at times. Highly Sensitive Empaths get thrown off by bright lights, loud noises, rough fabrics, or people crowding into small spaces. When empaths reach their limit, they can become introverted and reclusive. They are so deeply in touch with their feelings that the slightest thing can lift them to the heights of happiness or plunge them down into the depths of depression.

Empaths are often unusually sensitive to electricity and electromagnetic fields from light bulbs, stereos, and computers. As a result, they may psychically pick up thoughts or "feel" when someone is approaching long before others sense it.

Highly Sensitive Empaths are also often very creative people who may express themselves through art, writing, music, and dance. They also have above-average empathy for other people's problems and can be of great help.

Empaths are the healers and peacemakers of the world. They may do well in a helping profession, such as medicine or counseling.

Highly sensitive empaths have an uncommonly strong ability to sense others' moods, feelings, and thoughts. They are exquisitely aware of the world around them, including sounds that others don't notice, scents that others don't distinguish, and textures that others can't feel or touch. They notice the emotions and feelings of everyone around them. They may be so sensitive to others' moods, feelings, and thoughts that they can even feel when other people are anticipating their next words or movements.

Empaths typically have a strong ability to feel other people's emotions from an early age. They pick up on the subtle nuances of what others are thinking and feeling, even when those nuances are not being said aloud. Empaths may have an almost supersensitive sense of touch: their skin is more sensitive than average, which some empaths use to their advantage by unconsciously interpreting others' gestures and movements as simple touch sensations.

As they grow older, empaths realize that other people don't enjoy being around them, especially strangers. As a result, they tend to withdraw into their worlds and become more focused on their problems. When these feelings overwhelm, empathic people can become shy or frightened around others and avoid contact. They may stop seeking friendship or company as an escape, often retreating into solitary pursuits such as painting or writing poetry. They may even stop reading altogether.

Highly sensitive empaths can be incredibly insightful and see the world differently from most people. Their sensitivity is not a personality flaw but rather a unique and extraordinary trait.

The traits that Highly Sensitive Empaths possess are an evolved survival mechanism that has been passed down through thousands of years of evolution. Their senses are so keenly focused on the world around them that they can detect dangers such as impending tornados or earthquakes before anyone else. They can sense when a loved one is sick or injured, which is why they can be incredibly nurturing people who strive to help others with their emotional and physical needs. Highly sensitive empaths may have difficulty working in environments with fluorescent lighting, computers, or loud machinery.

Empaths are not Highly Sensitive Empaths; they do not experience every feeling of everyone that comes into contact with them. Due to these characteristics, Highly Sensitive Empaths find it difficult to develop their feelings because they always seem to mirror other people's feelings rather than have their thoughts.

Characteristics of a highly sensitive person:

1. Easily overstimulated.

This trait is often mistaken for shyness. It's not so much that a highly sensitive person can't talk to people. It's just that after a long day of socializing, they may need to go home and take a breather before reaching out to others in person or online. To expect this behavior from their friend or other empathic people, a highly sensitive person might view the highly sensitive person as rude or weak-willed. Although it is unrealistic to expect this behavior from every highly sensitive person, if a highly sensitive person says they prefer being alone and need some time to themselves before talking with others, they should not be judged for it. Other empathic people need to understand that it is ok for a highly sensitive person to need some alone time.

2. Forgetful

This trait is probably the most frustrating for friends and loved ones of a Highly Sensitive Empath. Often, a Highly Sensitive Empath will forget to call back a friend or family member who has left several messages for them. This is not because the Highly Sensitive Empath doesn't care about their friend or family member; they are so absorbed in what they are doing that they forget to call back.

3. Feelings easily hurt

Most empathic people find other people's words and actions incredibly blunt, but Highly Sensitive Empaths take everything people say to heart. It is not normal for a Highly Sensitive Empath to read a text message or email that someone has sent without physically feeling the pain. To make matters worse, empathic people are more likely to be hurt by their feelings than others. Often when someone says something hurtful towards them, it is not because they are angry but because they are hurt by what they have just heard. Additionally, when highly sensitive person is hurt by their feelings, they will often avoid social interaction entirely out of embarrassment and confusion.

4. Easily deceived

This trait may be heartbreaking for family and friends who deal with an empathic person daily. Empaths are incredibly selective when it comes to choosing their friends. Many people will be completely unaware of how loyal and nice a person they genuinely are. For this reason, Highly Sensitive Empaths choose to surround themselves with only other empathic people because they can't tolerate the feeling of being deceived by non-empathic people. The final thing that makes this trait so hard on a highly sensitive person is not knowing how to deal with their emotions and fears. People who have never experienced Highly Sensitive Empathy cannot understand what it's like for a highly sensitive person to be afraid of others' feelings, especially when they cannot figure out why they feel the way they do.

5. Trusting

Because Highly Sensitive Empaths are so easily deceived, they find it very hard to trust others. They are unaware of how they can seem judgmental towards people around them, and it isn't until they've been hurt that they realize that the root cause of all their problems is caused by the inability to trust other people.

6. Gets too involved in others' feelings

Often a highly sensitive person will feel the same feelings as another person in an attempt to understand what that person may be going through. This trait goes against being empathic, in which a highly sensitive person should be able to sense how they are affecting other people but not take that knowledge and use it against them. This can be extremely difficult for other empathic people who also want to avoid being hurt by others' feelings and understand those feelings better.

7. Helpless

Many empathic individuals have found that a great deal of the growth in their personal lives has come from developing tools to cope with the situation instead of waiting for someone to swoop in and rescue them. To help themselves better, they may think of ways to help others find their way out. This trait is extremely hard on Highly Sensitive Empaths because they can't cope with many emotions around them. They may find themselves in a situation where they are surrounded by people who are angry and arguing but have no desire to intervene because they don't like conflict and don't know how to deal with it.

8. Cannot take compliments

Highly Sensitive Empaths can barely accept compliments from others because their minds are so focused on what they feel that they cannot recognize their self-worth.

9. Gets drained easily

It's not uncommon for a Highly Sensitive Empath to feel drained after social interaction because of how much they absorb from others through their empathic nature.

10. Cannot read others' thoughts or emotions

This trait is probably the most frustrating for those close to an empathic person because there is no way to communicate with a highly sensitive person about the situation if it is true. It's important for other people who don't know what it's like to be an empath to understand that this trait can make a very painful situation even worse for those who are Highly Sensitive Empaths.

11. Cannot tolerate intense or loud sounds

It's normal for most people to get overwhelmed by the sounds of a big crowd, but for a Highly Sensitive Empath, that feeling of being overwhelmed is so intense and painful that they cannot stand to be in large crowds.

12. Extremely Creative

Highly sensitive people take every aspect of their surroundings, and their world becomes filled with intense emotions. Because of this, they are highly creative people who enjoy the arts. It's common for an empathic person to want to become a writer or an artist because it gives them the chance to express emotions through art.

How to be more empathic

Everyone is empathic. We can all be sensitive to our feelings and those of others around us. Yet, this capacity to feel is one of humanity's most precious gifts and one of its most fragile.

Most people strongly sense that empathy is good and that its presence in others helps ensure the well-being of society and our relationships. But many believe it's a burden that may be better for society to do without because its effects on behavior are too unpredictable and difficult to control.

Empathy is also a delicate thing to acknowledge, as it can take a long time to develop and requires us to put ourselves in another's shoes. This can be difficult for many people who may have been socialized (or bullied) into thinking that their feelings are peculiar or wrong or that their motives are suspect. It's not enough to say, "I'm empathic." We need to work at this with care and awareness that we can make mistakes.

Another reason empathy can be hard is because empathy needs more than just the ability to observe our feelings from someone else's perspective. Instead, we need to allow ourselves to feel the other person's reality and to be capable of acting with that in mind.

This can take practice, self-care, and continuous reflection on our feelings toward our fellow human beings. It is not easy because empathy is a highly sensitive skill than can be developed but also requires great strength, endurance, and courage.

If you manage to open up your heart and mind to feel what others are experiencing, it can become overwhelming at times. The chasm between your and their feelings may seem too wide for you to cross without losing yourself in their suffering. It can be easier to close down by withdrawing from the person and their problem.

We all have this capacity to shut down if we feel overwhelmed, especially those of us who have been hurt or shamed during our childhood for expressing our feelings. So understandably, trying to be empathic when so much suffering around us may sometimes seem worth it. Still, if we don't allow ourselves to feel, then we can only protect ourselves in a very narrow way, and we run the risk of feeling isolated and alone ourselves.

There are many ways you can build up your capacity for empathy.

* Take time to reflect on how you feel in your own life. Pay attention to the feelings that come up when you're in different situations and work out what makes you feel good and what makes you feel bad. When we don't look deeply at our own lives, we take on the lives of others without really understanding where they're coming from.

* Try to be aware of your motivations for doing things. For example, sometimes, we try to be good because we want others to like us or because it makes us feel superior. Little by little, try and look deeper into why you behave like this. Give yourself a chance to know your reasons for being the way you are.

* Think about the people in your life and their life. This can be especially useful if you are in a potentially toxic relationship, but whatever the situation, a little more empathy goes a long way. We're all more alike than we think, and even when something feels very personal, it's often driven by outside forces we know little about.

* Learn how to help someone in pain by noticing and directing their attention where they need it most. This may involve a great deal of practice and skill, but there are many ways you can learn how to help

another person who is suffering. For example, consider volunteering for crisis hotlines or doing online searches for other ways you might help.

* Work on the relationships in your life and be aware of how you're feeling at different times with each one. You can also try to notice how others feel about your relationships to see if any overlap or similarities can be addressed healingly.

* Take time for yourself to do things you enjoy doing, as well as try and put yourself in other people's shoes when you are out in the world. This will help you to see other people's feelings as clearly as your own. You'll be able to identify how others feel when things happen and how they think about the ways that they might behave in response.

* Being empathic needs more than just a set of basic skills; it is possible to allow yourself to feel another person's emotions deeply and at their deepest level, with no limits on your ability to act on them. This isn't easy, but it can be a real gift if you can get there.

* Remember that empathy is not a skill you're born with; you can develop it over time. But just as with any other skill, if you don't practice regularly, the muscles weaken, and your capacity to feel less. So to hone and maintain your empathic skills, work on them everyday in some way.

* Work on your self-care to ensure you have the resources you need to give from a space of generosity and compassion rather than from a place of vulnerability and fear.

* Don't be afraid to reach out for help when you need it. You can learn much about yourself by working with others on your empathic skills, but sometimes it just isn't enough on your own. Seek counseling or support groups, or find an empathic friend who will listen as often as possible. You'll feel better about it.

* Remember that empathy is not about feeling guilty about it but rather about doing something you care about with your whole heart and soul. Therefore, empathy is always a choice. This means we don't have to feel uncomfortable or guilty if we don't feel empathic toward someone – it just doesn't suit us right now.

* If you find you've shut down your empathy because it feels too intense to live with, remember that you can turn it back on again. You're not stuck like this or missing out on something special by doing so. It doesn't matter how long it takes for you to be able to reach out with empathy – the important thing is that you keep trying to live in a way that is truly in line with your values and who you want to be.

* If you want to experience a moment of feeling in your heart that feels like empathy, try a silent meditation in which you allow all thoughts and feelings from your body and mind to wash over you. This is a wonderful way to expand your sense of compassion and connectedness with the world.

The ability to be emotionally intelligent means being able to make the best judgments about people, events, and situations based on how they make you feel. It involves adapting your behavior in light of how others feel and understanding how they feel regardless of whether they show it.

In essence, emotional intelligence can be considered an ability to see things through another person's eyes.

Emotional intelligence is what allows us to read the feelings and motivations of others, and it is a huge factor in whether we can build strong and lasting relationships or not.

The development of emotional intelligence follows a similar progression as that of simply being empathic. However, whereas empathy is about giving to another person, emotional intelligence involves giving to yourself.

Without the right amount of self-awareness or the ability to make choices based on our inner wisdom, we cannot see things enough through somebody else's eyes. We can't see ourselves or ourselves in others, so we can't see what is going on.

The following provides a basic outline of the stages involved in becoming more emotionally intelligent. Note that this isn't a step-by-step guide for how to develop emotional intelligence but rather a discussion of the various facts that are important to know about this skill.

* Learn how to understand and use your feelings effectively. This takes practice and can be hard, especially when you're in an emotionally charged situation. But once you feel like you're getting closer to understanding yourself, you'll find your feelings don't surprise you anymore and are easier to understand when another person is feeling them too.

* Learn to notice the feelings of others. The things we do and say when we're feeling emotionally intelligent are completely different from what we do and say when we're not. So when you notice how other people are feeling, you'll better understand what they need or want from you or the relationship, which will help you further refine your emotional intelligence.

* Learn to understand your feelings concerning those of others. This is about constantly checking in with yourself about how you feel and why you feel that way so that your emotional intelligence doesn't go out the window when it's no longer needed.

Empathy offers us a chance to be fully human. It can be a wonderful gift and one of the most precious things we have as human beings. It's not easy to develop this quality but trying may offer us a chance to bring more joy into our lives and those around us, so it's well worth working at it.

The 5 steps of emotional intelligence.

Emotional intelligence is the awareness of and reaction to one's emotions and those of others.

Empathy is the ability to understand and share another person's feelings.

Intuition is the ability to sense a person's thoughts or feelings without any formal logical reasoning or prior experience with that individual.

Psychic abilities are supernatural mental powers/abilities with no scientific proof or evidence.

Some people have psychic abilities like ESP (extrasensory perception).

These five steps will train you to be an empath so that you can focus on emotions not just of yourself but also those around you and help make life easier for everyone through understanding their own emotions better - developing empathy for others.

Psychic abilities are the skills for empaths to pick up on feelings, emotions, and thought forms from different energies.

The 5 steps of emotional intelligence:

Step 1: Being aware of your own emotions.

This initial step is critical, but it cannot be easy. Just observing your feelings and finding out what you are experiencing can help you identify your emotions and also help you understand others more. Moreover, you sometimes ask yourself why this person is behaving the way they are - in which case paying attention to your own emotions can give clues about other people's emotional reactions.

Often, our first reaction to a situation is emotional and not intellectual. Identifying our first reactions can help us understand others' actions better.

Tip: Journaling works very well for people who have trouble connecting with their feelings. Writing down everything you think, feel, and sense helps you process your thoughts and feelings and learn new things about yourself.

Step 2: Being aware of other people's emotions.

"Smiling is an outward expression of inner happiness." - Sigmund Freud.

Once you have your own emotions under control, you can start paying more attention to others' emotions and adjust your actions on the fly depending on their emotional state.

Tip: Often, other people's emotions are based on their past experiences or those they have witnessed and understood only through their relationships with others. Sometimes people's behaviors can be the result of their feelings about themselves or the world in general for example; if a person is feeling too much fear or anger, it may manifest in some form of physical violence at someone else as another body shows signs of survival instinct due to fear and anger.

Step 3: Develop your intuition.

Building on the awareness of emotions, you want to develop your intuition which is the ability to sense thoughts and feelings that the person does not express. You can develop this ability by setting aside time where you are clear of distractions and focusing solely on your surroundings or training sessions. Concentrating on a sound, feeling, thought, or event surrounding you, you will notice small details that feel familiar, and new things will come to mind when focused on certain things.

Tip: Allowing yourself to be more open about your emotions can help with this step. Once you start feeling more comfortable in yourself, you will be able to allow feelings to flow more freely, and your intuition can pick up on these feelings and aid you in understanding others better.

Step 4: Use psychic abilities.

Psychic ability comes from the word psychic, which means "about the psyche." In this sense, it refers to any ability that allows them to perceive or interact with thoughts and feelings not expressed by the person.

It is important to remember that psychic abilities can lead to negative outcomes if the communication between an empath and the person with this ability is not established.

Tip: Developing these abilities does not have to be done alone. Help from others can greatly benefit both parties. Also, the more you do it, the easier it will become for you.

Step 5: Use feelings/emotions as a tool for understanding others.

This step may seem like an obvious one. Still, many people take an emotional approach based on ignorance and greed instead of their own emotions and those of others. They rely on them as a tool for understanding others better, thus making life easier for all involved.

This is the key step to becoming an empath because recognizing feelings and emotions as tools rather than feelings to be ignored will help in being more receptive to others.

Tip: Emotions are often used in stressful situations as a barrier to communicating with others but understanding how a certain situation affects you and how you react emotionally can be very helpful for those you seek advice from.

Empaths are seen as "healers" because they can understand others' feelings and be very empathetic but being an empath doesn't mean you have to heal people or fix them. The point is not to heal people but to learn how they feel so that you can understand them better and see their point of view easier.

It would be best to never decide how other people should act based on your emotions. However, it is a good idea to know how someone else feels because this will increase your understanding of the other person and help you improve communication with others in the long run.

Sometimes, empaths feel that their emotions control them because they can be so intense and overwhelming - but with practice, you will gain more control of your emotions, so it's possible for empaths to live a normal life.

You can also use your skills to protect yourself from emotional attacks from others. By understanding the emotions of others, you can learn how to not let other people affect you emotionally and how to deal with them in a way that makes the most sense. Emotional intelligence skills are the foundation of being an empath. They should be integrated into life daily by paying attention to your emotional needs and those of others around you.

Being an empath is one of the most rewarding and significant things one can do if one chooses to learn and apply these skills. They can help you better understand people as well as yourself. This understanding will open up many opportunities for you to interact with people in ways that benefit both parties.

There are various ways to develop your empathic abilities, but the first step is to be willing to put effort into understanding emotions and becoming more aware of your surroundings. Empathy is a complex skill that requires practice, patience, desire, and persistence, but once you have started down this path, it will open up many more possibilities for yourself.

Emotional intelligence stages are essential since they can develop their empathic abilities and better relationships with others through them. Once you realize that emotions are tools to be used and not something to be used against yourself or others, you will attain a greater level of understanding regarding how others think and feel.

Emotional intelligence is the ability to understand your own and others' emotions, accurately read and feel them, and comprehend other people's emotions. Empaths have a strong sense of empathy for others, which is an essential part of their daily lives when interacting with others. Therefore, developing your empathic abilities will greatly help you understand yourself.

With that being said, there are many ways in which you can improve your emotional intelligence skills or develop them further if you already have a strong understanding of what it means to be an empath. The following are common stages that can be used to better understand your abilities and improve your relationships with others.

Many people undervalue their empathic abilities as a part of their overall emotional intelligence. If you feel that you may be an empath, then it is important to give yourself a chance to understand these skills and work on them to make the most out of them.

Some people cannot empathize with others, meaning they cannot feel another person's emotions. However, this is one of the most basic forms of empathy and the most easily developed for those who wish to improve their empathic skills. Hence, it is worth considering before dismissing your abilities as weak or worthless.

There are many ways to develop your empathy skills so that you can feel more confident about your abilities and be able to better understand the emotions of others with practice and patience. The above stages are designed to help you better understand yourself as an empath, but there are many different methods of developing these skills, so if you don't quite agree with the stages above, that's fine as long as it works for you.

Suppose you don't think you're an empath yet but want to become one. In that case, it is important to consider practicing emotional intelligence by accepting that everything around us is connected on some level and that whatever happens affects us deeply. Many people think it is unusual or ridiculous to feel something for another person or even empathy for another. Still, the reality is that this is how life works.

Once you have accepted your ability to empathize with others, you will better understand yourself and others. As a result, you can understand the human experience on a deeper level and move forward in your personal and social growth.

How to find yourself and heal from empathic stereotypes

Are you highly sensitive? Do you often feel overwhelmed with the emotions and physical sensations of those around you? Do you take on everyone's feelings as your own, even when it is painful or uncomfortable to do so?

If this sounds like you, then chances are that at some point in your life, someone has called you "too sensitive," "too shy," or "just too much." They may have told you that if only you could be more like them, then life would be easy, and they would have much less work to do. But it doesn't have to be this way.

High sensitivity is not a handicap. Instead, it can be a gift - a tool that empowers you to get in touch with the world around you and see it as it is.

1) You are unique

Some people find it difficult to believe that every person on the planet is different. They think something must be wrong with those who cry at movies, have difficulty in social situations, or can feel their friends' emotions so acutely. They think we should all be alike and like them better than they do.

But when they hear that just about everyone feels different, they are relieved that maybe there's nothing wrong with them.

2) You can feel their pain

After all, if everyone else is sensitive, why can't you? The answer is that everyone can feel another's pain - but some people are more sensitive to it than others.

Having a heightened sense of empathy allows you to feel the emotions of others deeply and to sense the other person's suffering as though it were your own. It has also been shown that highly sensitive people can detect subtle changes in facial expressions, body language, and tone of voice, enabling them to understand another person's emotions accurately.

3) You have depth

In the long run, empaths often report that they are happier and healthier than others. Being highly sensitive is not a disadvantage. On the contrary, it can help you to:

* Have an increased awareness of your emotions and feelings and those of others.
* Be more creative as you live life more intensely.
* Become a healer, providing compassion and love to others in need.

Coming to terms with the fact that you are different can be very liberating! You don't have to pretend or win points to impress someone or fit in. You are born with sensitivity, the noblest thing you can be. It is a gift that you can use to help others, heal yourself and make your life rich, meaningful, and full of joy.

Understanding your sensitivity can create more harmony in your life by developing a more balanced perspective. For example:

* You often feel what others feel because you need human connection to survive, so it's healthier for you to accept this as part of your reality.
* Your empathic nature means that you are empathic to all people, not just those with similar experiences or needs like yourself.
* You are more likely to have less self-esteem.

As you can see, there is nothing wrong with sensitivity. Emotions are about connection and healing. They are a natural part of our existence, but sometimes this is not obvious to those around us.

The key is learning how to accept ourselves and how we experience the world.

Empaths who have accepted themselves as they are reporting that their lives are better because they have learned to live in their truths and express themselves freely.

One of the most important things you can do is to surround yourself with people who accept you and appreciate your sensitivity. Try not to put too much pressure on yourself, but if you find that others' expectations are getting you down, speak up for yourself.

4. You are not damaged

Divorcing yourself from your sensitivity is a common coping strategy played out by all people, not just empaths.

Many people who feel more sensitive to their environment often act in ways that are perceived as 'weird' or 'different.' For example, this may involve wearing dark colors, listening to sad music, and reading books with deep themes.

Empaths sometimes experience their sensitivity in a powerful, disempowering, and unhealthy way (for example, by feeling too overwhelmed by other people's emotions to have a healthy relationship with them). This can make some people think they are not okay and should be fixed.

But this is not the case at all. Empathy is a natural response to being alive. No one is damaged because they feel what they feel.

5. There is no right or wrong way to be

As you can see by now, being highly sensitive means being in touch with your inward self. This means that you are more reflective and sensitive to your environment, traumatic or otherwise. But contrary to popular belief, this is not a weakness; it's strength and resilience in the face of suffering and pain and human suffering.

Highly sensitive individuals are often not the ones you'd usually think of as 'strong.' Still, they can cope with adversity in their lives because they have a well-developed ability to feel pain and express it.

6.   You can still be good friends

You will find that empathic individuals experience more guilt, shame, anxiety, and depression than normal people. However, highly sensitive people often report that when they feel this way, they can focus on healing themselves while still being part of a healthy relationship with their loved ones. In addition, they tend to be more insightful and supportive of other people than their less sensitive counterparts.

And have you noticed how much easier empaths find it to forgive than other people? It's because they better understand why someone did something.

7.   You are not alone

Like I said in the beginning, it often appears that most people do not feel what you feel, making you feel like the odd one out. However, despite not having many empaths around, we are increasing.

We each have a different flavor, making our community unique and strong! But if you're like me, you may still doubt yourself. This is normal. Especially with something as sensitive as empathy, it can be hard to believe that we all are the same in this community.

Despite our differences, all empaths experience the same emotions, even if they express themselves differently. So when you feel down or lonely, remember that although your feelings may seem overwhelming, they are completely natural and part of the human experience. You are not the odd one; only your intuitive, empathic abilities set you apart from others!

8.   You can do something about it

If you have read this far, then you are probably convinced that being an empath is not a bad thing. Sure, sensitivity can cause some problems in your life, but knowing and accepting that you feel more deeply than others is the first step in changing how you deal with the world to become a more effective empath.

It only takes small steps to change how you use your empathy. Therefore, it would be best if you accepted yourself as an empath before building on this acceptance and integrating it into your daily life. For example:

- Accept that it takes time for you to make friends – don't feel like there's anything wrong with you because it happens so much.
- Stop beating yourself up for expressing your emotions so intensely. Instead, accept that you only do this to help others and yourself.
- Start with small changes. For example, tell yourself: "I can cope with the fact that I only want to talk about one topic" or "I can cope with feeling overwhelmed when talking to some people."
- Read a little more about how empathy works and how you can work with it better in your life!

9.   You don't have to be like everyone else

Empaths are the most loving, caring, and sensitive people on this planet and some of the strongest and most courageous. But don't think having these qualities means you have to fit a certain persona.

You can be yourself and know that others are like you. You can love your unique way of being alive!

Remember to take small steps to change your life to feel more empowered when dealing with others' emotions. And remember that you are a wonderful person for being so honest and strong!

10. Be true to yourself

Being an empath means accepting that you feel more deeply than other people in response to your environment. As we have seen, people who fall into this category tend to experience:

* Anxiety and depression
* Feelings of loneliness and isolation
* Anger and frustration

And yet many highly sensitive people show great strength and courage in facing these challenges. This is because they can channel their sensitivity into something powerful – empathy. Acknowledging that you are a highly sensitive person is the first step in changing how you deal with the world so that your sensitivity becomes an effective part of who you are.

Strategies to calm your senses and cope with pressure.

The Highly Sensitive Empath (HSE) is a type of empath with heightened senses. HSEs have an increased awareness of their surroundings, which can be overwhelming and overwhelming enough to send them into a downward spiral.

This book provides several strategies for balancing your sensory experiences, managing anxiety, and taking care of yourself when surrounded by people who don't understand your sensitivity level. The author also lists empathy skills anyone can use to make themselves feel better in these difficult situations.

HSPs are often called Super Sensitives because they have enhanced sensory perceptions and usually very high empathy levels- meaning that one thing they feel intensely is other people's emotions and needs.

Because of this, many HSPs find social situations to be very difficult, as well as people. However, there are many ways that a highly sensitive person can make themselves feel better during social situations, from learning to be more comfortable with uncomfortable emotions to developing the skills of a better listener. Some of the points in this book are useful for anyone, but HSP tendencies make it very important for HSPs to learn how to deal with these problems.

It's a misconception that HSPs are shy or even anti-social. This isn't always true, but many people think this because they assume everyone else is comfortable with things they aren't. They assume that all non-HSPs can handle going to large gatherings of people and being bombarded with different emotions, having certain smells in the air, and so on. This is not true, and HSPs need to realize how many people are like them and feel the same way they do.

Social anxiety disorder is a condition many highly sensitive persons suffer from, but it's not classified as any anxiety disorder in the DSMIV (psychiatry).

The difficulty that HSPs have in social situations results from having heightened senses, typically meaning an increased amount of empathy and other "energy" that can be overwhelming or unbearable. The DSM-IV lists 17 disorders involving excessive shyness, such as a social phobia. These are social anxiety disorders, and being highly sensitive does not fit these criteria.

Sensory processing disorder is a condition many HSPs suffer from, but it's not recorded in the DSM – IV (psychiatry). Therefore, there is no test for this, but it can also be treated by adjusting one's sensitivity levels.

Various strategies are useful in making HSPs feel better. These strategies can also be useful for any person, but they're especially helpful for social situations that may be difficult or make people uncomfortable.

Everyone has a different level of comfort in their skin, and there's no way to make yourself not have those feelings. However, some strategies help you become more comfortable with your and everyone else's skin.

Several of the points in this book focus on the idea of being a better listener. Think about what you're saying before you say it (try to pause before responding), and ask questions rather than telling people what to do or how to live their life.

The strategies for calming your senses and coping with pressure include:

1. Using a technique called "neurobics" or "neurotunes."

Neurobics or neurotunes are ways to stimulate your senses in a new way. For example, you can use music, art, or any other kind of activity that help you feel new things.

2. Focus on your five senses.

As an HSP, you are very sensitive to the world around you and yourself and what's happening inside you. So when you're in a social situation that isn't exactly fun, it's best to focus on your emotions and body for a little bit before going back into socializing mode again.

3. Finding new things is beneficial for everyone.

Finding new things can be beneficial for everyone. Even if you hate pink, it's good to think about what day's color might work for you. Whether shades of blue or green, many colors worldwide are good for people with HSEs to find comfort.

4. When everyone else is listening to music, use earplugs or turn them down.

When everyone else is singing and dancing in their way, you can use earplugs or turn them down so that your sensitive ears aren't being hurt by the noise from all of their songs and activity.

5. Don't make everyone feel bad for their problems.

If you're having a bad day or a hard time, don't talk about how things aren't fair or how "you hate the rain." Everyone deserves to feel good about themselves and where they come from.

6. Go out at night and find something that interests you.

Even if it's just watching the sunset, this is a positive thing for everyone to do because it makes people calmer and happier.

7. Be happy for every moment you have together.

The next time you're in a social situation, be happy for the moment – even if it's not perfect.

8. Don't worry about other people's reactions to you.

It's normal for people to have strong reactions when someone is different, but please don't worry about what others will think of you when they see you or how they feel about you. Moreover, HSPs need to be aware of what other people are feeling – even if it's scary or sad.

9. Wear colors that make you feel comfortable.

Wear colors that make you happy and feel good about yourself. This can make you feel happier and more confident than just wearing colors because everyone else is wearing them too.

10. Avoid social situations as much as possible.

If you don't like being in social situations, try taking a break or trying to avoid them altogether so that your mind doesn't get hurt from being bombarded with emotions and senses all at once.

11. Leave the area if the situation is too much for you.

Before you attend a social gathering or any event, try to prepare yourself for what might happen and what will be happening. Sometimes it may just be too much to handle, so don't feel you have to go unless you want something out of the experience.

12. Do things that make you feel good about yourself.

If there's something that makes you feel good about yourself, and it's within your budget, then by all means, do it and feel great about it!

13. Find a way to relieve stress in your life.

Try finding a way to relieve stress in your life – whether taking a break from social events or getting out of the house for a little bit. There are many different ways for you to take care of yourself and feel good about what your body needs.

14. Be realistic about how much you can do.

Please don't overdo it when trying to be social with other people because sometimes being too social isn't fun. Also, try to have realistic expectations about yourself and everyone around you since they are all different people with their struggles and triumphs.

15. Don't feel guilty if you need help.

If you need help with an event, don't hesitate to ask for it. It's okay to need help sometimes!

16. Keep the environment around you clean and tidy.

Keeping your environment clean and tidy can help you feel more comfortable with people. On the other hand, a messy or dirty environment can hurt your senses, so take the time to clean up or organize things before a social engagement.

17. Remember that everyone has different opinions and may not be right.

Remember that everyone has different opinions – even if they're right in your own opinion, it doesn't matter because their opinion is just as valid as yours (or anyone else's).

18. Don't be afraid to leave a social event or situation if you're overwhelmed by it.

No one will blame you for being unable to handle something, so leaving a social event or situation is okay if you need to calm down and feel better about yourself.

19. It's okay to talk about your feelings with other people.

It's normal for HSPs to have problems with creating distance between themselves and other people. Still, they need to figure out how they can be involved in more groups of people without overexposing their emotions and senses at the same time.

20. Find the balance between being in a crowd and having space for yourself.

Find the balance between being in a crowd and having space to yourself by going to different places or trying new activities instead of repeatedly doing the same old things.

21. Don't put too much pressure on yourself because it won't make you happy.

Everyone must remember that they deserve as much time as they need, no matter their emotional issues. Trying to push yourself too hard to be social doesn't help anyone – even if you're trying to help others or your self-esteem.

22. Don't use alcohol or other substances as a way to feel better.

Drinking alcohol and taking drugs will only encourage you to do more and more things that aren't good for you, which will end up hurting your mind even more in the long run.

23. Always keep your number of close friends at a minimum.

If there is someone who tries to be your friend when you don't want them around, then it's okay to log off of social networks and focus on the people you already care about because they're the ones who will make you feel better anyhow.

How to overcome anxiety and worry and develop social skills when you are a highly sensitive empath.

It's easy to become anxious, discouraged, and doubtful when the people around you seem confident, calm, and happy. You know something is wrong with that picture, but you can't put your finger on it. It's like always being the only sober person in a room full of drunk people. Their voices and actions are unclear; you can't make sense of anything.

What is it that separates you from the rest? Most people seem confident, outgoing, and friendly, but you feel different. You might say shy or quiet if asked, but inside, you're anything but those things. You may have even been told that you're arrogant or stuck-up because you tend to laugh at others' foolishness, and when they don't understand your witty humor, they get offended. Well, I'm here to tell you there is nothing wrong with being superior in intelligence, wit, and morality. It's better than feeling like a fool all the time because you become an imitator of fools.

That's not to say you're trying to be better than anyone else. It's just that you perceive others differently because you see through their masks. You know the difference between an authentic, sincere person and a phony. You know what it means to be yourself, to have your unique style, sense of humor, and taste in music. This can make it difficult for others to understand you, but fortunately, your time is coming when the world will realize how valuable you are and begin treating you accordingly.

First and foremost, know this about yourself:

You are a highly sensitive empath, and there is nothing wrong with that.

You have an amazing gift to offer the world because you can feel and see things others cannot.

You can feel auras or energy nonverbally.

These are the only physical senses you have, so you can't see or hear the world around you because you don't have eyes or ears. You must use your other five senses to perceive the world. But even though you should never try to stop being sensitive, it is good to learn how to conceal it from others and dull your emotional sensitivity. This is especially critical for advancing life and achieving your full potential as an adult.

If people are less emotional, they'll also be less judgmental and more open-minded towards people different from themselves.

Your heightened sensitivity allows you to pick up on subtle energies and feelings, thus giving you an advantage in terms of intuition and knowing what others are thinking. This can be a great tool for being a writer, artist, musician, or comedian.

There are positive ways in which your personality can develop. If you put effort into it, your unique gifts and talents will shine through so that people will come to appreciate them.

The best way to get started is by listing all the things that make you feel uncomfortable about yourself.

Therefore, these tips can assist in overcoming anxiety and worry and developing social skills when you are a highly sensitive empath:

1.   Realize that being different is a gift.

This will make you understand that you're in a position to influence others and add something missing from their lives. In addition, you'll also see that it's not a weakness to be different but a strength.

2.   Avoid negative people.

Know that you can only influence the world around you by being positive. Therefore, it's best to avoid negative influences because they will always try to pull you down with them. Unfortunately, there are times when you will have to put up with people who don't like who you are and even try to turn others against you. People like these are jealous because they wish they could be as confident as you. You might not understand it now, but when the power of your personality shows through, they will come to respect you and ask what they can do to get in on your good karma.

3.   Be proud of the things that make you feel insecure.

These are your strengths, and you should appreciate them because they make you who you are. Instead of trying to change yourself to fit in with other people, never forget how special you are as a person. For example, if certain things, such as loud noises or too many people in a room, bother you, it will be good to acknowledge this because no one else needs to know that they do. This can keep your sensitivities under wraps instead of having people constantly tell you how funny it is when something bothers you that doesn't bother them at all!

4.   Learn to embrace your differences rather than trying to hide them.

It would be best if you never tried to conform to the norms of society. This can lead you into a life of regret and unhappiness. The more you try to "fit in," the more likely you will become a conformist. Unfortunately, too many people try to be as dramatic, loud, and different as you are but often become frustrated with their lives because they can't live up to their expectations.

5.   Don't let others label you.

You don't need people to define who you are. Make it your mission to set the boundaries of your personality, and don't let others step along those lines. Even if they try to do so, stick to your guns by telling them that you can only be yourself, so there is nothing wrong with who you are and what makes you unique. You feel these things, not things others decide for you.

6.   Create a strong sense of identity.

Do what makes you happy, but remember that developing a strong sense of self-worth is important. Without a strong sense of self, you will think that your personality is not good enough, and you will doubt yourself. This will make you feel inadequate and cause stress in your life.

7.   Don't be anxious or afraid when you're around others.

Don't let other people control your emotions by bringing up things that bother you. If they say something to upset you, answer them with a question, "Why do you think I'm going to be upset?" You don't have to agree with their reasoning but answer them with a firm concern for their well-being because it's obvious they're worried about what you're going to do or say.

8.   Forget what people think of you.

Ask yourself: "What would I say if they asked me this?" For example, you can say a question to someone and then answer it yourself. You can have different opinions; your opinions don't have to match everyone else's. This is a good way to make yourself more confident in your personality and other people to better understand how you feel about things.

9.   Let everything go.

Don't hold grudges or be upset about things that happened in the past. Instead, please focus on the present because it's vital for growth.

10.   Be your own best friend.

Be your cheerleader and give yourself a lot of self-love. Building self-esteem from within is important because this is the only way to truly believe in yourself. As soon as you feel confident in who you are, other people will notice and be attracted to you because you can share your inner beauty with them.

11.   Take care of yourself.

Spend time caring for your basic needs such as eating proper meals, exercising, getting enough sleep, etc. If you fail to care for yourself, you may think you can't achieve anything. Of course, this isn't true, but it will be harder to be positive and happy if your physical body is not in good shape.

12.   Get enough sleep.

You will wake up feeling refreshed and less stressed if you get enough sleep at night.

13.   Be tolerant of others.

You need to realize that not everyone has the same level of sensitivity as you do, so they will not act or react the way that you would if a situation arose. This doesn't mean they have bad intentions because people have different ways of doing things based on their personalities, morals, cultural beliefs, and values. If you are honest and respectful, then others will be too.

14.   Be a good role model.

Think about how you want to be seen by others and make sure you live up to that ideal. If people think of you as a super-human who can do more than anyone else, they will automatically look up to you. Suppose they see you walking calmly with confidence and even having fun in front of them. In that case, they will feel comfortable around your personality, which is the only way to establish a good reputation. Otherwise, people might take notice of your behavior due to their judgmental nature but not because they like it or respect it, so they treat you differently because of it.

15.   Know your body and know your feelings.

Don't overeat because you think that you need it. This can lead to gaining weight unnecessarily, making you feel self-conscious and causing health problems. You should also think about how many hours of sleep you want before going to bed because this is important for good health, not just for the physical part, but it also affects the mind and will enhance your energy levels for other things.

16.   Have realistic expectations.

Life is unpredictable, so don't expect the world to change overnight. Instead, start small and work towards a specific goal instead of expecting overnight success.

How to create a peaceful work environment.

If you are highly sensitive, it cannot be easy to work in an environment that isn't pleasant. It's not uncommon for highly sensitive empaths to experience difficulty concentrating, depression, and anxiety that can lead to problems at work.

If you're an empath, it's easy to pick up on the negative energy of others, which will make you feel like your workplace is less than ideal. When you have a highly sensitive personality, you will feel more stressed out than others, even if your work is just as hard.

How can you create an environment where everyone is happy and healthy?

The following are some tips you might find helpful to help create a peaceful and positive working space so that you may focus better on the task at hand.

* Clean the office with natural products such as lavender or pine oil. This helps remove any negative energy left by others, so your mood stays happy and positive.

- Consider wearing a calming scent like lavender or peppermint oil while in your office. - Get rid of any unnecessary messy, or distracting items on the desk.
- Use a meditation room at work. Having a quiet place where you can concentrate and relax is beneficial to help shift negative energy from your workplace.
- Try meditation, breathing exercises, yoga, and aromatherapy to focus on the present rather than thoughts about the past or future.
- Meditate for at least five minutes at a time.
- Comfort yourself with lavender oil or vanilla oil when you find yourself feeling overwhelmed.
- Be mindful of what and how much you eat to avoid gaining weight.
- Eat healthy foods instead of caffeine and sugar, increasing anxiety, nervousness, and tension.
- Avoid being near people who are in your personal space.
- Choose to be with people who are calm and peaceful.
- Put a "do not disturb" sign on your office door if you need peace. This signal will help avoid interruptions when you work or study for short periods throughout the day.
- Be polite with co-workers but don't be afraid to explain that you would like to work quietly for a short period.
- Avoid spending a lot of time on the phone.
- Limit your interaction with people who are chatting, loud, or otherwise disruptive. If you want to talk about something, chat about a quiet activity such as sports or music.
- Take a break from work and gather your thoughts to refresh yourself and relieve tension.
- Don't believe everything you think. Try to logically analyze your thoughts instead of believing them automatically.
- Find ways to reduce stress in other areas of your life to feel more peaceful and decrease anxiety while at work.

If this rings true for you, here are some ways to create a more enjoyable work environment.

1. Make it known that you're highly sensitive

If your boss is a highly sensitive person and they know about your sensitivities, it's easier to make the workplace feel more comfortable. This may be as simple as telling them how you react to certain things so they know not to bother you with those things. For example, if you get bothered by the scent of perfumes or lotions, tell them that. It's better to tell them in private than as a group.

2. Use a calming scent

Use lavender oil in your office if your work environment is too chaotic and hectic. Even subtle scents of certain oils can calm an empath. If you're not feeling any difference at first, don't worry about it because it takes time for the effects to take place. Be consistent with using these scents so the positive energy will last longer.

3. Create a meditation room

If you have a chance to create your very own meditation room, make it a peaceful place for yourself. Use calming scents such as lavender, vanilla, or peppermint oil to reduce anxiety and stress.

4. Practice meditation

Meditation can help an empath lower their stress and anxiety levels. During this practice, you only focus on the present moment without thinking about the past or future. You can create your little niche in the workplace so you won't be disturbed daily. It's not about sitting in silence for hours but still having quiet time where you can be alone with your thoughts and clear them out before going back to work.

5. Eat healthily

To feel calm and relaxed at work, eating healthier foods is important, besides creating the right atmosphere. Avoid junk and unhealthy food that can increase anxiety and stress. Instead, feed yourself whole grains, vegetables, and protein like fish to help stabilize your moods.

6. Be less rigid with your surroundings

You should work at a place where you won't be bothered by co-workers but don't want to create an entire office environment controlled by rules just because of being highly sensitive.

7. Keep in mind what and how much you're eating

Since you need to eat healthy foods, consider that junk food will increase your anxiety and stress. Choose to eat healthier foods so that you stay calm while at work.

8. Avoid being near people who make you uncomfortable

If you feel you can't concentrate in your workplace because of people invading your personal space, avoid going to that place whenever possible. Try to stay away from your co-workers as a way to create more space for yourself at work.

9. Be less sensitive to disruptions

While it is great to be considerate of others, don't allow yourself to get all upset if someone is being loud, disruptive, or distracting. You must understand that people are different and can help you focus on your work. Instead of getting stressed out, find ways to redirect your thoughts elsewhere.

10. Be more open-minded with others

Don't be afraid to let others come into your life because it will not make you any less valuable. Everyone is unique in their way, and despite the inconveniences some people may cause, they still deserve your respect as equals.

11. Be more open with yourself

This is about personal development. Take the time and effort to learn how you can be a more compassionate person who cares less about society's rules and wants to live more harmoniously.

12. Refrain from being rude

As previously stated, you want your co-workers to respect you. They don't want to work with someone who is rude and doesn't appreciate them being there while they are working. Some people may seem rude because they're an empath, but it's just their nervousness talking, so don't be quick to judge them as rude people just because they're sensitive.

13. Create boundaries with others

It's understandable to be private at work, but a fine line between privacy and being too private can begin to be confusing. Try to create boundaries with your co-workers so they know where they stand while trying not to be mean or come off as rude.

14. Be honest with yourself

One of the best ways to reduce stress is by practicing mindfulness. When you're hyper-sensitive, you're easily affected by the people and environment around you, so it may take time to learn how to control yourself. That's okay but don't get frustrated over being in this situation. Instead, accept it for what it is and move on by practicing mindfulness daily.

15. Stay organized

Organized people know how important it is to remain calm at work. It's also a form of self-care as much as caring for others. You will also strengthen your creative side by being more organized so you can think more clearly and prevent stressful situations from arising.

16. Avoid being reactionary

Being reactive can make you feel unstable in the long run and create a sense of chaos when trying to concentrate in the first place. Try not to be reactionary and practice patience, kindness, and tolerance at work or with friends because that behavior doesn't benefit anyone during stressful times like work.

17. Avoid resentment

It's okay to be disappointed in others for not meeting your needs just because you're an empath. That doesn't mean you have to harbor feelings of resentment against them. Instead, try to forgive and forget so that there won't be any ill will between you and your co-workers.

18. Be mindful of how much time you spend online

Avoid spending too much time online as it can hamper your productivity and cause stress because social media makes you compare yourself with others. The next thing you know, you're getting frustrated with everything around you, and the results are far from positive.

19. Avoid being too connected to your phone

When you're hyper-sensitive, it's normal to get attached to your phone. Some people can't resist downloading new apps and games just because they crave more information on the latest app or game release, but it distracts them from the task.

20. Avoid social media

Social media can cause an overload of anxiety in the first place because you're constantly bombarded with a lot of information that is not necessarily helpful or necessary. You should avoid this kind of online activity whenever possible.

The next chapter will discuss Vagus Nerve. This is an important piece of the puzzle if you want to be more relaxed at work or anywhere in life. This nerve is located in the brain that helps with controlling behavior. You can easily become nervous or hyper-sensitive when your Vagus Nerve is out of whack. In this chapter, you will learn how to stimulate the Vagus nerve and how it works.

First, for the Vagus Nerve to work properly, you need to conserve energy by being aware of your body's needs. If you cannot maintain a tempo where you can focus on what is important in life, your mind will wander around with little concentration as everything seems to be a distraction.

Second, you need to remember that you're not just thinking about one thing when you are in the moment. Your thoughts are bouncing all over the place, and sometimes that can be frustrating because you feel like your thoughts overstep boundaries. The good news is there's a solution to this problem.

Third, develop a daily routine involving physical activity and eating balanced meals. You can also try taking supplements such as turmeric or goji berries that help with cognitive functions such as memory and concentration. The Vagus nerve is important because it gives us a sense of well-being and happiness throughout our lives, but it works in shifts depending on the circumstances or moods of the people around us.

VAGUS NERVE

AUTONOMIC NERVOUS SYSTEM.

The autonomic nervous system is a division of your body that controls and regulates involuntary actions. These actions function without any conscious control from the brain. For example, one involuntary action controlled by the autonomic nervous system is breathing. Breathing happens automatically and involuntarily. Another involuntary action is sweating, which controls body temperature.

The autonomic nervous system is viewed as having two divisions: the sympathetic nervous system and the parasympathetic nervous system. The sympathetic and parasympathetic divisions of your autonomic nervous system work together to ensure you are balanced within your body. For example, one set of nerves will make it, so you are hungry; another set will let you know you are full. This is why sometimes hunger can be overwhelming and hard to ignore, even when your stomach feels like it's about to burst or you feel nauseous from over-eating. This results from the sympathetic nervous system working against the parasympathetic system.

The parasympathetic nervous system has three main parts: the cranial nerves, spinal nerves, and sacral nerves. These parts work together to regulate involuntary actions within your body.

The cranial nerves are twelve in number, extending from different parts of your brain to different parts of your body. The head is controlled by the fifth cranial nerve, while the face and hands are controlled by the seventh, eighth, and tenth cranial nerves. The neck and shoulders are also controlled by separate portions of the tenth cranial nerve.

The spinal portion of your parasympathetic nervous system comprises 12 sympathetic nerves. These sympathetic nerves bring out some of your involuntary actions, such as breathing.

There are three sections to a sympathetic nerve: dura mater (stored in your skull), medulla oblongata (your spinal cord), and visceral nervous system (located in your abdomen). The visceral nervous system is the most important part of your parasympathetic nervous system. The visceral nervous system comprises your stomach, intestines, pancreas, kidneys, and other organs in the digestive tract. The vagus nerve is an example of a sympathetic nerve within this visceral nervous system.

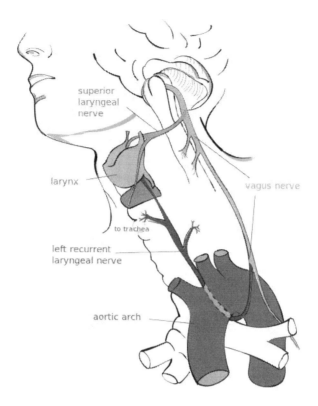

The vagus nerve is your tenth cranial nerve, but it also serves as a part of your parasympathetic nervous system. It controls functions such as chewing and swallowing food, organ activity within your digestive tract, and heart rate. The word "vagus" references a wandering action that this nerve takes after leaving the brain. It travels down your neck and into your chest. The vagus nerve goes to your liver, pancreas, stomach, spleen, and intestines. Getting to certain organs within the digestive tract, such as the stomach or intestines, takes a rather winding pathway that takes it back out of the body via an opening in the diaphragm.

The sympathetic nervous system comprises 12 nerves that extend from different parts of your brain to different parts of your body. The fifth cranial nerve extends from part of your brain called the hypothalamus to receptors in your eye. The sixth cranial nerve extends from the hypothalamus to receptors in your skin and face. The seventh cranial nerve extends from the hypothalamus to receptors in your muscles and face. The eighth cranial nerve extends from the hypothalamus to receptors in your lungs and vocal cords. The ninth cranial nerve extends from the hypothalamus to receptors in your heart, stomach, and intestines. The tenth cranial nerve extends from the hypothalamus to receptors in your neck, throat, and chest.

The vagus nerve is a unique structure containing sympathetic and parasympathetic nerves. It is an important part of the parasympathetic nervous system, but at the same time, it contains sympathetic or emergency nerves that allow you to respond to intense situations.

The emergency or sympathetic component of your vagus nerve is called the X-delta component of your vagus nerve. X-delta refers to the receptor's name, where impulses are transmitted into a sympathetic pathway within your body. The X-delta receptors are located in all areas of your body but are most numerous in the lungs and carotid sinus. These receptors are responsible for functions such as stimulating glands and muscles within your body during stressful moments. The most famous of these functions is sweating. The sweating response is generated from the over-accelerated heart rate and breathing to prepare your body for intense physical exertion. The X-delta receptors are responsible for causing you to sweat as a result of anxiety or stress.

X-delta receptor

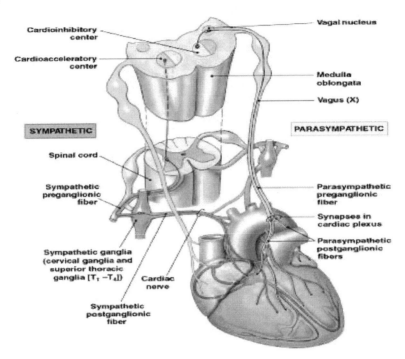

In addition to the sympathetic component, your vagus nerve also contains parasympathetic nerves called the L1 segment of your vagus nerve. These parasympathetic nerves are responsible for regulating functions such as heart rate, piloerection (body hair that stands up due to warming), and sweating. They also control gastrointestinal peristalsis, the contraction of muscles in your digestive tract.

X-delta receptors and L1 nerve fibers

The X-delta component of your vagus nerve and the L1 component of your vagus nerve are opposite in their actions. However, they both control a very similar response. The X-delta component is responsible for turning on your sympathetic nervous system, which increases your heart rate and causes sweating when you are anxious or stressed. On the other hand, the L1 component turns on your parasympathetic nervous system, which lowers your heart rate and allows you to relax when you are anxious or stressed.

Why is this important? Well, it can tell us a lot about how functions like stress and anxiety work in our bodies. The X-delta component causes you to sweat, get a racing heart, and breathe faster because it prepares your body for fight or flight. Your brain prepares you to defend yourself physically or run away from danger. The parasympathetic nervous system is responsible for relaxing your muscles and slowing down your breathing so you can be calm in the face of danger. If these responses did not occur when you were in danger, you would likely die. These bodily functions must occur without our awareness of them because if we considered every little action our bodies took during stressful times, we would be paralyzed by fear.

The X-delta component of your vagus nerve is responsible for these emergency responses by turning on your sympathetic nervous system. Without the X-delta component, you would have no way of dealing with intense physical situations that occur in life, such as running from a violent person or fighting off an attacker. If the X-delta receptors were not activated, you would be unable to sweat, you would have a very hard time breathing, and you would be unable to unclench your fists when angry.

When this response occurs without our awareness of it due to it being hardwired into our brains by evolution, it is called subliminal. What constitutes subliminal information to us is information that can be perceived by our subconscious or unconscious minds without our awareness. This includes any stimulus below our level of consciousness and requires a conscious response. This might include a smell, a sound, a sight, or even the feel of something around you. Subliminal messages are often hard to detect because they trigger the same response in our conscious and subconscious minds, so we may not be aware that we are responding to one when we would otherwise experience no response. Many scientific studies have examined how subliminal messages work on us, and there is no doubt that many of them cause a physiological response when exposed to them.

So how do subliminal messages get into our brains and cause such a physiological response without awareness?

Humans can take in information even if it is below our level of consciousness. For example, you can see something outside on the sidewalk or hear a noise or smell something that causes you to startle, but you will likely not think about it consciously. Many aspects of human behavior are thought to be hardwired into our brains due to this behavior becoming prevalent during our evolution. Therefore, subliminal messages are believed to be transferred onto the X-delta receptors and L1 nerve fibers by being stored in our unconscious minds. The X-delta receptors and L1 nerve fibers are responsible for reusing those messages and making them available to read.

Subliminal messages can come from many sources. The above explanation exemplifies how subliminal messages are delivered because it involves the X-delta receptors and L1 nerve fibers. The eye, for example, is another source of subliminal messages because we see things we don't realize. Subliminal advertisements on television or in magazines are also potential sources. They are delivered by the skin, consciousness, and other receptors via subliminal sentences that cause the same physiological response as seen with the X-delta receptor mechanisms described earlier.

When you see something, hear, smell, or feel something that causes a response in your body, it is called subliminal information. Subliminal information has to do with stimuli you can perceive but don't necessarily know. For example, take the following picture:

This picture probably caused a slight feeling of sadness in you because it contains human suffering and death. While this picture did not cause conscious thought to occur in your brain while looking at it, your unconscious mind perceived the image. It processed this image and the emotions associated with it and caused an unconscious feeling of sadness in your body.

The brain-body barrier.

There is a boundary that keeps your brain from getting involved with the bodily processes of your body. It's called the vagus nerve, and it's named for its function: to control involuntary muscles and regulate the speed at which they contract. The vagus nerve connects the brain to the heart, lungs, and stomach. All these organs directly connect to your brain, so rather than thinking about your digestive system during a test, clarify which muscle you are testing by pointing to it. If you think too much about your heart or lungs, you will get a response from them as a reflex.

This barrier is quite effective as other body areas are much easier to access for our minds. It works when we cut ourselves and bleed. Our brains recognize that our bodies need more oxygenated blood to help fight off pathogens and heal wounds, so we consciously will ourselves to hold our breath and tighten the muscles around our lungs. This causes a restriction in airflow as the diaphragm is pulled down, which restricts air intake. The vagus nerve plays a role in this process by subconsciously sending signals from the brain to constrict these muscles, even before we realize what's happening. If you're driving from point A to point B and you're cut off by a driver zipping in front of you, or your boss tells you he's giving your project to someone else, you're honking the horn. You're rarely annoyed by drivers who are going slow and in a line in front of your car.

Sex differences in heart rate variability. Another example is when we get upset with our significant other and yell at them. If we look at our heart rate, it increases and becomes more variable, which is a natural stress response. This is because we need more oxygenated blood for our muscles in a fight-or-flight situation. Think about the last time you were chased by a bear or knew you had to get across campus during an earthquake, and your heart rate was elevated -- it's because your brain was telling your body to prepare itself for action quickly to stay alive. Panic attacks.

The vagus nerve is a huge part of the brain-body barrier, but it's not the only one. The brain also has to be able to communicate with your muscles so that you can move and act efficiently. The problem with this communication is that as we age, it doesn't work as well as it used to. This is because our bodies and brains are changing, so our nervous systems have had to adapt for us to remain effective at our jobs, manage stress, and stay healthy. Think about this scenario: You're trying out for a new band in college and have a good chance of getting in. You're elated, but then you get to the tryouts and realize everyone else has had training. It's competitive, so you're stressing about whether you'll get in. The vagus nerve helps with this process by adjusting the muscles in your mouth to change how the brain perceives certain sounds. If someone asks you how your day is going, you will feel compelled to spit out a response without thinking about it. You can add a "fine" or "good" or whatever you want to reinforce your message, but the response will come out automatically.

If it weren't for this process, you would want to go home where you feel safe and warm after stressing out because you said something embarrassing in front of everyone. This is why we're compelled to respond to anything that's put in front of us -- it's our brains helping us move on from a stressful situation.

The brain-body barrier works by inhibiting signals and sending messages that help us perform tasks. It's difficult to do anything if you don't get a response from your body, so this is how the brain-body barrier keeps us safe from harm. But now we are growing older and natural changes are happening to our nervous system that causes problems such as clogged arteries, strokes, and dementia. The brain-body barrier is breaking down, which means that some of the signals it uses aren't working as efficiently as they used to -- remember when you get angry every time your partner walks by you? If a friend does something that upsets you, it doesn't take much for your stress levels to rise because your brain knows something negative is about to happen. It's a good thing, but when the cause is trivial and nothing bad happens, it can be very frustrating.

We need to take from this that natural processes are happening in your body and mind that you can't control. Some of them can help you stay healthy, but others can keep you from functioning at your best -- especially if you're terrified of being judged. This means that when you get nervous during a presentation or test, it's not because your body isn't working properly; your brain thinks something bad is about to happen and wants to prepare for it.

It's easy to blame the brain-body barrier for our problems, but not everything it does is bad. If you think about the last time your body was stressed and went to a social event, you probably ended up enjoying yourself. As you age, your brain is more active because it's adapting to allow you to do the activities you enjoy (which is why people over 60 are so happy with their lives). The vagus nerve correlates with this process, and when your brain can communicate better with your muscles, this also allows for more positive emotions like physical affection. In other words, we need to embrace many benefits of our brains' natural processes, especially if we're looking for a way to survive in today's society.

The brain-body barrier gets a bad reputation, and many misconceptions about what it does. We're going to go over some of the negative effects so you can understand how the brain-body barrier can make your life harder by not allowing signals. The brain-body barrier traps air in your arteries, which causes clogged arteries.

This happens when there's an issue with the signaling process between your diaphragm and your kidneys -- the kidneys have to filter blood constantly and send messages from the brain to let them know what's happening with our bodies. When the brain doesn't communicate effectively, your kidneys will allow more air into your bloodstream. This means your blood pressure won't be as high, and you won't have to worry about a stroke or heart attack. This is a good thing because you probably have high blood pressure when you sit down to do work (you're probably not moving around much when you're in class), but this can cause issues if you get angry or stressed out -- it can prevent the body from being able to exercise properly.

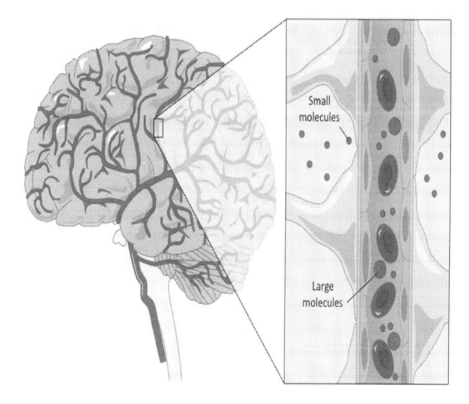

Cognitive decline can also occur because of an airlock in your arteries. Often we get frustrated when we don't remember things the way other people do. But when your brain has to filter out too many things from the environment, it has a hard time getting through all this information, and you'll find yourself forgetting things that you used to be able to do easily. Remember when you couldn't figure out how to turn your computer on? That's because there's an issue with your brain trying to communicate with your body about something important. What should have been easy is now a bit of a hassle because it's taking longer for your brain and muscles to communicate well.

How you're feeling is a result of these signals. Many people think that they can use willpower to control how they feel, and it's worked in other areas of their life, but it doesn't work here. The truth is that your body is doing what it was meant to do -- that's why some people can have the energy to climb mountains and jog for hours, while others can't even leave the house without getting tired. Your body is trying to communicate with your brain about something important, but your brain doesn't get the message because it's too busy thinking about things from the past -- like whether you'll be accepted into a new school.

The neurology of social engagement

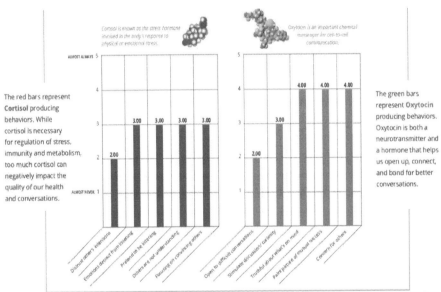

The vagus nerve is the tenth cranial nerve that travels inside the head and controls functions like heart rate, respiration, blood pressure, and digestion. It also plays a key role in initiating social engagement because its fibers pass through the brain stem. The vagus nerve detects changes in our surroundings, such as sound, touch, taste, and smell. This information then gets processed by other nerves, such as the parasympathetic nervous system, which innervates most of our organs, including the heart and lungs, resulting in increased heart rate and respiration.

The Vagus nerve offers a way to manipulate the parasympathetic nervous system through Vagus Nerve Stimulation (VNS). VNS is a treatment option for people with epilepsy or depression. It works by sending electrical pulses through the vagus nerve to stimulate it, and as a result, it positively impacts mood, alertness, and overall behavior. The theory behind VNS is that vagus nerve stimulation modulates activity in brain regions linked to regulating mood and behavior, such as the amygdala and prefrontal cortex.

In addition to managing stress, the vagus nerve also plays a key role in anxiety. Increased vagus nerve activity can lead to anxiety due to its connection to the amygdala and prefrontal cortex. Two parts of the brain deal with negative emotions, including fear and stress. Therefore, people who are prone to anxiety are less likely to respond positively to treatments like VNS because it is likely that VNS will increase their stress.

The role of the amygdala and prefrontal cortex in social engagement is not yet clear, but research has found that psychological treatment like VNS is successful in treating social anxiety when it is used along with behavioral therapy; however, improvements are only slight when used alone.

Social engagement-related disorders like social anxiety and autism are relatively recent, but they occur at a higher rate than expected, and their occurrence is rising. Research is continuously being done to understand their relationship with the brain, mostly focusing on the amygdala and prefrontal cortex. Current treatments for social anxiety are somewhat effective but insufficient in treating the disorder. There is a need for a better understanding of how these two parts of the brain interact with each other because it will aid in developing better treatments for people suffering from social anxiety.

The Vagus nerve is partly responsible for the fight and flight instinct; this is an instinctive reaction to stressful situations. A trigger for this reaction may be the smell of a stranger nearby or perceived danger, which leads to activation of the sympathetic system. This results in releasing chemicals like adrenaline, noradrenaline, and cortisol. These chemicals prepare the body to defend itself from danger. A consequence can be an increased heart rate, reduced blood flow to the digestive organs, and elevated blood pressure before running away from danger. The fight and flight response results from a strong autonomic nervous system response.

This response is important when it comes to social engagement because it is necessary to be able to interact with other people. The more we engage with people, the more the brain can develop communication skills. For example, a child can learn how to put objects into a box through observation, but they will never know how to use their imaginations and creativity if they do not engage in social interaction. They will never be able to be creative because they do not understand that there are different kinds of objects. This lack of understanding means that children's lack of cognitive development can lead to behavioral problems such as anxiety and an autism spectrum disorder.

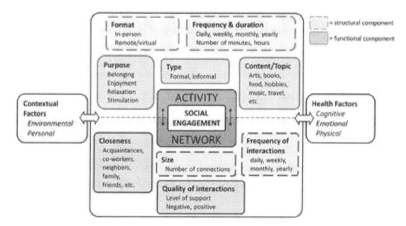

Keeping participation in society a priority for individuals who struggle with neurobiological and neurodevelopmental disorders is important. The importance of socialization has been proven through research. One study showed the effect of group-based interventions over individual ones in treating autism spectrum disorder. While some people may be wary of putting their children in social settings, they should be encouraged to do so and allowed to explore within their comfort levels. A child will not learn to engage socially unless they are allowed to engage socially, and if they are not given the opportunity, this area can be problematic later in life. Therefore, social engagement is key to a successful and healthy functioning brain.

Vagus nerve stimulation is useful for treating epilepsy and depression, but many people have concerns about its use, in addition to the fact that it is not approved for children. This neurostimulation has been valued as an effective treatment for years. Still, its acceptance has been limited by ethical debates such as the issue of personhood, questions of consent, and issues with some people's fear of being "zapped." The debate over consent points to the importance of obtaining patient consent and the ability to empathize with those who hesitate. These issues have caused some people to question whether the benefit of VNS outweighs any potential risk. Though the procedure has been in use for over a decade, little research has been conducted to study the long-term consequences of VNS. It may not be harmful, but it is also possible that VNS may cause psychological or physical damage through long-term use. Even though the procedure does not cause any physical damage, there are still concerns about memory loss and cognitive decline. How much brain plasticity exists for those who have received VNS? Can patients retain self-control under such stimulation? These concerns add to the controversy surrounding SNS and its effects on cognition, an area of research that doctors and scientists want to understand better.

VNS causes daily costs ranging from $1,000 to $1,500 per month. The costs are higher than the benefits of the procedure because it is still unknown whether or not it will improve a patient's quality of life. Since the FDA does not approve VNS for treating autism spectrum disorder, many insurance companies do not cover VNS expenses. Parents may pay for it out of pocket; applying for grants can help lower expenses for some families. The expense requires those who are considering VNS to consider the risks and benefits carefully before deciding on whether or not to have it performed.

The word "vigilance" comes from Latin, which means to stay awake. Vigilance is an important part of the fight or flight response and is, in most cases, helpful but can sometimes be problematic. It is useful in the case of protecting ourselves from danger, but it can also be a challenge when we are anxious and hypervigilant. When anxious or hypervigilant, we are constantly on alert; our minds are always running, even when nothing is wrong. Being vigilant sometimes makes us more prone to remembering things incorrectly.

The fear of missing a critical moment or being distracted by something irrelevant can disrupt daily life. In many instances, being overly vigilant can make a person feel more anxious and more likely to have an immediate negative response to stimuli.

Neuroplasticity is the ability of the brain to rewire itself through practice and training. A physically capable person can learn how to perform new tasks, such as running a marathon or playing an instrument on their own, but it takes additional years of experience to do this successfully. The brain is similar in that it takes training and practice for the individual brain to reach its potential. These training exercises help a person improve what they do and improve their skills. Through proper training, individuals can develop cognitive flexibility, which is the ability to shift attention.

An example of this can be seen in working memory. Working memory allows for the storage and manipulation of information that is being processed at the moment. It is crucial for problem-solving and other executive functions such as planning and inhibition, which are used in deciding where to focus attention. Training with spatial cues improves working memory because it allows a person to pick up on patterns that they normally would not be able to see. This is because people who lack spatial abilities are less likely to notice patterns around them or even see them without any kind of cue. People who struggle with this can be trained to pay attention to the space around them.

The brain constantly learns and can improve, if necessary, through practice and time. In the case of people who have had head injuries or strokes, their brains may have been damaged to varying degrees. When the brain is injured in this way, it needs more time to recover and heal than expected. Neuroplasticity allows for recovery by enabling the brain to move misplaced neurons or rewire unused connections between neurons. The plasticity of the brain allows individuals with mild memory problems to improve their memory skills and prevents further damaging effects from occurring due to aging or disease.

The twelve cranial nerves

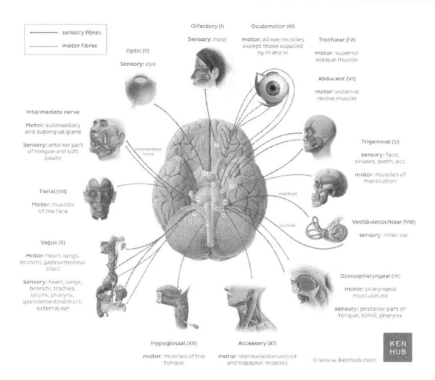

The twelve cranial nerves that run through the brain stem are attached to the vagus nerve, a bundle of nerve fibers running down the neck. This nerve plays a key role in our autonomic nervous system, which regulates body temperature, heart rate, and lung function. The vagus nerve is one of two cranial nerves related to speech (the other being the Inferior Ganglion), responsible for conveying sensory messages from the larynx and pharynx. Therefore, tumors can originate from or spread along this pathway.

Different cancers can damage cranial nerves due to invasion into or compression of the nerves. The cranial nerves that are most often affected are the vagus nerve and the trigeminal nerve.

There are 12 pairs of cranial nerves in humans. These nerves originate in the brain stem and exit through separate openings in the skull called foramina (singular: foramen). The cranial nerves control body functions that include sight, hearing, taste, smell, facial movements, balance, and other sensory stimuli related to vision and hearing, as well as motor functions such as speech, mastication (or chewing), and swallowing.

The vagus or tenth cranial nerve originates from the brain stem's medulla oblongata at the skull's base. It runs down through the neck and enters the thorax, where it splits to supply different areas of the body. The vagus nerve is important in controlling heart rate, lung, and digestive system functions. Damage to the vagus nerve can lead to a dropping heart rate, resulting in light-headedness, fainting, and dizziness. Damage to this nerve can also cause a drop in blood pressure, which may lead to tachycardia (rapid heartbeat) and an irregular heartbeat that can lead to syncope (fainting).

The vagus nerve helps to regulate the digestive system. It carries signals from the digestive tract to the brain, allowing a person to monitor body processes and digest food. The vagus nerve is also used in speech and is responsible for communicating feelings such as crying, laughing, and tasting sensations.

Therefore, the twelve cranial nerves include:

1. Facial

This nerve consists of the facial nerve (CN VII) and the inferior alveolar nerve (CN V3). The facial nerve transmits information from the face, eyes, forehead, and scalp to the brain. The inferior alveolar nerve transmits information from the mandible and maxilla to the brain. It is essential since the nerve supplies the facial muscles and is linked to the motor mechanisms of chewing, speaking, swallowing, and blinking.

The facial nerve may be damaged when underlying tumors spread and press on it. This can lead to drooping of the eyelids, perioral numbness or weakness, hearing loss (if connected to the ear), or facial pain. Moreover, a tumor that presses on the facial nerve may cause a loss of sensation in the face called hemifacial anhidrosis. Tumors or infections may damage the inferior alveolar nerve. Infections such as tooth abscesses, gum disease, and osteomyelitis can damage this nerve and subsequent tooth pain or difficulty chewing.

2. Optic

This nerve consists of the optic nerve (CN II) and the ophthalmic branch of V1 (a branch of the trigeminal nerve). It transmits information from the retina to the brain. Therefore, damage to this nerve can lead to visual impairment due to blindness, visual field loss, or double vision. In addition, damage to the optic nerve can cause involuntary actions of the eyes without conscious control, such as blinking, squinting, and eye movements. Therefore, this nerve is essential since it allows us to see.

The optic nerve can be damaged by tumors that spread and compress the nerve or by infections and inflammation. Moreover, it may be damaged when tumors develop in the eye and spread along the optic pathway.

3. Olfactory

This nerve consists of the olfactory nerve (CN I) and the vomeronasal or Jacobson's nerve (CN IX). It transmits information from the olfactory bulb in the brain to the nose. A tumor that presses on this nerve may cause a loss of sensation in one or both nostrils, and it may also lead to changes in smell due to damage to olfaction areas on either side of the nose. In addition, it can spread to other parts of the body.

The olfactory nerve may be damaged by tumors that press on the nerve or by infections. Tumors may also spread to this nerve in people with certain autoimmune disorders and certain types of cancer.

4. Oculomotor

This nerve consists of the oculomotor nerve (CN III) and the trochlear nerve (CN IV). It transmits information from the brain to muscles responsible for eye movements, such as adduction, abduction, elevation/depression, and circumduction. It also sends information on pupil diameter to the brain. Therefore, damage to this nerve can lead to double vision or blindness. Moreover, it can spread to other parts of the body.

The oculomotor nerve may be damaged by tumors that compress or press on it or by infections and inflammation. In addition, tumors with compressive or infiltrative growth patterns may damage this nerve as they grow outward into surrounding tissues or toward deeper structures. Moreover, it may be damaged when tumors develop in the eye and spread along the optic pathway. The trochlear nerve may also be damaged by tumors such as acoustic neuromas and meningiomas that grow into or adjacent to the nerve.

5. Trigeminal

This nerve consists of the ophthalmic (CN V1), maxillary (CN V2), and mandibular (CN V3) divisions. It transmits information from the brain to muscles responsible for chewing, biting, swallowing, and other motor functions of the mouth. Therefore, damage to this nerve can lead to facial weakness or numbness on one side of the face (hemifacial atrophy). Moreover, it can spread to other parts of the body.

The trigeminal nerve may be damaged by tumors that press on this nerve or by trauma (such as a blow to the head). Moreover, it may be damaged when tumors develop in areas such as the base of the skull or the brain and spread along the trigeminal pathway.

6.   Abducens

This nerve consists of CN VI and V2 (a branch of CN V1). It transmits information from the brain to muscles responsible for eye movements, such as abduction, adduction, and upward gaze. Therefore, damage to this nerve can lead to double vision or blindness. Moreover, it can spread to other parts of the body.

The abducent nerve may be damaged by tumors that press on this nerve or by trauma (such as a blow to the head). Moreover, it may be damaged when tumors develop in areas such as the base of the skull or the brain and spread along the route of CN VI.

7.   Trochlear

This nerve consists of the trochlear nerve (CN IV) and the superior oblique muscle (CN III). It transmits information from the brain to muscles responsible for eye movements, such as elevation, depression, and abduction. Therefore, damage to this nerve can lead to double vision or blindness. Moreover, it can spread to other parts of the body.

The trochlear nerve may be damaged by tumors that press on it or by trauma such as a blow to the head. Moreover, it may be damaged by tumors developing in areas such as the base of the skull or the brain and spreading along CN IV.

8.   Interosseous

This nerve consists of CN XI and XII. It transmits information from the brain to muscles responsible for finger movements, such as abduction and adduction. Therefore, damage to this nerve can lead to the inability to move fingers in certain ways or loss of sensation in them. Moreover, it can spread to other parts of the body.

The interosseous nerve may be damaged by tumors that press on it or by trauma (such as a blow to the head). Moreover, it may be damaged when tumors develop in areas such as the base of the skull or the brain and spread along CN XI and XII.

9.   Deep peroneal (or tibial)

This nerve consists of the deep peroneal nerves and the extensor digitorum longus muscle. It transmits information from the brain to muscles responsible for foot movements, such as dorsiflexion, plantar flexion, and eversion. Therefore, damage to this nerve can lead to various problems with movement in the foot and ankle due to permanent weakness or paralysis on one side of the body or foot. Moreover, it can spread to other parts of the body.

The deep peroneal nerve may be damaged by tumors that press on it or by trauma (such as a blow to the head). Moreover, it may be damaged when tumors develop in areas such as the base of the skull or the brain and spread along the deep peroneal nerve.

10.   Vagus

This nerve consists of the vagus nerve (CN X) and various visceral nerves. It transmits information from the brain to various body parts, such as the pharynx, heart, lungs, and stomach. Therefore, damage to this nerve can lead to hoarseness or problems swallowing (due to damage to the pharynx), heart problems that may lead to heart failure or irregular heartbeat(due to damage to the heart), difficulty breathing (due to damage to the lungs), and upper abdominal pain (due to damage to the stomach). Moreover, it can spread to other parts of the body.

The vagus may be damaged by inflammation or tumors that involve this nerve or by trauma (such as a blow or a car accident). Moreover, it may be damaged when tumors develop in areas such as the base of the skull or the brain and spread along the vagus nerve.

11. Hypoglossal

This nerve consists of the hypoglossal nerve (CN XII) and the muscles of the tongue and palate. It transmits information from the brain to muscles responsible for tongue movements, such as protrusion, retraction, and elevation/depression. Therefore, damage to this nerve can lead to the inability to move the tongue in certain ways or loss of sensation. Moreover, it can spread to other parts of the body.

The hypoglossal nerve may be damaged by inflammation or tumors that involve this nerve or by trauma (such as a blow or a car accident). Moreover, it may be damaged when tumors develop in areas such as the base of the skull or the brain and spread along CN XII.

12. Visceral (responsible for vomiting)

This nerve consists of CN IX, X, and XI. It transmits information from the brain to muscles responsible for vomiting (similarly to the role of the vagus nerve). Therefore, damage to this nerve can lead to vomiting due to damage to the brain or stomach. Moreover, it can spread to other parts of the body.

The visceral nerve may be damaged by inflammation (such as gastritis) caused by tumors that press on it or by trauma (such as a blow or a car accident). Moreover, tumors may develop in areas such as the base of the skull or the brain and spread along various parts of these nerves.

Cranial Nerve	Function	Origin	Destination	Foramina
Olfactory	Olfaction	Olfactory epithelium	Telencephalon	Olfactory F
Optic	Vision	Retina	Optic chiasm and midbrain	Optic F
Oculomotor	EM, P	Ventral mid-brain	Muscles: superior, medial, inferior rectus, inferior oblique, levator palpebrae superioris, ciliary	Superior orbital fissure
Trochlear	EM	Dorsal mid-brain	Superior oblique muscle	Superior orbital fissure
Trigeminal	S, M	Pons	Masticator muscles Pons (sensory)	Superior orbital fissure, F rotundum, F ovale
Abducens	EM	Pons	Lateral rectus muscle	Superior orbital fissure
Facial	S, M, P, taste (anterior 2/3 of tongue)	Pons	Facial expression muscle, lacrimal and salivary glands Pons (sensory)	IAC, stylomastoid F
Vestibulocochlear	Hearing, balance	Pons	Medulla, pons, cerebellum, thalamus	IAC
Glossopharyngeal	S, M, P, taste (posterior 1/3 of tongue)	Medulla	Muscles of speech and swallowing Parotid gland Medulla (sensory)	Jugular F
Vagus	S, M, P	Medulla	Throat, lung, viscera Medulla (sensory)	Jugular F
Accessory	M	Medulla Spinal cord	Soft palate, throat, neck muscles	Jugular F
Hypoglossal	M	Medulla	Intrinsic tongue muscles	Hypoglossal canal

What is the vagus nerve?

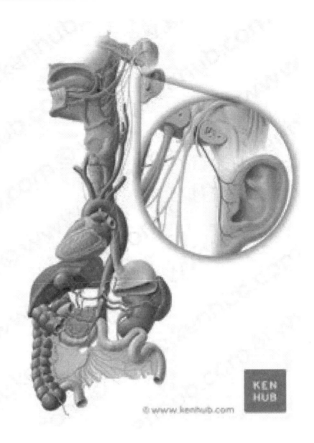

In the simplest terms, the vagus nerve is a long nerve that runs from your brain stem to your abdomen. It's part of the body's parasympathetic nervous system and helps you relax after a stressful day.

The best way for most people to release tension in their bodies is by lying down with their head on a pillow, using deep-breathing exercises, or even just walking for 20 minutes. In other words, you rely on your vagus nerve to calm down after exercising, or stress levels are high.

The parasympathetic nerve helps your body rest and recover from a stressful day, and the vagus nerve is where you relax and restore yourself after you've had a stressful day.

One of the main nerves in your body runs down from your brain stem to your abdomen. It's called the vagus nerve because it originates in the brain stem and moves through the neck and down to the heart and the abdomen. It has two parts to this process: one part to help control swallowing and the other part that helps govern digestion. It also sends signals for your heart rate to slow down and for the sphincter at the bottom of your esophagus to relax (allowing food to back into your mouth).

The vagus nerve is responsible for triggering your relaxation response. It helps you breathe deeply, which leads to a calm state of mind. It slows down the heart rate and lowers stress hormones in the body. Deep breathing works via the vagus nerve. So if you're trying to calm down, speak slowly and breathe deeply; those are simple exercises that trigger it.

The vagus nerve is also responsible for helping you release stress. It slows down the heart rate, relaxes the muscles around your esophagus and stomach, lowers blood pressure, and improves glucose levels in the bloodstream.

Many people are unaware of the vagus nerve's role in their lives. They haven't discovered that they could relax and relieve tension by using simple relaxation techniques such as deep breathing or sitting quietly. So we're going to talk about the vagus nerve now.

There are two types of the vagus nerve: the afferent and efferent vagus nerves.

The afferent vagus nerve sends signals to the brain that allow a person to experience feelings of satiation after eating, leading to decreased appetite. It is activated by the hormone ghrelin, which works on the hypothalamus. The efferent vagus nerve helps control food movement through the digestive tract and also helps control heartbeat by slowing it down. The efferent vagus nerve sends signals from the gastrointestinal tract to the Vagus Nerve Bud in the brainstem, which passes information onto different areas of your brain, including those related to appetite control and digestion. It's also responsible for lowering your heart rate. The vagus nerve is sometimes called the "wandering nerve" because it moves through so many parts of the body.

The cranial component, or "cranial nerves," of the vagus nerve includes the Facial Nerve: This nerve controls voluntary movements of muscle related to facial expression, including smiling and frowning.

Vagus Nerve: Consists of two parts—one that provides sensation to the neck and throat area and one that deals with the movement of muscles related to swallowing food and liquids. Both parts are important for normal functioning in these areas.

Vestibulocochlear Nerve: Provides functions related to hearing and equilibrium (balance).

Glossopharyngeal Nerve: Provides control of motor function for muscles related to swallowing.

Brain Stem: Provides important functions related to the brain, including auditory and visual function and consciousness. Approximately 1 million fibers of the vagus nerve innervate the gastrointestinal tract. They are excitatory, mainly affecting secretion, motility, and sensation. Vagal innervation of the gut is via both sympathetic (thoracolumbar) nerves, activating effects on muscle and secretory cells in the gut, and parasympathetic (cranial) nerves, which mostly have inhibitory effects. In addition, two main branches of the vagus nerve innervate different parts of the gut. The larger of these two branches, the deep vagus nerve (VDR), runs along the bottom of the esophagus and then splits into a superficial vagus nerve and a long thoracic vagus nerve. These nerves are located close to each other. Your face is covered with a massive network of nerves called cranial nerves. This network gives you your eyes, ears, mouth, and nose, but it also helps control your digestive system by sending signals from your stomach to your brainstem and from there to other regions of your body.

Characteristics of vagus nerve include:

a. Efferent vagus nerve is a long, primary neuron originating in the CNS and terminating at muscle or glands.
b. Efferent vagus reaches most organs.
c. Efferent vagus has both motor and sensory functions (gustatory, auditory, cardiac, and tubular functions).
d. Afferent enters through the dorsal root ganglion (trigeminal) and leaves the spinal cord via the dorsal root.
e. Afferent vagus has sensory modality only (smell).

f. The afferent/efferent segregation is not sharp – there are motor points on both sides of the trachea and sensory points on both sides of the stomach.

g. Vagal fibers join the cranium and sacral plexus at the level of the medulla.

h. The visceral motor nuclei are located in the medulla, PNS, and spinal cord (mainly at sacral levels).

The Vagus nerve is a mixed nerve which means that it has both sensory and motor branches. Motor branches of the vagus nerve (3–6) innervate muscles of the pharynx, larynx, trachea, and esophagus so they can control their movements – except epiglottis, which is innervated by the superior laryngeal branch of the hypoglossal nerve. Sensory branches of the vagus nerve (7–9) provide taste sensation on the epiglottis and pharynx, general sensation to the larynx, and sensory input from the esophagus.

The vagal nerve has two major branches: the short cervical ventral rami and the long thoracic ventral rami, which innervate the viscera of the thorax, abdomen, and pelvis.

Vagus nerve innervation of serosal surfaces is in dermatomal order: tracheobronchial tree (C3-4), bronchial tree (C4-5).

Vagus nerve projections to abdominal viscera are as follows: coronary arteries, splanchnic nerves (S2-S4), mesenteric plexus, vas deferens, and the testis.

The vagus nerve is involved in eating behavior by triggering the satiety center in the hypothalamus to signal the cerebral cortex of your brain. If a person were to eat all they wanted but they remained hungry and overate, they would most likely eat too much in one sitting (this is called binge eating). If a person were to eat when they are full, people call this "satiated": this is the behavior of people with anorexia nervosa or bulimia nervosa.

The vagus nerve is also involved in controlling heart rate and blood pressure. The vagus nerve is a bridge between the gastrointestinal tract and the brainstem and a conduit for food to reach other parts of your body. Research has shown that patients who have undergone vagotomy have high blood pressure, delayed gastric emptying, decreased heart rate, and increased blood cholesterol levels. The vagus nerve is one of the most fundamental pathways for afferent information about our bodies' internal state and relationship to the external environment. When we are hungry, signals from our stomach travel to our brain via this pathway which initiates eating behavior. When we are physically active and begin to get tired, signals from the periphery travel to our brain via the vagus nerve. This results in the initiation of restful behavior. We can control this pathway via a simple hack: research has shown that chewing gum can improve your homework performance and athletic performance (e.g., increased stride length during running). Chewing gum increases saliva production, which signals your body that it is not in danger of starvation.

The Vagus nerve is responsible for the primary motor function of cranial nerves IX, X, XI, and XII and a taste sensation in the posterior one-third of the tongue.

The Vagus nerve innervates many organs, including the heart (pulse and contractility), lungs, bronchi, thymus, spleen, pancreas, liver, and stomach.

The Vagus nerve is also connected with the chemoreceptors of the olfactory pathway and mediates chemosensitivity to food-related stimuli. A Schiller–Fuchs reflex can be elicited in monkeys and some humans by application of a local anesthetic to the vagus nerve near the jugular foramen.

Historical recognition of vagus nerve.

The Vagus nerve (from Latin "vagus," meaning "wandering") is a paired cranial nerve that lies in the neck. It carries sensory information to and from the viscera or visceral organs, mainly carrying signals from the heart, lungs, and major arteries. Leonardo da Vinci named the vagus nerve in 1493, which Harvey Cushing rediscovered in 1878.

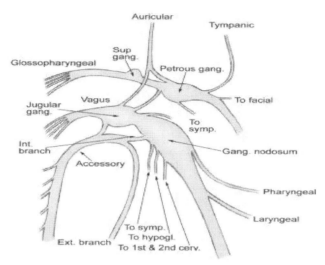

On the surface of the neck, in the groove for the jugular vein, is a large nerve, about as large as a crow quill. It arises from the medulla oblongata and passes downward, lateralward, and backward, distributed to all neck parts. It has been called the Nervus vagus (the wandering nerve). It is distributed to all parts of the head, face, and neck except the lips, palate, and glans penis. It supplies the muscles of the palate, the pharynx in general, the larynx, and all muscles of the face except one – this is by a branch from the cervical plexus. The vagus nerve is also responsible for activating the vocal cords, therefore causing speech to be possible. It is also the nerve that controls the external ear canal and foramen.

It innervates blood vessels, which are mostly in the abdomen and limbs. Also, it has preganglionic parasympathetic fibers that synapse in the ganglia of the superior cervical ganglion on its way out from the medulla.

The vagus nerve has three branches—the pharyngeal, superior laryngeal, and recurrent laryngeal nerves. In addition, some anatomists name a fourth branch—the sympathetic cervical nodes. The superior laryngeal nerve is the main nerve to provide the larynx muscles with motor innervation. The pharyngeal nerve supplies most of the plexus. It is also responsible for laryngeal nerve palsy. It runs through the cervical ganglion and sends projections to the superior cervical ganglion and the pre-tracheal muscles of the neck and larynx.

The pharyngeal nerve probably arises from the recurrent laryngeal nerve or the glossopharyngeal nerve. In humans, it passes downward and forward, downward and backward, lateralward and lateralward, forward again, and backward.

In mammals (including humans), both afferents from the vagus nerve and efferents to its motor nuclei are known as axons. Efferent fibers originating in the medulla and the brainstem carry signals to the lungs and heart. The reflexes mediated by the vagus nerve are collectively known as the "vagal reflexes" or "vagal responses." These reflexes are studied under the name of "vagal regulation," focusing on gastrointestinal secretions, motility, and respiratory function.

The vagus nerve produces parasympathetic effects on the heart and torso. It increases heart rate, slows the heart's pace, and lowers blood pressure.

The vagus nerve also controls a reflex that causes the larynx muscles (laryngeal reflex) contraction. When this occurs, it restricts airflow from the lungs to ensure that only air from the mouth passes through the nose. This reflex is mediated by a reflex arc formed in response to the stimulation of sensory nerves located within the larynx—the glossopharyngeal nerve.

Historically, carotid sinus massage was used to stimulate the vagus nerve and cause the larynx to become paralyzed. This action would temporarily cause a person to stop breathing, causing the person to faint. Today, a cardiac arrest is induced instead by stimulating the vagus nerve through an electrode on the surface of the heart, a method known as cardioversion.

The vagus nerve plays an important role in the digestive system. It slows down gastric motility and increases gastric emptying, allowing for more effective digestion. This is accomplished by contracting the abdominal muscles and releasing neurotransmitters (serotonin, acetylcholine, and adenosine) that relax smooth muscle in the intestines, increasing motility. It also controls the release of gastric juice during eating and food digestion by slowing down peristalsis.

The vagus nerve is responsible for increased heart rate and blood pressure, which are at their lowest when one is asleep or unconscious due to a drop in sympathetic activity. This means that one's blood pressure and heart rate will decrease greatly, even fainting in an unconscious state. The vagus nerve is also responsible for opening the airway during a cough, allowing air to pass through the trachea.

Many diseases and conditions can have a negative effect on the vagus nerve, especially degenerative diseases of the brain such as Parkinson's disease or amyotrophic lateral sclerosis (ALS). Vagus nerve involvement with symptoms is commonly seen in chronic obstructive pulmonary diseases (COPD) patients, such as bronchitis or emphysema. Vagus nerve dysfunction can also be encountered in neurodegenerative diseases or strokes. It can also be damaged by some forms of surgery, such as cervical or thoracic spinal fusion.

Vagal nerve stimulation is a treatment for depression that has not responded to other treatments. It was approved for use in the United States by the Food and Drug Administration in October 2007 for patients who have not responded to at least one antidepressant medication. Initial results appear promising, but long-term outcome data are not available yet.

The vagus nerve plays an important role in controlling milk letdown during breastfeeding. It stimulates milk ejection and contractions of the breast (breastfeeding).

Some also believe the vagus nerve to be one of the weak links in the heart's electrical conduction system, responsible for slowing down the heart rate. More than 100 reported cases of cardiac arrest among medical students during surgical procedures (cardiac arrest during surgery), which has been attributed to decreases in vagal tone. The action may not be instantaneous and will take time to produce full effects. Researchers attribute this effect to the vagal inhibition of cardiac motility, which inhibits impulses from reaching the atria and slowing down the heart rate.

The vagus nerve can be injured from medical procedures, particularly during thoracic surgery. Commonly, the nerve is injured during thoracic surgery or repairing of the spine. Vagus nerve injury is difficult to diagnose as many signs, and symptoms are nonspecific as to origin.

Inhibition of one vagal effect (or its opposite) can cause bradycardia—a slowed heart rate; however, over-stimulation of the vagus nerve may lead to tachycardia—a fast heart rate. In patients with vagal denerva-tion syndrome and certain other pathological conditions, bradycardia is the norm, and tachycardia is seen only at times of great stress.

The vagus nerve, which contains parasympathetic fibers to the heart, regulates both phases of the cardiac cycle, namely diastole (relaxation of heart muscle) and systole (contraction of ventricular muscle). Thus, it is also called "the heart nerve."

How to stimulate the vagus nerve.

Vagus Nerve: A nerve that is one of the nine pairs running to and from the brain. It offers a branch to all body organs. The vagus nerve can be stimulated through a position for meditation known as sama vritti (equal breaths).

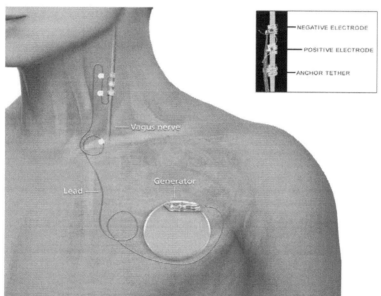

The main function of the vagus nerve is to control blood pressure by relaxing the tone in large vessels and increasing the tone in small vessels. Active also stimulates sluggish activities like heart rate, digestion, and respiration.

Stimulating this nerve will have many positive effects on your health, such as improved heart-rate variabil-ity and increased ability to respond more appropriately during stress episodes or surges.

It will also calm your nervous system and reduce levels of C-reactive protein, a biomarker for inflamma-tion. Some research has indicated that vagal stimulation can play a role in panic disorder, posttraumatic stress disorder, obsessive-compulsive disorder, and other mental illnesses. In addition, a study in male mice showed that stimulating the vagus nerve decreased food intake, suppressed body fat storage, in-creased energy expenditure, and abolished diet-induced obesity.

The Vagus nerve is one part of our parasympathetic nervous system which is responsible for resting or healing the state of our bodies (digestion, sex, etc.). The sympathetic nervous system is the other part of the parasympathetic nervous system responsible for our fight-or-flight response. So stimulating only the vagus nerve leaves us in this calm state where we cannot produce any action to defend against stressful situations. We are just sitting ducks waiting for something to come and kill us.

This position is more than just stimulating a nerve. It stimulates your nervous system to naturally produce chemicals that will help heal and balance out your whole body's nervous system instead of completely ignoring it.

The vagus nerve runs from the base of your brain to your abdomen. It temporarily puts your body into parasympathetic mode, which is responsible for stimulating "rest and digest" responses. This will help to switch you into a more relaxed state.

Vagus Nerve Stimulation: To stimulate the Vagus nerve to sit in any comfortable position, take slow breaths through your nose and slowly exhale through an open mouth after each inhalation (called Sama vritti).

This should be done for at least 15 minutes and up to an hour at a time. You can also listen to a guided meditation (see below) while practicing this yoga technique, making the process easier.

If you find it hard to focus on your breathing or are distracted, try to bring your focus back to your breath. You can do this by counting each inhalation and exhalation (one breath- one count or two -one or two-one).

Inhale 1, Exhale 2, and so on.

If you are using guided meditation, try to keep your mind focused on what the voice is saying, but if it wanders again, return your focus back to the voice.

Once complete, stretch out all your muscles, such as your arms and legs. This will help return everything to normal once more after being relaxed.

Therefore, these tips can guide how to stimulate the vagus nerve:

a. Practice good posture (as a yoga beginner, learn about postures before the practice)
b. Try to keep the spine straight, especially when seated and lying
c. Always try to breathe using your diaphragm (the floor of your chest should move outward when you inhale and inward when you exhale). This will activate the vagus nerve and help with proper oxygen intake/carbon dioxide removal from your blood.
d. And finally, to stimulate the vagus nerve correctly and safely, you need to maintain a healthy diet and eating habits so that your body can easily absorb all necessary nutrients and be maintained healthy at all times. Taking in nutrients like minerals, vitamins, and antioxidants will keep your body from becoming deficient.

Moreover, you should also be aware that there are two types of neurotransmitters (neurotransmitters are chemicals that nerves release and are used for sending signals between nerve cells).

The digested food travels to the stomach when you eat a meal, breaking it down into glucose. The insulin hormone is released by the pancreas and begins to convert glucose into the energy the brain needs to process short-term memory. This is called insulin resistance (IR). This leads to type 2 diabetes. Insulin resistance occurs when there is an excess of insulin in your bloodstream.

When you are IR, it is not just your brain that suffers. It also makes your body vulnerable to becoming insulin resistant, in general. This means that you will be more susceptible to type 2 diabetes and heart disease.

The same happens when your body becomes deficient in other minerals and vitamins.

Therefore, when you eat a meal or snack, you should always choose foods high in nutrients instead of foods high in calories without any nutritional value.

Therefore, the best foods are:

i.   Fruits and vegetables (organic)
ii.   Whole grains such as brown rice and oatmeal (preferably organic)
iii. Nuts (preferably raw)
iv.   Healthy fats such as fish and olive oil (organic)
v.   Legumes
vi.   Calcium-rich foods like milk and cheese.
d.   If you are exercising, you should ensure calcium intake is at least 1200 mg.
e.   Drinking any form of caffeine during the day will significantly reduce the amount of sleep you get over the course of a 24-hour period, so try to limit this as much as possible.
f.   Try to eat foods with high water content, such as fruits and vegetables.
g.   Sugary foods have been associated with many negative health effects, including obesity, heart disease, and cancer. Avoid these like the plague.
h.   Stressful events can impact levels of cortisol or stress hormones. High levels of cortisol have been associated with high cholesterol and heart disease. For example, if you are stressed, you may be eating more foods that contain sugar to make up for the increased need for calories in your body (to power through the day's stress). These sugary foods should be consumed in moderation, and try to eat healthy fats whenever possible.
i.   Exercise will help you lose weight and increase your energy level. This is because, after a strenuous workout, your body burns glucose more rapidly, which is a sign that insulin is working properly in your body.
j.   Lastly, sleep is important to your overall health and should be taken seriously. After all, as we mentioned earlier, sleep is one of the ways that neurons in your brain communicate with each other.

Sleep can be very damaging to your health if you don't get enough of it (which indicates that there are a lot of neurotransmitters working in your brain that are not being utilized properly). Suppose you are constantly stressed out and have a lack of sleep over the years. In that case, this can lead to a wide variety of health problems such as memory loss and cognitive decline (though none of these issues will happen overnight --it may take several years for symptoms to show up).

Therefore, to stimulate the vagus nerve, you will have to ensure that you do not suffer from any deficiencies. The best way to achieve this is by maintaining a healthy diet. You need to break your sugar, coffee, and caffeine addiction while using vagus nerve stimulation. You can replace your coffee or soda with green tea, which contains L-theanine, a natural amino acid that improves mental alertness without any side effects such as jitters or sleeplessness because it is relaxing. And if you are addicted to sugar, you should try to avoid it as much as possible.

In addition, when it comes to exercise, you should make sure that you are pushing your body hard enough that it will have an effect on the fat and muscle in your body. One of the easiest ways to do this is by exercising with a heart rate monitor. You can buy heart rate monitors online or in a store.

Don't forget to drink lots of water during exercise. And when it comes to eating healthy fats, olive oil and fish are great sources, while avocados and nuts are also good sources of healthy fats.

When you try to stimulate your vagus nerve, you should also ensure that you get the proper nutrients in your diet. This is because the vagus nerve is a highly underrated part of our body that requires proper nutrition to help it function at its optimum level. As we mentioned earlier, the vagus nerve turns carbohydrates into energy while removing fat from the blood stream and regulating blood pressure, heart rate and blood sugar levels (this happens by releasing certain neurotransmitters). One of the most important aspects of improving your health concerning the vagus nerve is avoiding any deficiencies as much as possible.

Functions of the vagus nerve.

* Brain

The Vagus nerve works in the brain through the cranial nerve X. It affects the regulation of different parts of the brain and has an effect on mood. The brain can be stimulated by the vagus nerve through the brainstem and vagus nerve. The brain and the vagus nerve communicate via neurotransmitters such as acetylcholine, dopamine, and serotonin. Moreover, the vagus nerve also has a connection with the sympathetic nervous system. The sympathetic nerve is activated when we are stressed or in danger. When the brain

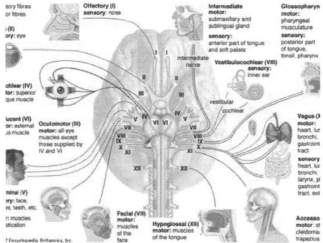

perceives a threat, it will also stimulate the sympathetic (fight or flight) nervous system, and this changes our blood pressure and heart rate so that we can defend ourselves from any real danger.

* Neck

The vagus nerve begins in the brain stem in the medulla, then descends down into the neck, and is connected with many structures such as the heart, lungs, and stomach. The effect it has on these structures depends on which branch of the vagus nerve it is stimulating. The neck is a very important part of our bodies as it is connected with many vital organs, and the vagus nerve is the connection between the brain and these organs. Examples of structures that are affected by this nerve are the heart, stomach, lungs, and digestive systems. Therefore, the vagus nerve has a big effect on the function of these organs.

* Sensory functions

The vagus nerve is connected to the motor neurons in the brain and spinal cord. This means that the nerve helps us with our sensory functions. The sensory systems are important because they help us understand how our bodies are working and how we can take appropriate actions based on this information. For example, it is important for us to know what our heartbeat sounds like so that we can react appropriately if we notice any problems with our heartbeat (such as when we feel our heartbeat is too fast or too slow). The vagus nerve also affects other areas of the body such as saliva, stomach acid, and kidney function. Therefore, the vagus nerve is important in helping us to maintain our body functions, and it also keeps us healthy.

- Special sensory functions

The vagus nerve helps to regulate our breathing and heart rate. This helps us to remain calm, even when we are in danger. The vagus nerve also helps to control body temperature and blood pressure which are important when we are under threat. For example, if you are feeling stressed due to an exam or you were told that you had cancer, your heart would start racing, and you're breathing fast: These effects would lower your body temperature so that it wouldn't be so high as it is under stress. The sympathetic nervous system can activate the fight or flight response. When this happens it will change the blood pressure so that there is more blood being pumped around the body, therefore, increasing the oxygen supply. This makes us breathe quicker to supply our brains with more oxygen so that we can defend ourselves. The vagus nerve helps to control these effects of the fight or flight system.

- Motor functions

The vagus nerve is also connected to the motor neurons which help us move. This can be used to help us when we are in danger. When we are stressed, the vagus nerve can cause paralysis of our limbs so that we cannot move and therefore will not be able to defend ourselves. This paralysis is temporary, and it wears off when the danger has passed.

The vagus nerve helps to control these effects of the fight or flight system.

The vagus nerve is not just one nerve but a collection of sensory, motor, and parasympathetic neurons that begin at the brain stem. The vagus nerve is a mixed nerve. The motor component of the vagus nerve arises from neurons within the nucleus ambiguous. These motor neurons are cholinergic and project to the thoracic and abdominal viscera, causing them to contract in a braking fashion; this slowing response generates an "anti-gravity" effect on the visceral organs. Parasympathetic innervation of the heart arises from cells in the central nervous system, including those that also innervate smooth muscle tissues in other parts of the body: these cells are known as "cardiac companion cells".

- Pharynx

The Vagus nerve crosses the pharynx leaving it on the right side. The vagus nerve innervates the pharynx, which is responsible for swallowing (the passage of food and liquid via the mouth into the esophagus) as well as regulating breathing. Therefore, the vagus nerve is important in swallowing because it stimulates the muscles required for this process. In addition, the vagus nerve also improves the breathing mechanism.

The brain stem is the most important part of the central nervous system. It is located at the base of the brain, and it consists of three parts: the medulla oblongata, pons, and the tegmentum. The brain stem controls basic functions such as consciousness, body temperature, and heart rate as well as bodily movement. The vagal nerve plays an important role in some of these basic functions including heart rate and body temperature regulation. In addition to this, when we are in danger, our brains will activate our sympathetic nervous system, but there isn't anything that can stimulate our parasympathetic nervous system (parasympathetic control of our heart and digestive systems).

- Larynx

Vagus nerve – The vagus nerve innervates the larynx, in particular, the vocal cords. When the vagus nerve is stimulated, it causes a small reflex which causes vocal cords to close. The closure of the larynx creates a reflex that raises blood pressure and also lowers heart rate. Therefore, some functions of this nerve are stress related as we often feel an increase in pressure in our necks when we are under stress. Thus, the vagus nerve is a vital part of our body as it is involved in our breathing, speaking, and swallowing.

The vagus nerve has many other functions that are not related to the fight or flight response but are still important for our overall health such as regulation of the respiratory tract and heart rate.

- Recurrent laryngeal nerve

The vagus nerve is numbered as the tenth cranial nerve. The vagus nerve is located in the neck, and it is responsible for controlling some of the body's most important functions: breathing and swallowing. The recurrent laryngeal nerve is responsible for these two processes.

The larynx (or voice box) is at the top of the trachea leaving your skull to enter your chest through your throat. The larynx ensures that air enters your lungs. This helps you to keep oxygen in your blood when we are not exercising or eating so that you can continue fighting for breath against an attacker or when you are under huge amounts of stress. The larynx is not just important in helping to save our lives but also in helping us to speak.

The recurrent laryngeal nerve is one of the nerves which arise from the vagus nerve. It supplies the muscles of the larynx and its derivatives. The recurrent laryngeal nerve supplies all the intrinsic muscles of the larynx except for the cricothyroid muscle, which is innervated by a branch from C1 (first cervical segment).

The pharynx is made up of two tubes that run from our nose and mouth to our stomach (and even smaller tubes on top leading from our nose to our lungs). When we swallow food and water, it passes through these passages.

- Vocalis inner laryngeal nerve

The vocalis inner laryngeal nerve branches from the vagus nerve and supplies the muscles of the larynx. The vocalis inner laryngeal nerve is activated by the vagus nerve, and when it is active, it causes paralysis of some muscles of the larynx. Moreover, it causes the adduction of the vocal folds.

- Parasympathic functions

The skin of the neck is made up of a network of nerves that supply sensation to the surface area above and below the surface of our skin. These nerves are responsible for pain. For example, when you have a toothache, this is because you have an infection in your body that has affected your nerve endings on the skin (just like any other part of your body), so when you touch this area, it causes pain in that part of your body. The vagus nerve helps to control these effects of the fight or flight system.

Polyvagal theory

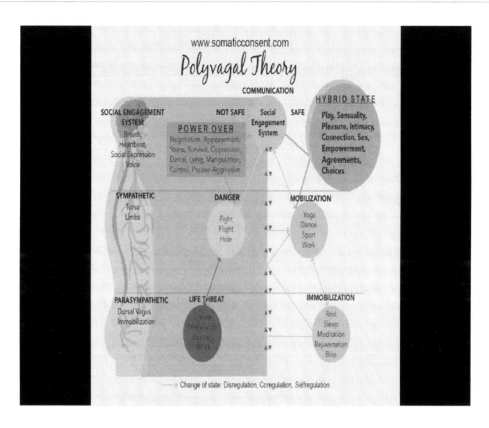

The polyvagal theory is a biopsychosocial model that integrates autonomic nervous system functioning, social engagement behavior, and speech-related breathing patterns. The theory postulates that these three components of the body's response to stress are regulated by an evolutionarily ancient system in mammals called the vagus nerve. It is thought that this system evolved from the sympathetic nerve system, which is responsible for amplifying the effects of stress throughout the body. This system consists of two separate circuits: the parasympathetic and the sympathetic.

The parasympathetic nervous system is activated when a person is relaxed and in a passive state, such as when lying down or seated. It regulates the functions of glands and organs, such as the heart, lungs, and digestive tract. These functions are in "rest-and-digest" mode during periods of rest or sleep.

The sympathetic nervous system is activated when an individual is engaged in an intense and immediate response to stress, such as by fighting or fleeing. This system maintains the body's active state during periods of stress.

The polyvagal theory proposes that the interaction between these two systems influences how an individual copes with life's daily stresses. For example, in a person who experiences chronic anxiety or whose parasympathetic circuit is poorly regulated, the threat, fear, or emotions resulting from stress are amplified via the sympathetic system, and there is little chance that this person will reach a relaxed state that could restore their ability to handle stress.

The polyvagal theory is effective for treating individuals with depression and panic disorders. In addition, clinical trials it has been shown to help improve the treatment of pain and disorders such as asthma and PTSD.

The vagus nerve is one of the cranial nerves in the nervous system. It arises from fibers from the brain that arise from parts of both sides of the brain called the cortex (including frontal lobes). In humans and wolves, this nerve begins in a bundle that includes fibers originating from each side of the brain.

It runs in a direction lateral to the spinal column (away from the body) and passes through a bifurcation at about level C4 or C5. These are called "conduits for vagus."

* Common problems related to cranial-nerve dysfunction:

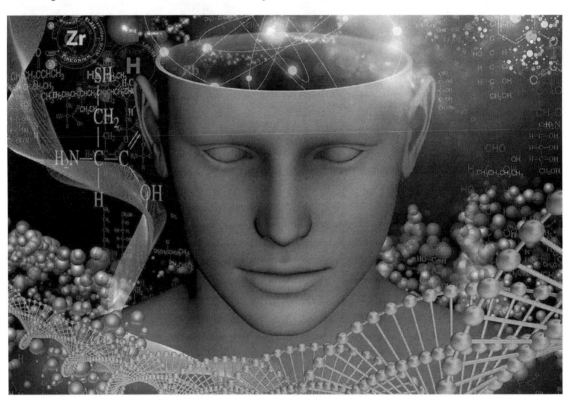

The problems that can arise from cranial nerves include the following:

a. Brainstem Compression

The brainstem is a collection of structures at the top of the brain. It controls basic reflexes and functions like breathing, heart rate, and coordinating movement. When problems arise in a part of the brainstem, these reflexes can be disrupted and function poorly. For example, if part of the brainstem gets compressed by a blood clot or tumor, there may not be adequate control for breathing or heart rate. This condition is called cauda equina syndrome (CES).

CES can be caused by several conditions, like spinal disc herniation (a bulge on a nerve that compresses the spinal cord) or inflammatory diseases of the vein that supplies blood to the brainstem (such as multiple sclerosis). It's also related to cases in which tumors are pressing on nerves and causing problems with breathing.

When there is compression in the brainstem, other functions may be affected. For example, if one of the cranial nerves is compressed below the level where it leaves the brainstem, it won't function properly.

b.   Cranial Nerve Injuries

Cranial nerve injuries can affect the function of any one of the cranial nerves. For example, a severe head injury can injure the brainstem and damage any one of the cranial nerves that are passing through this area. The most common cause of cranial nerve injuries is traumatic injuries such as car accidents and falls.

c.   Cranial Nerve Tumors

Several types of tumors can occur in parts of the brain in which some parts of the brainstem lie. These tumors can be benign (non-cancerous), like meningioma (cancer of the membranes that cover the brain and spinal cord), or malignant (cancerous). In these conditions, the nerves may also become compressed and damaged.

d.   Hydrocephalus

Some children are born with an excessive amount of fluid in the brain. This condition is called hydrocephalus. It's most noticeable when children are young and may be treated by surgically draining excess fluid out of the brain so that it can reabsorb into the ventricles of their brains (the spaces inside their heads where cerebrospinal fluid collects). There are times, however, when this condition is difficult to treat and can be fatal. Hydrocephalus is also called "water on the brain."

e.   Spinal Cord Injury

Damage to a person's spinal cord can break communication between the brain and the rest of the body. This damage can occur from a fracture in the spine that disrupts neural fibers that project from part of the spinal cord called a gray column. Since both sides of this structure work together, any damage here will affect both sides of the body and result in weakness or paralysis.

g.   Brain Abscesses

A brain abscess is an infection inside the skull that travels through one or more small openings in the bones of that area (a sinus). Infection most often causes this condition from bacteria entering the skull through a wound on the skin or a dental abscess. A skull fracture located near these openings may also be a contributing factor. The infection can travel up into the brain and cause damage.

h.   Carotid Arteriosclerosis

In carotid artery disease, "scarring" occurs at the base of the neck, where it meets the aorta (the body's main artery). This "scarring" (atherosclerosis) can lead to narrowing and serious problems with blood flow through one or more of these arteries, which can cause strokes and heart attacks.

To prevent carotid artery problems, treatment is directed at decreasing the risk factors. These include:

Other causes of compression in this area include a brain tumor or abscess. This type of pressure can lead to symptoms including difficulty talking, difficulty swallowing, and changes in vision that mimic a stroke.

18.   Panic disorder- A panic attack is a sudden episode of intense fear that occurs for no apparent reason and lasts for several minutes or even hours. During these attacks, there are symptoms like palpitations, sweating and trembling, shortness of breath, and dizziness. The person may believe they have a heart attack or stroke.

* Emotional issues

This type of anxiety disorder is related to an unresolved conflict expressed throughout the body. For example, a traumatic event from the past may cause emotional reactions when it comes up as a trigger in everyday situations or activities. It's common for sufferers to have physical health issues such as chronic headaches, digestive problems, difficulty sleeping, and loss of energy that may not be directly related to emotional conflicts. Sometimes people with panic disorder suffer from physical health issues, but their emotional struggles interfere with their ability to effectively treat these issues.

One of the major functions of the vagus nerve is to relay messages between the brain and the body. A problem with this nerve can cause various issues related to this communication system. For example, if there's a problem with sending signals to and from the brain, it might be difficult for someone to feel their body or any sensations they are experiencing. This can lead to emotional reactions aimed at getting attention or helping with recognizing physical sensations. This may be expressed through anxiety, anger, and irritability. In addition, being "out of touch" with your body can cause emotional reactions when events occur that feel scary or distressing (for example, in a panic attack). Vagus nerve problems can also affect how someone experiences emotions. For example, someone with a vagus nerve problem might experience a surge of adrenaline when in danger, resulting in feelings of panic or arousal.

It's not uncommon for people to develop conditions that affect their vagus nerve and relate to worrying and anxiety. For example, the tilt table test can evaluate balance issues by having patients lie on a tilt table under stable conditions. If problems are found in this area, they can be caused by various factors, including many medical conditions such as diabetes or Parkinson's Disease, as well as some psychological ones such as anxiety, depression, and post-traumatic stress disorder. Some medications have also been linked to this condition (like nicotine and neuroleptics).

What happens if the vagus nerve is damaged?

The Vagus nerve is the longest cranial nerve that connects the brain to the abdomen. It sends a branch that goes to the heart in addition to going south of the diaphragm and up to the chest.

The Vagus nerve's function controls motor function. Still, it also controls important processes such as regulating blood pressure, causing coughing and swallowing saliva, helping respiratory organs work better with emotion regulation, and it helps control our heart rate.

It affects not only all these processes but also our ability to see, hear, speak or understand language because all of these functions are controlled by one vagus nerve.

This nerve also may decrease our sexual function because it is needed for orgasm.

The vagus nerve connects the brain to the body through the phrenic nerve, which is connected to the diaphragm. This vagus nerve, in addition to being needed for breathing and heart rate control, is also important in many other ways.

The vagus nerve controls many processes in your body, and without it, those processes will not be able to work properly. For example, without its operation, it would be difficult for you to have a normal heart rate or the ability to eat and drink normally.

If the vagus nerve is damaged, it may activate the sympathetic nervous system. This system is responsible for raising your blood pressure and heart rate. It also stops you from making the digestive juices in your stomach that help you digest foods properly. These functions are not only important for people who are injured or sick, but they are also vital to everyday life.

The vagus nerve connects the brain to the body through the phrenic nerve, which is connected to the diaphragm. This vagus nerve, in addition to being needed for breathing and heart rate control, is also important in many other ways.

The vagus nerve controls many processes in your body, and without it, those processes will not be able to work properly. For example, without its operation, it would be difficult for you to have a normal heart rate or the ability to eat and drink normally.

If the vagus nerve is damaged, it may activate the sympathetic nervous system. This system is responsible for raising your blood pressure and heart rate. It also stops you from making the digestive juices in your stomach that help you digest foods properly. These functions are not only important for people who are injured or sick, but they are also vital to everyday life.

Therefore, the following effects can be experienced if this nerve is damaged:

1. Increase in blood pressure and heart rate

Blood pressure and heart rate are both controlled by the sympathetic nervous system. If we damage this nerve, the brain will send signals to our sympathetic nervous system, which will then cause our blood pressure to be regulated, and our heart rate will increase.

2. Decrease in ability to breath

The vagus nerve connects the brain to the body through the phrenic nerve, which is connected to the diaphragm. This vagus nerve, in addition to being needed for breathing and heart rate control, is also important in many other ways.

The vagus nerve controls many processes in your body, and without it, those processes will not be able to work properly. For example, without its operation, it would be difficult for you to have a normal heart rate or the ability to eat and drink normally.

If the vagus nerve is damaged, it may activate the sympathetic nervous system. This system is responsible for raising your blood pressure and heart rate. It also stops you from making the digestive juices in your stomach that help you digest foods properly. These functions are not only important for people who are injured or sick, but they are also vital to everyday life.

3. Difficulty breathing during sleep

If your vagus nerve is damaged, you will experience difficulty breathing during sleep. As a result, you will wake up more frequently from sleep and have a lower level of quality your sleep. You may also experience chest pain when sleeping and even have higher blood pressure levels in your body at night.

4. Difficulty swallowing saliva

If the vagus nerve is damaged, it can decrease the saliva you swallow during your day compared to other people because it controls the muscles in your throat so you can swallow properly. This helps with swallowing foods and drinking water.

5. Difficulty seeing and hearing during certain times of day

The vagus nerve connects the brain to the body through the phrenic nerve, which is connected to the diaphragm. This vagus nerve, in addition to being needed for breathing and heart rate control, is also important in many other ways.

The vagus nerve controls many processes in your body, and without it, those processes will not be able to work properly. For example, without its operation, it would be difficult for you to have a normal heart rate or the ability to eat and drink normally.

If the vagus nerve is damaged, it may activate the sympathetic nervous system. This system is responsible for raising your blood pressure and heart rate. It also stops you from making the digestive juices in your stomach that help you digest foods properly. These functions are not only important for people who are injured or sick, but they are also vital to everyday life.

6. Difficulty speaking and understanding language

If the vagus nerve is damaged, it can decrease your ability to speak and understand language because it controls many of your speech functions, such as breathing and heart rate control, as well as language functions in the brain, such as vision, hearing, and recognition.

7. Difficulty swallowing and eating normally

The vagus nerve connects the brain to the body through the phrenic nerve, which is connected to the diaphragm. This vagus nerve, in addition to being needed for breathing and heart rate control, is also important in many other ways.

The vagus nerve controls many processes in your body, and without it, those processes will not be able to work properly. For example, without its operation, it would be difficult for you to have a normal heart rate or the ability to eat and drink normally.

If the vagus nerve is damaged, it may activate the sympathetic nervous system. This system is responsible for raising your blood pressure and heart rate. It also stops you from making the digestive juices in your stomach that help you digest foods properly. These functions are not only important for people who are injured or sick, but they are also vital to everyday life.

8. Trouble swallowing foods and eating properly

If the vagus nerve is damaged, you may have difficulty swallowing certain types of foods like those that require large amounts of chewing since the food will not be properly mixed with saliva or it will not be mixed correctly due to complications from changes in the esophagus caused by damage to this nerve.

9. Vomiting during sleep and severe nausea

The vagus nerve connects the brain to the body through the phrenic nerve, which is connected to the diaphragm. This vagus nerve, in addition to being needed for breathing and heart rate control, is also important in many other ways.

The vagus nerve controls many processes in your body, and without it, those processes will not be able to work properly. For example, without its operation, it would be difficult for you to have a normal heart rate or the ability to eat and drink normally.

If the vagus nerve is damaged, it may activate the sympathetic nervous system. This system is responsible for raising your blood pressure and heart rate. It also stops you from making the digestive juices in your stomach that help you digest foods properly. These functions are not only important for people who are injured or sick, but they are also vital to everyday life.

10. Difficulty swallowing saliva

If the vagus nerve is damaged, it can decrease the saliva you swallow during your day compared to other people because it controls the muscles in your throat so you can swallow properly. This helps with swallowing foods and drinking water.

11. Trouble speaking and understanding language

If the vagus nerve is damaged, it can decrease your ability to speak and understand language because it controls many of your speech functions, such as breathing and heart rate control, as well as language functions in the brain, such as vision, hearing, and recognition.

12. Tingling, numbness, and pain in the face

If the vagus nerve is damaged, it can decrease your ability to speak and understand language because it controls many of your speech functions, such as breathing and heart rate control, as well as language functions in the brain, such as vision, hearing, and recognition.

13. Loss of balance when walking or standing still

The vagus nerve connects the brain to the body through the phrenic nerve, which is connected to the diaphragm. This vagus nerve, in addition to being needed for breathing and heart rate control, is also important in many other ways.

The autonomic nervous system's three circuits.

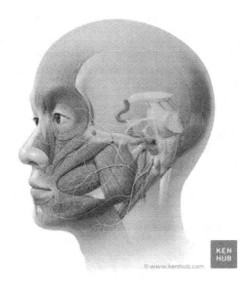

More than any other part of the body, the vagus nerve is responsible for regulating our digestive and respiratory systems. It helps control what we perceive as emotions, from fear to anger. It's also involved in regulating our heart rate and blood pressure, maintaining the heart rhythm, and controlling major organs like your liver.

Another important function of this nerve is memory storage — it connects back to our hippocampus, which plays a significant role in long-term memory formation. This means that when we are under stress or experiencing an emotional event, one circuit of this nerve can release neurotransmitters that lead to increased activity on the other two circuits, leading to euphoria or terror, respectively.

The three circuits are essential since they are interactive and depend on each other for optimal function. This includes all the circuits of the autonomic nervous system, including the enteric nervous system.

In this book, we are going to focus on circuit one. This is often referred to as the fight-or-flight response, which separates humans from all other mammals. This is a powerful circuit, and it can be overwhelming and debilitating when we become stressed.

Along with learning about the first circuit, we will also look at some tools and strategies for managing stress levels in your life. Because without them, you will never truly reach that state of peace you desire and need.

These autonomic nervous system's circuits include:

a.   sympathetic nervous system

The sympathetic (fight-or-flight) response is our main tool for dealing with stress when it is overwhelming or harmful to our survival. The sympathetic (fight-or-flight) response is triggered when the brain detects an "alarm" that something is wrong — as in, "something bad" has happened or might happen very soon in the future. So what does that mean? It means that something bad has happened or might happen very soon in the future, which could threaten your survival. So what do you do? You withdraw, fight, and defend yourself.

We are here on this earth to survive, and the fight-or-flight response is a very effective tool that we use to protect ourselves. It is our "escape-and-defend" system when we need it most. When called upon, the body produces an immediate surge of adrenaline and cortisol -a hormone that prepares us for protection from threats. This is also called the "startle reflex."

Our bodies create this partly because of positive feedback loops inside our brains. When the stress is over, this system overreacts and produces two hormones, adrenaline, and cortisol. They are hormones meant to be released in stressful or dangerous situations. While cortisol may have a purpose in short spurts during an emergency, prolonged exposure can have undesirable effects.

"It is important for people to become aware of their fight-or-flight response. It is a survival reaction that activates our heightened awareness of danger, increasing blood flow and metabolism in the areas of the body associated with danger. This is especially true of the heart, skeletal muscle, and gut. It will wear out if we do not use this protective mechanism for long enough periods.

b.   Parasympathetic nervous system

The parasympathetic nervous system has a calming effect on the body. It helps to restore balance to the body and mind. This is activated when an "alarm" isn't detected about danger or stress.

This has two major effects:

- Cortisol levels are reduced
- Heart rate, blood pressure, and respiration slow down

This system also has other effects, like activating the digestive processes, including releasing enzymes and hormones that stimulate the pancreas to secrete insulin and glucagon. While this positively affects our bodies, it can lead to problems if not used properly. Therefore, it's best to use the parasympathetic nervous system as much as possible.

The two components of the parasympathetic nervous system are:

1) Cranial nerves (CN) III, VII, IX, and X — release neurotransmitters that act on the heart, lungs, and digestive system.

2) Somatic nervous system — this is the one we will focus on here.

The Somatic Nervous System

This system senses what your body feels and sends messages to the brain, which then sends signals to your muscles. It uses feedback loops, such as stretch reflexes, so the brain receives information about how things affect you.

The sympathetic nervous system is triggered by a change in sensations in the body that indicate stress, threat, or danger. The parasympathetic nervous system works to get us back into balance again after being released from stressful situations. It's not a conscious response, so it's usually unconscious.

c. enteric nervous system

The ENS is composed of an extensive network of neurons that control your body's internal system, with millions of neurons within this system. While it is a part of your peripheral nervous system, it is considered autonomous. This means that its functions can operate independently of your brain and spinal cord.

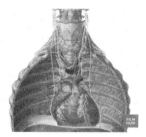

It is made up of two parts:

These neurons control several activities, including:

- Digestion
- Motility
- Absorption
- Secretion

It's connected to the sympathetic and parasympathetic nervous systems, so these three systems are interconnected. Moreover, it has one end connected to the brain and the other to the rest of your digestive tract. This means that it can help control both processes in your body, which is vital for it to perform optimally.

In this circuit, we will focus on learning how this system controls gut function. This will help you understand how your body functions in digestion and, more importantly, allow you to understand why things work the way they do.

The ENS consists of two parts:

1) Dorsal ganglion — this is where neurons from your sympathetic nervous system connect and control your immune system. It also helps control blood pressure.

2) Pedunculopontine nucleus — this is the part of your ENS that controls your gut.

The PN is made up of neurons that control the following functions:

- Both the sympathetic and parasympathetic nervous systems
- Gastroenterology
- Motility
- Secretion (including saliva)

When it comes to digestion, it's usually referred to as the enteric nervous system. It's a very small system that runs through your entire gastrointestinal tract from mouth to anus. It is composed of two parts:

1) Dorsal nerve plexuses — these are located in various areas within your gut, from mouth to anus.

2) Ganglia — these create a network composed of afferent and efferent fibers, which means they can either receive information or send messages.

When you are born, the PN contains more cannabinoid receptors. It uses endocannabinoids as a neurotransmitter. As you age, it decreases in these receptors but increases in substance P receptors.

This system serves as your body's main regulator for the following activities:

- Digestion — helps control all gastrointestinal functions and is responsible for maintaining homeostasis. This refers to when something becomes balanced again after being disturbed by some factor outside your body.

Homeostasis and the autonomic nervous system.

The Vagus Nerve is a part of the Autonomic Nervous System, which innervates both the Sympathetic and Parasympathetic. It controls the rate of blood vessels pulsing in the gut, heart, and digestive systems.

It is involved in controlling lactation and menstruation cycles. Vagus nerve stimulation is used to try to control seizures.

The Vagus Nerve has branches that go into a multitude of organs, including:

Heart, lungs, stomach, intestines, kidneys, liver, spleen, thymus, and kidney's adrenal glands.

It is a diagnostic tool to look at the heart's health. One of its branches goes into the heart and becomes a branch of the Sympathetic nervous system. When there is something wrong with the Vagus Nerve, it will not be sending information to the Sympathetic nervous system.

This will cause the heartbeat to slow and possibly stop, which could lead to death if not treated. The Vagus Nerve can also be used as a treatment for severe seizures (eclampsia and tonic-clonic).

It is used in surgery when it comes into contact with blood because it can cause clotting; otherwise, it is safe to use.

The Vagus nerve is also used as a diagnostic tool to examine the heart's health.

One of its branches goes into the heart and becomes a branch of the Sympathetic nervous system. When there is something wrong with the Vagus Nerve, it will not be sending information to the Sympathetic nervous system.

This will cause the heartbeat to slow and possibly stop, which could lead to death if not treated. The Vagus nerve can also be used as a treatment for severe seizures (eclampsia and tonic-clonic). It is used in surgery when it comes into contact with blood because it can cause clotting; otherwise, it is safe to use.

The Vagus Nerve is a critical part of the Autonomic nervous system. The Autonomic Nervous System is the part of the nervous system that acts through the nerves. The branches of the nerve that go into different organs make up its Parasympathetic and Sympathetic sides. It is located in the brain's central core, located between the two hemispheres, and goes to both sides.

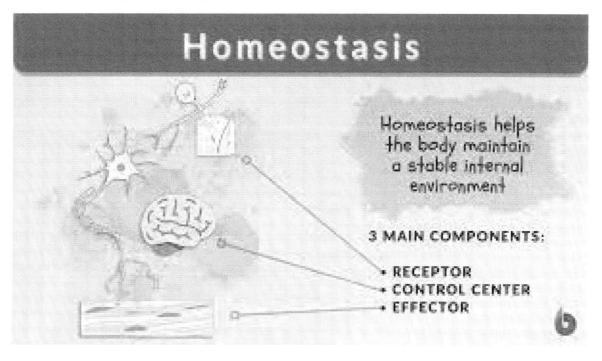

Homeostasis is the ability of the body to maintain a stable internal environment. It is affected by the Autonomic Nervous System. Homeostasis is controlled through homeostatic receptors in a process known as negative feedback. The body will have an ideal temperature, a normal pH level, and a steady heartbeat rate. When there is any change to these three key factors, then it will send out signals of change to other parts of the body that are responsible for maintaining homeostasis. This can happen on its own or with another signal from outside forces.

Homeostatic receptors have a mechanism of action that regulates changes in the central nervous system. When there is a change in the body's normal homeostatic substances, they will trigger signals that travel along the vagus nerve. These signals travel with the vagus nerve to other body parts, such as the heart and lungs. Suppose an organ has not received these messages from its cells. In that case, it will automatically receive a signal from another part of the body when it does not have a homeostatic receptor for them on its own.

To function, various organs and systems need certain chemicals normally found in blood or tissue fluids. The organs and systems must maintain homeostasis of all these chemicals. Chemical and Hormonal signals can affect the function of other organs.

Electrical imbalances within the autonomic nervous system can affect how we interact with our environment. If there is an imbalance in neurotransmitters, homeostasis will not be maintained. For example, depression is caused by a chemical imbalance within the nervous system that affects neurotransmitters in the brain.

The Autonomic Nervous System mostly regulates itself through feedback loops that allow it to remain stable. The Autonomic Nervous System consists of two parts. The Parasympathetic and Sympathetic Nerves.

The brain has two sets of nerves: the Sympathetic and the Parasympathetic. The nerves are responsible for many of their actions, whether a fast or a slow response. If there is no nerve activity, the body can still function, but a slow one can lead to death.

The vagus nerve is sometimes called the longest nerve because it runs from the brain to other organs in your body; this includes parts such as the Heart, Lungs, and Stomach's digestive system.

Therefore, the Autonomic Nervous System carries out homeostasis through:

a. Negative feedback -The nerve impulses the organs and systems receive will automatically stop any chemical or hormonal signals at the right time to maintain homeostasis.
b. Positive feedback - The Autonomic Nervous System can regulate itself through many different pathways, but most deal with minimizing chronic stress on the body.
c. A combination of negative and positive feedback - When the Autonomic Nervous System can maintain homeostasis, it will function properly because the chemical and hormonal pathways that control organs and systems will run smoothly.

The Autonomic Nervous System is a very complex system that works almost miraculously to keep the body functioning.

The Autonomic Nervous System regulates itself, but there are times when it might need help from outside influences to maintain homeostasis. Some of the main causes of malfunctioning can be:

a. Head injury - The amount of blood flow to the brain can change following a head injury, which can affect the Autonomic Nervous System, causing malfunction.
b. Heart disease - Heart disease can affect the Autonomic Nervous System because it affects the oxygen supply to your entire body.
c. Parkinson's Disease - The brain's dopamine pathways are affected by Parkinson's disease, which can affect the Autonomic Nervous System, causing malfunction.
d. Diabetes - Type 1 and Type 2 diabetes can cause malfunctioning of the Autonomic Nervous System by increasing chemical imbalances.
e. Liver Disease - Liver failure can also cause malfunctioning of the Autonomic Nervous System because it affects its ability to regulate chemicals that control such processes as breathing and blood pressure.
f. Severe Trauma - Severe trauma can also cause malfunctioning of the Autonomic Nervous System because it affects the chemical pathways that control your organs and systems.

g. Infection - Infections can also cause malfunctioning of the Autonomic Nervous System by affecting the chemical pathways that control your organs and systems.

h. Brain Injury - Brain injuries can also cause malfunctioning of the Autonomic Nervous System because it affects the chemical pathways that control your organs and systems.

i. Other illnesses - Other illnesses can also affect the Autonomic Nervous System, causing malfunctioning because they affect other parts of your body, such as the heart or lungs, through chemical imbalances.

j. Drugs - Drugs can also cause malfunctioning of the Autonomic Nervous System by affecting chemical and hormonal pathways that control organs and systems.

The Autonomic Nervous System is a very complex system that works almost miraculously to keep the body functioning. The system's three main components are Sympathetic Nerves, Parasympathetic Nerves, and Homeostatic Receptors. When you combine these three main components in one system that self-regulates itself, then it allows your body to do many things on its own such as: regulating heart rate and blood pressure, controlling digestion, controlling breathing, etc.

The Autonomic Nervous System is responsible for regulating many body functions, such as heart rate, blood pressure, and digestion. This system continuously monitors and adjusts these functions to keep them within a normal range.

This system can be broken down into two parts: the sympathetic and parasympathetic systems. The sympathetic and parasympathetic nervous systems are not working all the time simultaneously; they are always one or the other. One part working while the other part is resting helps regulate your body's functions to remain balanced.

The Autonomic Nervous System regulates many body functions, which it controls through feedback loops involving negative and positive feedback mechanisms.

The autonomic nervous system has a wide range of functions. Some parts of the brain are stimulated by it, such as:

a. Cerebral Cortex
b. Limbic System - The Limbic System is located deep within the brain and regulates emotion, memory and learning, behavior, and motivation
c. Hypothalamus – The hypothalamus controls all pituitary functions such as body temperature regulation; hunger, thirst; sleep cycles; sex drive, and emotional responses
d. Spinal Cord and Nerves – The spinal cord is the main communication pathway between the brain and body.

Five states of the autonomic nervous system.

The autonomic nervous system comprises two divisions—the sympathetic and the parasympathetic systems. The sympathetic activates organs that release neurotransmitters, while the parasympathetic inhibits organs that release neurotransmitters.

The enteric (or ventral) vagal nerve lies between the brain and the stomach. It is responsible for regulating heart rate rhythm, among other things, as well as visceral functions like digestion. Its activity can be detected in other body parts by a change in heart rate or blood pressure.

The five states of the ANS include:

1. Sympathetic response

The sympathetic response is activated during periods of stress and rapid physical activity. It increases heart rate and the force with which the heart contracts. It relaxes the smooth muscles of the bronchi, allowing the airways to dilate. The skeletal muscles are activated by sympathetic fibers, increasing their tone and making them contract more forcefully. The pupils of the eyes dilate, and perspiration increases. Blood flow is directed toward major muscle groups and away from organs not involved in physical activity (the "fight-or-flight" response). Moreover, the blood is shunted away from the skin into the muscles, making it pink and warm. The end result of this activation is more energy.

Therefore, this response is essential since it provides the vital energy required for "fight-or-flight" situations. The hypothalamus and the brainstem control the sympathetic system. The effect of this response is mediated through the release of various hormones into the bloodstream.

2. Parasympathetic response

The parasympathetic response (also called the "rest and digest" response) activates organs that release neurotransmitters while inhibiting organs that release neurotransmitters. Specifically, this system increases the activity of the salivary glands, stomach, and intestines. It also inhibits respiration and digestion, making your belly relax, increasing blood flow to the muscles, and decreasing it to the skin. The pupils of the eyes constrict, secretions decrease, and heart rate slows down. Therefore, this system is responsible for restoring energy spent during activity in times of rest or relaxation. This response aims at preserving energy.

The hypothalamus and the brainstem control the parasympathetic response. The effect of this response is mediated through the release of various hormones into the bloodstream.

This response is vital in waking and certain aspects of consciousness (alertness). It promotes digestion and absorption, relaxes smooth muscles throughout the body, helps maintain a healthy immune system, and keeps blood glucose levels within a normal range. This system also plays an important role in sexual arousal.

As you will see in the next section, the parasympathetic response is associated with subjective feelings of calmness and relaxation. The parasympathetic system is called the "rest and digest" system because it conserves energy for future demands. When this system is activated, it reduces heart rate, lowers blood pressure, and dilates pupils.

The enteric (or ventral) vagus nerve supplies the gastrointestinal tract and activates an increase in peristaltic action within its walls. In addition, it regulates the secretion of gastric acid and pepsinogen (an inactive form of pepsin). When this nerve is activated, gastric motility and gastric secretions are increased. The vagus nerve is central to controlling blood pressure by the brainstem.

This nerve also regulates the contraction of muscles in the esophagus and stomach and relaxes them when it decreases activity. The vagus nerve is considered a major component in the gut-brain axis regulating digestion. It coordinates other organ activities, like breathing, heart rate, muscle movement, and mood.

3. Reticular Stimulation

The third state of the autonomic nervous system is termed reticular stimulation. It occurs when a stimulus activates a large area of several sensory fibers that come into contact with the same nerve endings—the proprioceptive afferents to the CNS (central nervous system). The efferent fibers from these sensory afferents then pass through many ascending tracts, synapses, and interneurons, all in rapid succession to arrive at their point of origin.

For example, the Alpha1 (α1) receptors on the blood vessels will respond to stimulation from a drug that blocks the inhibitory effects of acetylcholine at that point in the body. When this happens, acetylcholine will be released through the parasympathetic system, and it will cause vasodilation at this point of origin.

The term reticular stimulation is derived as an analogy to one's thoughts: one has many thoughts, but they are organized in such a way that they can be grouped into complex thought patterns called "patterns" or "schemas."

A certain stimulus (like food or drink) will activate several receptors along the course of their afferent fibers back up to their origin point. This will lead to a series of afferent impulses that then converge and send one single efferent impulse through a descending pathway (or "reticulum"). However, the efferent fibers do not all arrive simultaneously at their point of origin.

They will sometimes arrive so rapidly that they cannot be distinguished. This is called coactivation. Furthermore, synchrony is associated with these impulses, an effect called common excitation (or shared excitation).

Reticular stimulation can also refer to the complex network of ascending axons with which these afferent fibers travel. The network consists of individual parallel or serial nerve pathways or tracts that form the ascending reticulum. Some are sensory tracts, while others are part of the motor system.

This reticular stimulation is responsible for the effect of sedation that one may feel due to opiates (or opioids) or other drugs. These drugs have a high affinity to either α1-adrenergic receptors on blood vessels or κ-opioid receptors on nerves within the CNS (central nervous system).

The former mechanism can cause vasodilation, a lowering of blood pressure, and a reduction in pain. Moreover, the latter can cause sedation, mood changes, and dysphoria with prolonged use. However, when both these mechanisms work simultaneously to produce this effect, they tend to be additive in their effects.

4. Sympathetic Stimulation

Sympathetic stimulation refers to activating the sympathetic division of the autonomic nervous system. This response is also known as fight or flight. It prepares an organism for dealing with a threat by activating various physiological systems, including cognitive and behavioral changes. These changes allow the organism to respond effectively to a threat, typically by fighting or running away from it.

A stressor that can lead to this sympathetic response is typically one that threatens an organism's well-being and causes fear, which then triggers this response through the brain's limbic system. For example, a loud noise or impending collision can trigger this response. This response will cause various physiological changes, including increased heart rate and blood pressure, faster breathing, and higher glucose levels in the bloodstream.

Exercise can also trigger sympathetic stimulation (such as sprinting to escape danger). It is vital in the "fight-or-flight" response of the nervous system. However, if stimulated for too long, it can have harmful effects (such as hyperthermia).

The sympathetic stimulation can also cause constriction of the bronchi in the lungs, which helps to increase the force of contraction during exhalation (EVC).

5. Immune response

The immune response is the reaction of an organism to invasion by pathogens. It involves both non-specific and specific responses. The non-specific response consists of the body's natural, inborn defenses; it is found in plants and animals, and fungi (such as yeast). These defenses include physical barriers such as the skin, chemical barriers such as acids and enzymes, and biological barriers; for example, inflammatory responses and the production of antibodies.

The non-specific response does not involve the activation of specific immune cells but rather the activation and mobilization of various other cell types to restrict the spread of pathogens.

The specific response is a more targeted immune reaction that activates certain white blood cells, or lymphocytes, to destroy foreign substances. This adaptive reaction prepares the immune system for future challenges by producing memory T and B lymphocytes.

This section discusses two types of responses: nonspecific responses and specific responses (both cellular). The nonspecific response is not as effective as the specific response.

6.   Nonspecific response

The nonspecific response is the most common type of immune reaction and involves both humoral and cellular immunity. It responds to foreign or otherwise threats by activating special white blood cells (antibodies) to recognize the invader. These antibodies are made in the immune system's B-cell lymphocytes, which reside in the bone marrow (or lymph nodes).

For this reaction to occur, a "foreign" substance must first activate these white blood cells. This substance is usually a molecule from an invader.

This can be achieved by administering two different types of drugs: A drug that initiates the B-cell reaction. The molecule that initiates this response must be specific for the particular invader and not for another substance (such as a chemical or drug). This is called "antigenic specificity." The second drug can inhibit this response. It has no antigenic specificity, but it delays the reaction.

The three neural pathways of the ANS.

The autonomic nervous system (ANS) is composed of two opposing systems that control the constriction and dilation of blood vessels. The ANS is a subsystem of the peripheral nervous system, which controls unconscious activities in organs such as digestion, circulation, respiration, and urine production. The ANS regulates body functions necessary to sustain life by controlling heart rate, breathing rate, salivation levels, and perspiration rates.

The ANS includes two opposing systems. The sympathetic nervous system operates through the release of norepinephrine, constricting blood vessels and increasing the heart rate. The parasympathetic nervous system operates through the release of acetylcholine, which widens blood vessels and slows down the heart rate. Both systems are responsible for maintaining body functions necessary to sustain life. The ANS is a subsystem of the peripheral nervous system, but it also receives input from several glands (e.g., pituitary) via hormones secreted into the bloodstream by those organs. These hormones are called autocrine or paracrine hormones. The peripheral nervous system is composed of nerve bundles that transmit impulses to and from our organs. The ANS acts on two opposing systems to control blood flow, heart rate, and other functions.

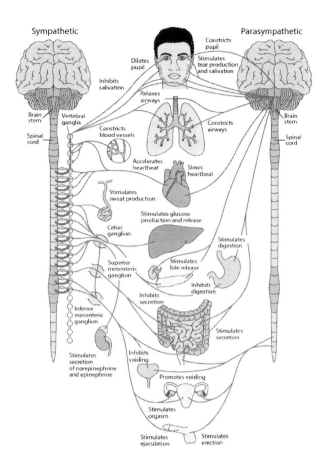

1. The autonomic nervous system

The sympathetic nervous system operates through the release of norepinephrine. This action causes constriction of blood vessels using alpha motor neurons (α-neurons) (sometimes called the "suck" pathway). The α-neurons serve as the muscles of the vascular system, causing blood vessels to constrict by firing action potentials called "myocardial contractions" (MCPs) that shrink the diameter of blood vessels.

The parasympathetic nervous system operates through the release of acetylcholine. This action causes dilation of blood vessels using cholinergic neurons (sometimes called the "push" pathway). These neurons slow heart rate by causing blood vessels to open up rather than contract.

The Vagus nerve is a paired nerve that extends from the medulla in the brain down to thoracic vertebrae T1–T9 and lumbar vertebra L3. The nerve branches into the left and right vagus nerve in the thoracic and lumbar regions of the spinal cord. Each vagus nerve continues into the abdomen, supplying many of the viscera with nervous projections.

The Vagus Nerve carries fibers from sympathetic and parasympathetic pathways to organs in the chest cavity and abdomen. The autonomic nervous system controls bodily functions such as digestion and breathing that are not under conscious control. As its name implies, the ANS is controlled by the autonomic nervous system, which sends impulses from the brain to organs in the body that control these functions.

The ANS is composed of two opposing systems called sympathoadrenal and parasympathetic. In this diagram, sympathetic fibers are shown in black, and parasympathetic in white.

Each system of nerves has inputs from most major glands that secrete various hormones into the bloodstream. These hormones are called "autocrine or paracrine." The function of hormones secreted by glands is affected primarily by neural input from central and autonomic nerves. The peripheral nervous system is composed of nerve bundles that transmit impulses to and from our organs. The ANS acts on two opposing systems to control blood flow, heart rate, and other functions.

The autonomic nervous system (ANS) is a subsystem of the peripheral nervous system that regulates internal organs' functions. The ANS has several components that work together to ensure a regulated and steady output of nerve impulses to the organs they supply. These components ensure cardiovascular homeostasis, gastrointestinal motility, respiratory control, urination, and kidney function.

A simplified diagram of the ANS is shown in figure 2. The sympathetic nervous system includes nerves that receive stimuli from the hypothalamus and pass information onto the thoracolumbar center (T2–L2).

2.   The sympathetic nervous system

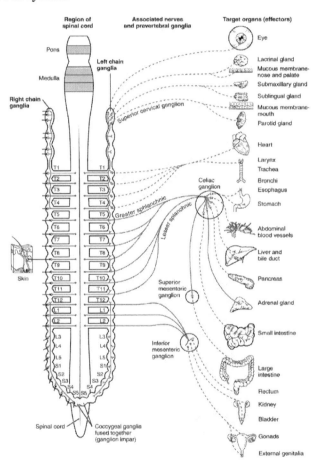

If either of these two systems fails (i.e., if they are dysfunctional), a compensatory pathway is triggered. This compensatory pathway is called the parasympathetic nervous system, sometimes called the "rest and digest" pathway.

For example, if the sympathetic nervous system fails to function properly, then the patient will experience restlessness. The "rest and digest" pathway compensates for this by causing the release of hormones into the bloodstream that cause relaxation of the smooth muscles of blood vessels, thus increasing their ability to open wider.

This is known as negative feedback regulation: a signal across a biological interface such as a nervous system (or other) receptor or "feed-forward." When used in the physiology-the flow of ions through phospholipid membranes in cell membranes (for example), this feedback is not exactly "negative." Still, it can be described as a faster than normal/desired cancellation of an excitation signal. Negative feedback regulation is used to achieve homeostasis- the state of a system that has constant conditions and maintains itself as best in that environment.

Physiological homeostasis requires the nervous system to regulate the flow of nutrients and other substances. This is achieved through a negative feedback regulation feedback mechanism because the nervous system can shut down sympathetic responses at the start or end of a burst to minimize these effects. At first, this seems counterintuitive, but homeostatic regulation does not always lead to a positive result, as it does with anabolic steroids, where increased muscle mass leads to negative outcomes such as loss of skin elasticity, tendon strength, and joint stability due to steroid-induced atrophy.

3. The endocrine system

The endocrine and autonomic nervous systems (ANS) work in tandem to help an organism maintain homeostasis. The ANS is part of the peripheral nervous system, which connects the central nervous system to every body tissue. The central nervous system has two divisions, the brain, and spinal cord, which are not physically connected to any other body part. It is thus a closed loop, a network that creates and stores information. The brain thus can retain information while constantly receiving new information from outside systems such as the ANS, immune system, and sensory organs.

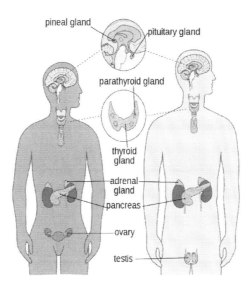

The ANS helps control many physiological processes by regulating the actions of smooth muscles, cardiac muscles, and glands. It also interacts with the endocrine system to create homeostasis. The ANS comprises two subdivisions: the sympathetic nervous system, responsible for stress and "fight or flight" responses, and the parasympathetic nervous system, which has a general relaxing effect on the body.

The ANS plays an important role in maintaining the balance between opposite or contrary forces in a biological system. For example, it controls blood pressure by constricting arteries and expanding veins in response to certain stimuli.

In this way, it maintains blood pressure within an acceptable range that can vary during daily life (e.g., in stress response) but is kept constant within the limits of a normal day-night cycle.

The ANS regulates blood pressure by increasing peripheral resistance and decreasing cardiac output. It also reduces blood flow to the skin and sweat glands by dilating arterioles.

These changes increase blood pressure (BP). The balance between the parasympathetic and sympathetic branches determines whether BP increases or decreases. For example, veins are constricted during sympathetic stimulation so that less venous return can occur, thus decreasing stroke volume and cardiac output. This then results in an overall decrease in BP. Similarly, veins are dilated during parasympathetic stimulation to allow for increased blood return to the heart, increasing cardiac output, and BP.

The ANS system plays a role in blood glucose maintenance. When consumed, glucose must enter the liver and be converted into glycogen. This is done through gluconeogenesis in the liver and epinephrine-mediated activation of glycogen synthase in the muscle cells. Suppose more glucose is needed than can enter the peripheral tissues through glycogen synthesis or epinephrine-mediated activation of glycogen synthase occurs. In that case, this excess must be stored as fat tissue by fatty acid oxidation in adipose tissue.

The sympathetic nervous system and the parasympathetic nervous system both play a role in regulating glucose homeostasis. When carbohydrates are consumed, insulin is released from the pancreas, and insulin causes an increase in glucose transport into muscle and adipose cells. The sympathetic nervous system causes an increase in epinephrine, which increases glycogen synthesis. Epinephrine also helps decrease fatty acid oxidation.

The ANS controls blood pressure and heart rate through the sympathetic and parasympathetic divisions. Both divisions influence blood vessels by causing them to constrict or dilate. The parasympathetic division increases heart rate while decreasing the force of contraction; it decreases BP by decreasing peripheral resistance through vasodilation of blood vessels.

The two-hybrid circuits of ANS.

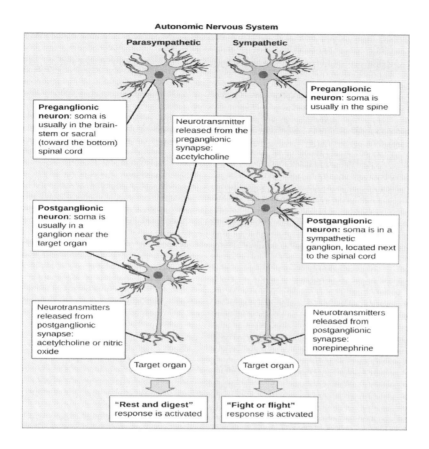

ANS circuits pass electrochemical signals from the vagus nerve to the nucleus or the solitary tract in a somatomotor neuron, an arm or leg muscle. The neurons in these circuits are excited by sensory input of a stimulus, such as a touch, vibration, temperature, sound, and taste. The vagus nerve receives input from several senses and sends output to an ANS circuit that will initiate an autonomic response when it receives an appropriate signal.

The ANS consists of a cluster of vagus nerve endings located in the brainstem's medulla oblongata, along with sympathetic preganglionic neurons that innervate local tissues. These two neuronal pathways can function independently or in combination to trigger various autonomic responses.

Claude Bernard first described the ANS in 1859. The dual electrical stimulation of the vagus nerve causes muscle contraction that is not directly innervated. This action can be reproduced artificially by stimulating the vagus nerve and the motor nerve of a small muscle, such as the thigh or finger.

The ANS belongs to the autonomic nervous system (ANS). The ANS is part of an internal organ part of our autonomic nervous system; it is located in the brain stem and contains neurons that control our bodily functions. These functions include:

The somatic (somatic) vagal pathway innervates and controls effects on the heart, lungs, gastrointestinal tract, bladder, ureters, and male genitalia.

The visceral (visceral) vagal pathway innervates and controls effects on smooth muscles in many body parts.

The two pathways of ANS consist of a cluster of vagus nerve endings located in the brainstem's medulla oblongata, along with sympathetic preganglionic neurons that innervate local tissues. These two neuronal pathways can function independently or in combination to trigger various autonomic responses.

The somatomotor (somatic) vagal pathway consists of afferent and efferent neurons that work together to initiate a parasympathetic response. The somatomotor pathway is used to facilitate a change from a state of alertness to relaxation; the goal is to reduce the heart rate and decrease blood pressure. There are two particular types of somatomotor neurons. One type, termed a vagal afferent neuron (VA), sends signals to the medulla oblongata and targets both the vagus nerve and sympathetic preganglionic neurons. Both pathways contain a mixture of static and dynamic fibers, so the process is not always smooth. For example, cardiac output can be increased or decreased by the simple act of breathing or coughing.

The efferent (efferent) vagal pathway consists of parasympathetic preganglionic neurons that control end organs. The efferent pathway can produce forced expiration in response to multiple afferent inputs to both pathways (autonomic braking).

The sympathetic preganglionic neurons originate in three areas, the thoracolumbar trunk, the intermediolateral cell column of the spinal cord, and a few other areas. The preganglionic sympathetic neurons that control this pathway are divided into two types. One type termed adrenergic (adrenergic) neurons sends postsynaptic signals to muscle fibers via alpha- and beta-adrenergic receptors. The second type, cholinergic (cholinergic) neurons, use muscarinic acetylcholine receptors to stimulate vagus nerve receptors. This pathway tends to be blocked by anticholinergics such as atropine.

The motor (motor) vagal pathway consists of pre- and postganglionic neurons that act upon skeletal muscle and glandular tissue, as well as additional effects. The preganglionic neurons originate in the spinal cord. The postganglionic sympathetic neurons target skeletal muscle, glandular tissue, heart, blood vessels, and end organs via nicotinic acetylcholine receptors.

The ANS consists of a cluster of vagus nerve endings located in the brainstem's medulla oblongata, along with sympathetic preganglionic neurons that innervate local tissues. These two neuronal pathways can function independently or in combination to trigger various autonomic responses.

Therefore, the two-hybrid circuits of ANS include:

1. Somatomotor circuit (or visceromotor circuit):

The vagus nerve endings are located in the medulla oblongata, along with sympathetic preganglionic neurons that innervate local tissues. These two neuronal pathways can function independently or in combination to trigger various autonomic responses. Moreover, the somatomotor circuit (or visceromotor circuit) consists of afferent and efferent neurons that work together to initiate a parasympathetic response. The somatomotor pathway is used to facilitate a change from a state of alertness to relaxation, and the goal is to reduce the heart rate and decrease blood pressure. In addition, the vagus nerve fibers are some of the longest known in the human body. This circuit allows the vagus nerve to play a part in many different organ systems. Therefore, the somatomotor circuit consists of a variety of different underlying mechanisms, such as:

a. Triggers of the parasympathetic nervous system:
i. Beginning of activity:
ii. Opioid drugs (tolerance/dependence):

b. The sympathetic nervous system:
i. Sympathetic nerves innervate the aorta and the blood vessels, which can raise blood pressure; therefore, when a parasympathetic neurotransmitter is released, it causes vasodilation and lowers blood pressure.
c. The somatomotor circuit controls every organ in your body; however, the heart is the most important organ in this circuit due to its control by nerves and hormones that are regulated by this circuit.

2. Visceral circuit:

A cluster of vagus nerve endings located in the medulla oblongata, along with sympathetic preganglionic neurons that innervate local tissues. The two neuronal pathways can function independently or in combination to trigger various autonomic responses. Moreover, this pathway consists of parasympathetic preganglionic neurons that control end organs. The efferent path consists of parasympathetic preganglionic neurons that control end organs.

The ANS consists of a cluster of vagus nerve endings located in the brainstem's medulla oblongata, along with sympathetic preganglionic neurons that innervate local tissues. These two neuronal pathways can function independently or in combination to trigger various autonomic responses. This circuit controls every organ in your body; however, the heart is the most important organ in this circuit.

Therefore, the visceral circuit includes:

a. The vagus nerve endings are located in the medulla oblongata, along with sympathetic preganglionic neurons that innervate local tissues.

The two neuronal pathways can function independently or in combination to trigger various autonomic responses. Moreover, this pathway consists of parasympathetic preganglionic neurons that control end organs. Therefore, this circuit controls all your organs, including the heart, brain, and stomach.

b. The parasympathetic preganglionic neurons that control end organs.

The efferent path consists of preganglionic sympathetic neurons that innervate the heart, blood vessels, and end organs via nAch receptors. Moreover, these preganglionic sympathetic neurons originate in three areas, the thoracolumbar trunk, the intermediolateral cell column of the spinal cord, and a few other areas; therefore, nerves from the sympathetic pathway have targets to muscles and glands as well as fiber systems such as:

i. The parasympathetic preganglionic neurons that control end organs.
ii. The visceral circuit controls all your organs, including the heart, brain, and stomach.

The visceral circuit controls all your organs, including the heart, brain, and stomach; however, nerves innervate the GI tract and lymphatic system to regulate them.

This circuit is related to the gastrointestinal tract because it is activated whenever you eat, and if the motor circuit is misfiring, you may have trouble swallowing.

The ANS controls every aspect of your body because it activates all your organs and sends signals to them to function according to their purpose. The visceral muscles help us maintain our posture, keep us upright, and eat and breathe. Moreover, the visceral muscles include:

1. The phrenic nerve:

The vagus nerve controls the parasympathetic function of the diaphragm, the main muscle involved in breathing. The diaphragm is a large dome-shaped muscle that separates the thoracic cavity from the abdominal cavity. It contracts and relaxes to alter the air volume in both cavities and assist breathing. Therefore, it is composed of two muscles:

2. The esophagus:

i. The visceral nervous system consists of all of your internal organs. In contrast, the somatomotor nervous system consists of all other organs except your abdominal organs (such as the heart, lungs, and diaphragm). However, the ANS is responsible for stimulating or inhibiting the muscles of the esophagus, which are one group of visceral muscles.

Therefore, the ANS controls your internal organs through three different pathways that can function independently or in combination to trigger various autonomic responses. Moreover, the ANS consists of a cluster of nerve endings in the medulla oblongata and sympathetic preganglionic neurons that innervate local tissues. The two neuronal pathways can function independently or in combination to trigger various autonomic responses. Furthermore, this pathway consists of parasympathetic preganglionic neurons that control end organs; therefore, these three neurological circuits are essential for all physiological processes and are involved in many clinical disorders.

The vagus nerve controls the parasympathetic function of the diaphragm, the main muscle involved in breathing. The diaphragm is a large dome-shaped muscle that separates the thoracic cavity from the abdominal cavity. It contracts and relaxes to alter the air volume in both cavities and assist breathing.

What is biobehavior?

Behavior is the actions of living beings and their reactions to internal or external stimuli.

Biobehavior is the study of system-level behavior in an individual. It deals with how that system integrates its behaviors across all levels, how it responds to stimuli, and how it can alter itself due to experience. Biobehociorists are interested in understanding what drives behavior by examining feedback loops between biology and environment (or between environment, cognition, and behavior).

Biobehavior may be described in two ways: 1) as a system-level behavior or 2) as the integration of psychological, biological, and social-cultural variables.

System-level behavior refers to the individual behaviors that comprise an entire behavioral unit. The term "biobehavior" suggests a focus on macro behavior—the overall functioning of a living being at all three levels: 1) the internal physiological, cognitive, and emotional states; 2) the interactions between internal conditions and external stimuli (such as food availability or tool use); 3) social interactions with other individuals within the unit (such as aggression or nurturing).

Biobehavior integrates the individual's biological, cognitive, and social-cultural processes. At the micro level, this integration involves identifying the unit's behavioral repertoire (the behaviors it performs at all levels) and then describing how it responds to environmental stimuli or experiences. Micro behavior is about finding "the balance between demands of internal physiological states on the one hand and external stimuli and opportunities on the other." The unit's response is a function of its life history, genetics, developmental history, neurophysiology, psychology, culture, and past experiences. At the mesos level, individuals within a system communicate with each other to gain access to resources (such as food or mates). At the macro level, individuals within a group coordinate their behavior to form larger groups.

All levels interact. Therefore, the description of micro behavior must also include Mesos and macro behaviors. The term "biobehavioral system" is thus a holistic approach to describing a living being at all three levels: physiological, cognitive, and social-cultural processes.

Biobehavior is complementary to neuroscience, which studies brain function or neural mechanisms in isolation from the organism or environment (i.e., in artificial systems). Biobehavior, in contrast, focuses on the integrated system.

Biobehavior also differs from sociobiology, which focuses on the adaptive advantage of behavior without regard to an organism's internal processes or neural mechanisms. In contrast, biobehavior is interested in why organisms change due to experiences and how they respond to internal and external stimuli in real time. Biobehavior doesn't simply explain how organisms adapt to their environment but also how they alter their environment due to their behavior.

The term "biobehavior" was coined by O'Donnell (1948). He used it to describe the relationship between human being and their environment. It was introduced into a research context by Vittorio Gallese in 2000. Gallese coined the term "biobehavioral system" to describe a living organism in its totality, with its psychological, neural, social-cultural, and biological components. The concept gained popularity among neuroscientists to draw attention to how internal processes (such as one's beliefs or emotions) influence behavior. Gallese first used the biobehavioral system (Gallese et al. 1996). Since its introduction, it has been applied extensively by neuroscientists and scholars across fields of psychology, sociology, anthropology, and neuroscience.

In his review of biobehavioral systems, Gallese makes the case that biobehavioral systems fundamentally differ from traditional reductionist models of scientific research (such as the physiochemical or genetic model), which focus exclusively on the external environment, internal physiology, or neural mechanisms. In contrast, the biobehavioral model of Cacioppo & Berntson attempts to understand the organism as a "complete situated activity system" in which "internal processes and the environment dynamically influence one another through the moment-to-moment processes of encoding, representing, and producing behavior."

Biobehavioral narrative analysis is a research methodology designed to "highlight relational patterning that can illuminate multiple layers of human experience." It is a collaborative practice that relies on small groups to build biobehavioral narratives. It integrates qualitative research methods such as thematic analysis, discourse analysis, and grounded theory with neuroscience methods such as EEG readings or fMRI scans.

Biobehavioral narrative approaches are useful for identifying complex patterns of interrelated experiences that traditional quantitative methodologies may overlook. When we analyze a group of people, we can uncover how their interpersonal relationships shape one another's behavior and cognitive processes.

Biobehavior is used in case study research to describe the relationships between an actor (individual or group) and its environment, including culture, social class, historical context, and other circumstances.

The biobehavioral approach has been criticized for what is perceived as a widening gap between the understanding of brain mechanisms and their behavioral manifestations. Some argue that it is easier to study concrete, observable behaviors than it is to study relatively intangible cognitive processes. For example, Antonio Damasio has argued that behavior can be studied in controlled laboratory conditions. In contrast, an understanding of decision-making or emotional regulation requires the influence of multiple individual and environmental factors. Another concern is that biobehavior relies too heavily on subjective reports from the actor being studied, which could be affected by memory bias or other reporting errors.

Characteristics of biobehavior:

a. In biobehavior, there are two research directions: from physiological processes to cognitive and social-cultural processes and from cognitive and social-cultural to physiological processes.
b. Biobehavioral research aims to study the whole psychological process in a unified way. When people talk about the brain, they refer to biochemical processes and physical mechanisms, but they do not talk about how these biochemical processes influence people's behaviors and thoughts. Suppose we want to conduct a true study of psychological and cognitive processes. In that case, we will have to go beyond this kind of analysis and include the physiological systems.
c. Although there are many studies of physiological processes in isolated organisms, such as plants or lower animals, few studies include physiological and ecological (non-physiological effects) components in their talk about the system being studied.
d. There are also very few studies that focus on the neural mechanisms of a living organism. Although people have made great advances in understanding the neural mechanisms at work in lower animals, they have had less success in explaining how brain function influences higher organisms, such as humans.
e. Finally, many people like to talk about psychological and behavioral processes as if these processes were independent of biological systems and processes. However, virtually all psychological and behavioral processes are influenced by biological functions (physiological ones). Even cognitive or social-cultural functions are affected by physical or biochemical processes. The recognition of the importance of these relationships is particularly important for research on living organisms, especially human beings.

Biobehavioral systems study human psychological processes in the context of the mind-body problem, emphasizing the active relationship between behavior and physiology. The biobehavioral approach is a theoretical framework that seeks to provide a more comprehensive understanding of human behavior by accounting for the interactions and interrelations between the cognitive, neural, social-cultural, and biological levels of analysis. It examines how these elements dynamically interact with one another through a process of ongoing feedback loops.

The biobehavioral approach focuses on how psychological processes and their corresponding substrates (i.e., neural, biochemical, and genetic) are co-developed throughout an individual's lifespan (lifespan development). This approach recognizes the simultaneous influences of biological systems on human behavior and the complex developmental processes that shape biological systems over time.

The origins of biobehavioral systems theory stem from the work of American psychologist Walter Cannon. In the 1920s, Cannon published "Organization for physiological homeostasis as a basis of behavior," which argued that all organisms are in a state of physiological disequilibrium with their environment and that they constantly adjust this equilibrium through the action process (activity). However, it was not until the post-World War II cognitive revolution that this theoretical approach became more widely recognized. In 1950, psychologist William James Dillon published "An Introduction to the Physiology of Behavior," which became one of the first texts formalizing Cannon's behavior theory into a coherent theoretical framework.

A biobehavioral perspective advocates a shift in focus from decomposing the mind into different levels (such as cognitive, social, or biological) to exploring how the mind and body work together to produce behavior. Vittorio Gallese coined the term to describe a "total system approach" to psychology and neuroscience. Biobehavioral systems are believed to be constructed by information originating from neuronal structures that interact very disorganized with other stimuli, such as internal states, emotional processes, and cultural contexts.

Effects of activity in the ventral vagus circuit.

Antagonistic effects on heart rate and respiratory frequency (decreasing both). Activation of the neuroendocrine system, mediating relaxation in response to sympathetic activation

The Vagus nerve is a major nerve that controls much of the activity in the ventral vagus circuit. The circuit is responsible for regulating blood pressure, heart rate, and many other vital processes. Cause of death due to Vagus nerve damage includes cardiovascular collapse, apnea, and shock. Treating certain types of epilepsy through surgical removal or destruction of portions of this pathway has been attempted but with mixed results.

Brainstem projections from the nucleus ambiguus to the hypothalamus are involved in the neural control of responses to stress and are called Amygdala modulation by Peripheral Activation (AMPA). Vagus nerve stimulation inhibits AMPA and causes a decrease in heart rate, suggesting that efferents from the ventral vagus nerve inhibit sympathetic activity.

Other studies found that electrical stimulation of the vagus nerves effectively reduces heart rate and blood pressure when administered to humans implanted with pacemaker electrodes for treating heart failure.

The Vagus Nerve modulates immune cell activity by secreting several different cytokines. The Vagus Nerve innervates various macrophages, mast cells, and lymphocytes. The effects are mediated by releasing IL-1, IL-6, TNFα, and GM-CSF. When administered to mice with experimentally induced colitis, vagus nerve stimulation promoted M1 activation and decreased Th17 differentiation without altering normal colonic homeostasis. Vagus nerve activation also increased the number of circulating CD8+ cytotoxic T cells and NK cells. Other reports suggest that the vagus nerve can alter the phenotype of DCs by increasing MHC-II and CD40 expression while decreasing co-stimulatory molecules ICAM-1 & B7.

Increased vagus activity has been associated with cardiovascular disease, including atherosclerosis and heart failure. The mechanism involves altering blood flow to the heart by altering baroreflex activity. In one mouse study, mutant mice homozygous for a disruption in the "Gpr88" gene significantly reduced atherosclerosis incidence and improved cardiac function after myocardial infarction. One explanation for the improvement is that nerve stimulation cannot only alter the normal rhythm of the heart but also can alter the autonomic tone of the dam.

Stimulation of vagus nerves has been reported to increase the secretion of endorphins, with an increase in beta-endorphin up to 9 hours after stimulation. The specific receptors involved are currently being tested.

Vagus nerve tumors are rare but include carcinomas (10%), astrocytomas (1%), and oligodendrogliomas. Most are located in areas innervated by white matter and non-motor cranial nerves: olfactory nerves, oculomotor nerves, facial nerves, and trigeminal nerves. They are treated with surgery and radiotherapy. The survival rate is surprisingly high; one study found a recurrence rate of approximately 6%.

Vagus nerve stimulation has been used to relieve neuropathic pain, such as diabetic neuropathy and postherpetic neuralgia, and to treat depression. A Cochrane review found that it was effective for neuropathic pain, but there was insufficient evidence for the effectiveness of vagus nerve stimulation for depression.

In a randomized controlled trial, vagus nerve stimulation was more effective than placebo for reducing chronic spinal cord injury-induced neuropathic pain intensity in two of three experimental groups (overall effect size = 0.25). When more than one technique was used, vagus nerve stimulation was more effective than a cervical and dorsal rhizotomy.

Vagus nerve stimulation has been used in patients with epilepsy. In one study, about half of the patients were completely free of fits for five years, and ten of the sixteen had no fit for four years. In another study, patients treated with vagus nerve stimulation sustained reduced seizures. They were over 90% seizure-free after two years, while those not using vagus nerve stimulation were primarily controlled by valproate or phenytoin.

Vagus nerve stimulation has also been studied for its effect on post-traumatic stress disorder (PTSD). In one small randomized controlled trial, a higher dose of vagus nerve stimulation was found to be more effective than isoflurane anesthesia at reducing PTSD symptoms such as hyperarousal and flashbacks.

Vagus nerve stimulation has been used for chemotherapy-induced neuropathy. One double-blind study found that, in patients undergoing chemotherapy for colorectal cancer, vagus nerve stimulation reduced the number of hot flashes, improved quality of life, and decreased fatigue in 63% of the patients. A Cochrane review found insufficient evidence supporting vagus nerve stimulation as a replacement for or adjunct to conventional methods for treating chemotherapy-induced peripheral sensory neuropathy.

Vagus nerve stimulation is used as a muscle relaxant. This is often achieved through a transcutaneous method by stimulating the vagus nerve through electrodes implanted at a distant site called an activator station.

Therefore, the effects of activity in the ventral vagus circuit include:

a. The parasympathetic thrills originate from the nucleus ambiguous, pass via the Wallerian tract, and terminate in the superior cervical ganglion, where the fibers cross to form the recurrent laryngeal nerve.
b. Stimulation of the vagus increases glutamate secretion by inhibiting kainate-type substances with vagotomy or bilateral nucleus ambiguous lesions.
c. With continuous stimulation, there is an increase in excitatory transmission at both distal and proximal levels of thalamocortical synapses and an overall excitatory effect on the cerebral cortex (cf - The vagus nerve modulates cortical activity)
d. The interaction of both phasic and tonic components of the vagal afferents with both phasic and tonic components of the cortical afferents modulates cortical activity
e. The sustained activation of cortical neurons damages the synaptic connections.
f. Cortical Hyper-reactivity: (for pain, fatigue, motor disturbances, depression)

Vagus nerve stimulation has also been used to stimulate the respiratory muscles. In one randomized trial, 20 patients were treated with high-frequency vagus nerve stimulation for six weeks to alleviate their chronic obstructive pulmonary disease (COPD). Twenty-five percent had a decrease in airflow at rest, and 50% had an improvement in forced expiratory volume in one second (FEV1).

g. Vagus nerve stimulation has been used to stimulate the respiratory muscles. In one randomized controlled trial, 20 patients were treated with high-frequency vagus nerve stimulation for six weeks to alleviate their chronic obstructive pulmonary disease (COPD). Twenty-five percent had a decrease in airflow at rest, and 50% had an improvement in forced expiratory volume in one second (FEV1).
h. It has been observed that the onset of action is within a few days and tends to stabilize after two weeks.

i.   In supraventricular tachycardia (SVT) cases, vagus nerve stimulation is beneficial in converting the heart rhythm from SVT to normal sinus rhythm.

j.   It has been observed that vagus nerve stimulation can improve cardiac output, mean arterial pressure, and stroke volume in patients suffering from myocardial infarction by increasing the vagal tone.

k.   Vagus nerve stimulation is also known to enhance food intake by stimulating gastric secretion, motility, and secretion of pancreatic juices resulting in better digestion and absorption of nutrients

In a small study, vagus nerve stimulation improved the ability of patients with spinal cord injury to tolerate various stimuli, including hypoxia and hypercapnia.

Post-traumatic stress disorder (PTSD) has been found to be associated with hyperactivity in the amygdala, a brain region involved in fear learning and memory, and decreased activity in the ventromedial prefrontal cortex associated with extinction learning. Vagus nerve stimulation has been found to decrease the activity of the amygdala and improve extinction learning of PTSD symptoms.

At least two patients with Tourette syndrome have been treated with vagus nerve stimulation. Both were in their fifties and had the most severe form of the disease; both showed improvement in symptoms after treatment. Neither had responded to any other treatment, but both showed significant improvement only when vagus nerve stimulation was used in addition to anti-psychotically drugs.

Diabetes-associated neuropathy may be successfully treated by a pacemaker-like device implanted in the chest that sends continuous electrical pulses to the left vagal nerve. Wearable devices, such as hearing aids, have been designed to stimulate the vagus nerve. Various vagus nerve stimulators are commercially available from several companies that offer these devices for therapeutic and diagnostic applications.

Effects of activity in the dorsal vagus circuit.

The dorsal vagus nerve is the longest cranial nerve, which sends branches to the stomach, lungs, and other viscera. In humans, it is sometimes called the pneumogastric nerve.

The dorsal vagus nerve is comprised of afferent fibers that carry sensory information and efferent fibers that relay motor commands to the muscles of the stomach, gallbladder, and intestines.

The dorsal vagus nerve plays an important role in regulating digestion. When stimulated by a gastrointestinal input (e.g., intestinal distention), it causes smooth muscle contraction in those organs to enhance their peristalsis and expelling functions.

The efferent motor commands in the dorsal vagus nerve reach the viscera after they cross the spinal cord via synapses in the paragigantocellular reticular formation. Those fibers are part of a reflex arc that involves afferent and efferent fibers from the nodose ganglion to relay sensory information about blood pressure, respiration, and swallowing.

The nervous connections between viscera and brain function in areas like satiety and appetite. Vagal afferents send signals to the area postrema, located at the base of the fourth ventricle in the brain. The area postrema is an important brain structure because it is rich in neurons that sense changes in blood composition, such as pH or glucose levels, and relay that information so the brain can respond. For example, those neurons send signals to the hypothalamus when they sense a change in glucose levels to elicit an appropriate response—either to get food or store energy by decreasing metabolism.

Activity in the dorsal vagus circuit can inhibit the sensation of nausea when stimulated through the area postrema after peripheral activation. Activity in this circuit can also suppress food intake by modulating centers responsible for hunger and satiety and affect autonomic control over heart rate, bronchial reactivity, and airway resistance. Vagal afferents from the dorsal vagus nerve send signals to the nucleus tractus solitarii (NTS) in the brainstem, a connection point of neural pathways that control cardiovascular, respiratory, and gastrointestinal functions. The dorsal vagus first synapses on NTS neurons before it sends signals to areas that control food intake and satiety.

The activity in the dorsal vagus circuit can also affect respiratory control during sleep-breathing disorders such as chronic obstructive pulmonary disease (COPD). Patients with COPD experience difficulty breathing during sleep because they have shallow breathing and because they experience micro-awakenings during the night. Those micro-awakenings are associated with arousals from sleep and periods of hyperventilation followed by apnea. The dorsal vagus nerve is part of the pathway that relays neural signals to control respiratory function, such as snoring and breathing during sleep.

In an experiment, the activity in the dorsal vagus nerve was stimulated in healthy subjects to test its effects on breathing during sleep. In response, the autonomic nervous system sends efferent commands to increase airway resistance, slow down breathing rate, and prolong expiration time. Those changes in breathing resulted in decreased apnea episodes and better blood oxygenation. Those changes occurred without stimulating other reflex pathways (e.g., via carotid body stimulation). The activation of the dorsal vagus nerve made healthy subjects respire at a slower rate during sleep and did not affect breathing during wakefulness.

The dorsal vagus nerve is important in keeping people alert and in good health. People who lack enough activity in the dorsal vagus circuit can experience symptoms such as pain and depression because they cannot respond to those signals sent from peripheral organs, resulting in maladaptive eating patterns that contribute to weight gain by increasing appetite.

The dorsal vagus nerve is an important target for treating several conditions, including gastrointestinal, heart, eating, urinary, and movement disorders.

There are a variety of different disorders that can involve the dorsal vagus nerve. Some of them include:

a. Disorders related to the dorsal vagus nerve
d. Disorders that can cause damage to the dorsal vagus nerve
e. Diseases affect areas in which the dorsal vagus nerve plays a role
g. Conditions of unknown cause
h. Other conditions, where more research and answers are needed
i. Bibliography

Several clinical trials are being performed to treat dorsal vagus nerve conditions. One of them is to test if electrical stimulation of the dorsal vagus nerve in patients with severe depression can reduce depressive symptoms and improve mood. Another one is to use electrical stimulation of the dorsal vagus nerve with a gastric pacemaker to treat obesity. Another clinical trial uses an implanted device that stimulates dorsal root ganglion cells to treat pain from diabetic neuropathy.

Some of those disorders can be treated by stimulating activity in the dorsal vagus nerve or by directly implanting electrodes on that nerve. The electrical stimulation is done to reverse the symptoms of the disorder. For example, intestinal paralysis caused by C. difficile infections can be reversed when patients are given electrical stimulation to the area postrema to stimulate peristalsis and relieve constipation. When a serious illness like cancer causes intestinal paralysis, or when patients are under stress, electrical stimulation to the area postrema can be sufficient.

The dorsal vagus nerve can also be used as an alternative method of treating some pains from diabetic neuropathy. In patients with diabetic neuropathy, nerves in the peripheral nervous system that originally stimulated muscles so that muscles contract and relax are damaged. That type of nerve damage results in pain and weakness, resulting in compression of nerves in the neck or other areas. The dorsal vagus nerve normally supplies those nerves on the neck with signals that tell them to contract muscles so that patients experience relief from pain. To treat pain and weakness caused by diabetic neuropathy, electrodes can be implanted on the dorsal vagus nerve at the base of the neck or in other areas to provide signals from a small generator.

When patients are given electrical stimulation to their dorsal vagus nerve over time, they become more sensitive to that electrical stimulation, resulting in reduced symptoms caused by the dysfunction of other organs. For example, patients with irritable bowel syndrome who are given electrical stimulation over six months' notice improved digestive function after treatment.

When it is unable to properly send signals related to swallowing and eating food, patients can experience dysphagia—difficulty swallowing that could result in aspiration pneumonia and death.

The dorsal vagus nerve that innervates the heart has a dual function. When activated, it slows down the heart's beating by inhibiting the firing of neurons that control heart rate (called pacemaker cells). On the other hand, it increases the force of contraction by controlling muscarinic receptors in cardiomyocytes. It also functions as a third-order sensory nerve and innervates the peripheral nervous system, which controls bladder and bowel activity. The tract of nerves central to the control of cardiac rhythm and autonomic nervous system activity is known as the vagus nerve. This has led to its being called both the parasympathetic and sympathetic nerves. People with damage to their dorsal vagus nerve usually have little or no control over their heart rate.

Many structures within the spinal cord are interconnected with one another through a very wide network of nerve fibers, almost like an intricate net that spans from above down to below. The dorsal vagus nerve is one of the most prominent connections that extend from the brain to the spinal cord. The connection between these nerves and the rest of the nervous system is called a nerve root.

The dorsal vagus nerve has many branches and endings, some of which are important for it to function in its normal purpose. There are two main branches, called cranial and caudal median nerves. The median cranial nerve runs from the brain stem as a branch of the fifth cranial nerve (trigeminal). It then runs along with other nerves from the brain stem to reach its target on the back of the head just below the ear lobe.

The other main two branches of the dorsal vagus nerve are the caudal median nerve and the caudal vagus nerve. The caudal median nerve is also called the vagic or cranial vagus nerve, which is located just above the thyroid gland and continues to reach its target on a small tissue on the back of the brain stem. It then continues towards a large portion of the brain known as pons and medulla oblongata.

The functions of these two branches are different in contributing to the overall action of the dorsal vagus nerve.

Therefore, the activity in the dorsal vagus circuit includes:

a. Decreased heart rate (pacemaker cells)
b. Increased force of contraction
c. Decreased force of relaxation (muscarinic receptors)

d. Increased parasympathetic tone to heart.
e. Decreased sympathetic tone to heart
f. Decreased intestinal motility (kidneys, bladder, and intestines)
g. Decreased secretion of gastrointestinal hormones related to motility and absorption
h. Increased secretion of pancreatic enzymes by pancreas
i. Increased secretion of gastric acid by stomach
j. Increased secretion of biliary acids by liver
k. Decreased secretions of hormones from adrenal medulla, pancreas, and thyroid gland
l. Increased secretions of gastrointestinal hormones related to digestion
m. Stimulation of the dorsal ventricular dilatation in the brainstem, which results in decreased blood pressure (baroreceptor activity)
n. Stimulation of carotid body activity—increased breathing rate (reduces CO_2 levels) and increased oxygenation of blood (reduces acidosis).

Somatopsychological problems.

This is when you feel a headache, itches, your neck hurts, or pain at the back of your head. People with somatopsychological problems experience their bodies as a source of distress.

Somatophobia's effects on social life can make it very difficult for those who suffer from this disorder. The solution to overcoming this disorder will require additional time and energy that interfere with daily activities.

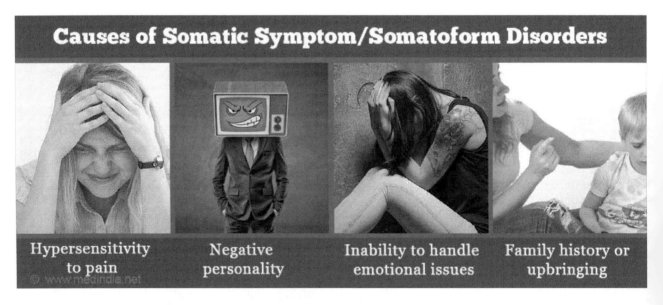

The vagus nerve entrainment may help alleviate somatopsychological symptoms in people with vagus nerve entrainment problems due to its relaxing health benefits. Still, it should not be relied upon on its own.

Since the vagus nerve is a calming nerve, it is a useful tool for pain management. The vagus nerve is also related to digestion since it helps move food along the gastrointestinal tract.

People with somatopsychological problems, on average, have difficulties in starting and maintaining conversations. However, people with vagus nerve entrainment may find it easier to communicate due to its ability to relax the body through tension.

Since the vagus nerve plays a role in warm and cold systems, it can be an important tool in certain medical applications, such as researching temperature control concerning potentially life-threatening diseases.

The vagus nerve is related to the solar plexus, which plays an important role in controlling the body's temperature. This may be related to sensitivity to cold and hot temperatures.

In addition, the vagus nerve also plays a role in relaxing the body. This can help people with somatopsychological symptoms since tension is common in somatopsychological disorders.

Situations requiring patience and focus on mental tasks are also common among people with somatopsychological problems. The vagus nerve entrainment may help relieve stress due to the muscle relaxation it entails.

Another way that vagus nerve entrainment may be beneficial to people with somatopsychological problems is when it comes to dealing with physical pain. The vagus nerve helps process painful stimuli in the body by sending signals processed by the brain.

Vagus nerve entrainment may also improve a person's focus on physical activities due to its ability to relax muscles and reduce stress. In addition, it also improves sensation and movement coordination when performing certain tasks.

Therefore, people who have difficulty focusing on certain tasks may find it easier to use vagus nerve entrainment as a relaxation technique before performing tasks requiring focus.

The vagus nerve plays a role in managing stress because it helps regulate the amount of oxygen that reaches the brain. This can be useful for people with an overactive nervous system.

Vagus nerve entrainment can be used to improve blood and bone circulation, which are related to improving sleep quality. This is important since excessive sleepiness can cause somatopsychological problems.

Vagus nerve entrainment can also benefit people suffering from diabetes since it improves blood glucose monitoring and body temperature regulation.

In people with diabetes, the vagus nerve is often damaged. This can be alleviated by vagus nerve stimulation. Vagus nerve entrainment can help maintain the vagus nerve's function so that it is not further damaged if it has not been affected by damage before.

Vagus nerve entrainment may also be effective in those who experience pain during nervous stimulation due to its calming benefits. This can be especially helpful for reducing the severity of migraines and tension headaches since these are common somatopsychological symptoms affecting many people.

Therefore somatopsychological problems include:

a. Discomfort in your body

Discomfort in your body can be in the form of pain, a common symptom in various diseases such as arthritis and other inflammatory diseases. Pain is often treated with over-the-counter or prescription medicines since it may be caused by a medical condition such as muscle strain or injury that needs further attention from the doctor.

Its characteristics include:

* recurrent, widespread pain
* diffuse, intermittent pain
* mild to moderate intensity of pain
* sensitivity to cold and heat

This discomfort can be in the form of itching or any other type of physical discomfort. It is often found on the surface of your skin, which varies from person to person. This can depend on how sensitive your skin is, but it is generally believed that people with dry skin suffer from this more than those with oily skin. These types differ in how the treatment is provided using different products, including creams and lotions that help relieve the symptoms associated with discomfort in your body.

b. Feeling dizzy

Feeling dizzy can be caused by factors such as a change in altitude, standing up for long periods without moving, and changes in atmospheric pressure due to weather changes. Dizziness can also be caused by several medical conditions that require immediate attention from a healthcare provider such as heart disease, low blood pressure, poor nutrition, pregnancy, and vertigo.

Its characteristics include:

* feeling unsteady on your feet
* seeing things spinning around you
* feeling that the world is spinning around you
* difficulty focusing your attention on something when standing still or lying down

It is characterized by a feeling that you are moving even though you are not or that objects in your surroundings move, even if you are standing still. Aside from this, it can also result in nausea and vomiting. This can happen after getting out of bed or turning suddenly due to motion sickness, motion-sickness-inducing stimuli such as the following seasickness, watching vehicle movement while riding in a car or boat, and reading or watching television while traveling.

c. Headaches

Since headache is a common symptom of several diseases, it can be treated with prescription medicines such as pain relievers. However, if the cause of the pain is in your nervous system, then vagus nerve entrainment may be beneficial.

Its characteristics include:

* usually felt in one part of your head
* usually feels like "a band around your head" that gets worse with any movement or activity. This can cause a feeling of pressure and sometimes may make you feel nauseous. It can be associated with both tension and migraine headaches.
* intensity of pain is low to moderate
* onset is gradual
* frequency of headaches increases with age.

According to the website mentioned above, migraines are characterized by a rapid, pounding pain that covers one side of the head and sometimes extends down your neck and into your back, usually accompanied by severe visual disturbances. They can also be accompanied by temporary loss of vision and sensitivity to light. Onset can occur minutes to days before the headache, lasting a few hours after its occurrence.

A migraine headache is associated with 5-14 days of attack frequency per month unless stated on this website's page about migraines.

d.   Numbness

Numbness is a symptom of peripheral vascular disease, carpal tunnel syndrome, and diabetes. It is characterized by tingling, numbness, or loss of feeling in the hands and feet. This can happen when walking and standing up too quickly. Numbness can also be caused by changes in atmospheric pressure due to weather changes or altitude changes.

Its characteristics include:

* tingling or numbness in your hands and feet
* can sometimes be accompanied by weakness or muscle spasms
* usually feels as if the circulation is impaired.

e.   Pain with movement

Pain without movement is a common symptom caused by arthritis and fractures that may require medical attention from a healthcare provider. Pain with movement may affect someone's ability to move effectively since it can cause stiffness in muscles and joints when moving them.

Its characteristics include:

* pain in your joints or muscles
* pain with exertion or movement of your joints and muscles
* the pain worsens with movement but rarely goes away on its own.

f.   Loss of appetite, weight loss, and fatigue

Loss of appetite can be caused by several diseases, such as diabetes, gastrointestinal disorders, cancer, pancreatic cancer, and hypothyroidism. These may also occur after a traumatic event such as surgery or other types of injury. Loss of appetite is also one of the most common symptoms experienced by patients suffering from depression, which is characterized by long-term sadness or depression that can have causes that are not physical, such as anger and frustration.

Its characteristics include:

* lack of appetite and poor appetite
* often occurs when a person is in bed or even on the couch watching television, causing you to feel guilty about giving up your favorite food and unable to bring yourself to eat it.
* may or may not cause weight loss

Stress and sympathetic nervous system.

The sympathetic nervous system is often called the "fight or flight" response. When something triggers, the adrenal gland releases a stress reaction from the brain, adrenaline, and cortisol. This hormone enables you to respond quickly and appropriately when faced with a challenge or danger. One way that your body is affected by this reaction is through your stomach and intestines — you may notice that hunger disappears, bowel movements slow down, food moves slower through your stomach, or bolts of pain shoot down your esophagus.

Some people can't make cortisol in response to stress and may lack the ability to respond with a fast-acting fight or flight response that would enable them to survive. These people may experience chronic stress or even depression. The body can adapt to chronic stress, but this adaptation may be unhealthy. Some symptoms of stress are reduced appetite, cold hands and feet, fatigue, difficulty sleeping, and tendencies to overeat or eat foods high in sugar.

Stress is often worsened by social isolation, which makes it difficult for you to deal with negative emotions and hard to face the things that are going on in your life. You may find that you go through a period of stress each day when faced with something difficult, like dealing with a bully or being bullied yourself. If you live alone and are isolated from friends, family, and other people, depression can result from stress.

Feeling stressed is natural; it's part of life. But when stress is chronic or serious, it can lead to health problems. A chronic overreaction to everyday stressors — a pattern of intense or persistent worry, anxiety, and tension that might not seem like something you have control over — is the most common form of mental illness in the United States. Over one-third of adults in this country report having symptoms of clinical depression within the past year.

In addition to impacting our health, chronic stress can also take a financial toll on families. People who report chronic stress are more likely to miss work and have lower salaries. They are also more likely to divorce or become separated from a spouse and have fewer financial resources. If you live alone, you may use up all of your "social capital," which can lead to social isolation and stress.

Stress can affect many aspects of health and well-being, including chronic pain, heart disease, high blood pressure, high cholesterol, anxiety, depression, breathing problems, sleep disorders, gastrointestinal complaints (such as nausea), migraines, immune system problems, lack of concentration, weight issues, poor memory. Cortisol also makes people more prone to other chronic diseases.

When you're under stress, you may find that you're tired all the time and aren't able to fall asleep at night. You may have trouble concentrating, especially if you are under mental or physical stress. If you suffer from chronic pain, the adrenal glands may be at work making chemicals that make pain worse instead of better. This is a vicious cycle of thought and feeling, leading to an adrenal gland reaction that leads to symptoms in the body that worsen the pain.

The stress response in the body is primarily mediated by the sympathetic nervous system, which stimulates the heart to beat faster and raises blood pressure. The body also releases norepinephrine, a chemical that mobilizes the brain and body for "fight or flight" activity. Cortisol is released from the adrenal cortex in response to stress, increasing glucose levels to provide energy for the muscles so they can be prepared for action. However, if the muscles are not engaged in action, they will instead put the glucose into fat cells — thus contributing to weight gain. On top of that, cortisol also increases appetite and decreases metabolism.

Cortisol has other effects as well. It sensitizes pain receptors and promotes inflammation. It contributes to feelings of apathy or depression. It suppresses immune function and growth processes, leading to an increased risk for illness or cancer. It may even cause a decline in the thinking skills you need for survival.

This stress response must have a "shut-off valve" because if it were to continue unchecked, it would destroy your health! When you are fleeing from a predator, for example, cortisol levels rise but fall again when there is no longer any danger.

On the other hand, cortisol levels don't always fall back down when they should. Thus you may find yourself experiencing a constant state of fight or flight. If you are always looking for danger, your body may be unable to completely shut down that adrenaline reaction.

If you can't fall asleep at night or wake up in the morning with a feeling of dread, that's a message from your body. It tells you something is wrong and needs to be dealt with. If problems during the day cause the same reaction, these messages can pile up without resolution and make it harder for your body to return to a state of equilibrium and rest. Chronic insomnia can turn into a vicious cycle of insomnia, leading to more stress, less sleep, and even more stress.

The stress response is not necessarily negative. It can be good when it alerts you to a potential threat or danger. However, if you are always in fight or flight mode, this can lead to problems. The battle-ready state is more likely to lead to a lack of sleep, chronic health problems, and weight gain than survival.

What would happen if you turned off your stress response? Well, some people often become very quiet after they stop stressing over a situation. You may even see them looking in the mirror and saying things like: "I've given up!" or "There's nothing I can do!"

Paradoxically, this is more stressful than dealing with the source of stress. It is one thing to deal with a bully in person and another to feel helpless. Some people go into denial and say that the bullying doesn't bother them, or they make excuses for the bully. These reactions are often worse than the stress response itself because they add to the load on our bodies and keep us from doing something about it.

When you live in an environment where bullying is routine, the stress response can be very useful. It may not allow you to handle the situation by yourself, but it will have had a positive effect — allowing you to do something about it.

The most important thing is to avoid being constantly angry or overtired. If you have made a serious effort, given up enough time, and couldn't get away from your bully or situation, this will come naturally as long as you give your body what it needs — rest.

If you're one of those who has a hard time getting over stressful situations, it may be time for you to take charge! The first step is learning how your body responds under stress. You'll find out what isn't healthy for you and what you need to do to fix it. You'll also learn the difference between stress and emotions.

Relationship between stress and sympathetic nervous system:

a. If a person is exposed to stress, he/she produces more adrenaline.
b. Adrenaline is released from the adrenal medulla.
c. Adrenaline causes the sympathetic nervous system to be stimulated.
d. Sympathetic nervous system stimulates heartbeat and raises blood pressure; Simultaneously, it stimulates the part of the adrenal cortex, which releases cortisol into the bloodstream, reaching its peak 20 minutes after release.

Therefore, if you are experiencing high levels of stress day in and day out, your adrenal glands are probably overworked and exhausted; hence your immune system cannot work at its best. As a result, you will be prone to infections and other health problems.

e. You will also be likely to catch up with a cold easily.

To sum it up, if a person is experiencing high levels of stress and does not know how to get rid of it, they should talk to the doctor and find out how to reduce their stress. They should also talk to an expert who can help them understand how to best deal with their stress, helping them to release all that pressure. This way, they will enjoy a healthy life and stay as fit as possible.

The fight-- or fly reaction.

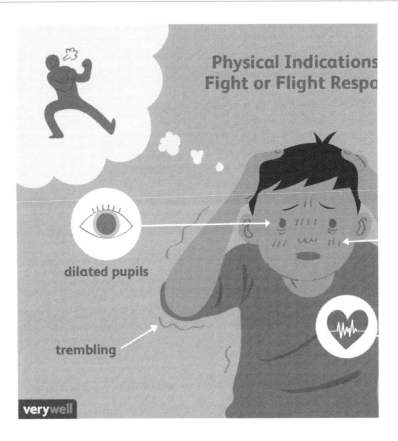

Fight or fly reaction is a term used when referring to the reaction of the vagus nerve to danger and other stimuli. The vagus nerve is a large cranial nerve that starts in the medulla oblongata of the brain stem and descends through the neck, chest, abdomen, diaphragm, spleen, and pancreas. Its role includes aiding in heart rate control via modulation of parasympathetic activity from thoracic spinal cord circuits (the "cardiac" vagus) as well as maintaining intestinal tone via stimulation of preganglionic sympathetic fibers from enteric ganglia (the "enteric" vagal).

The vagus nerve works by inhibiting the over-action of other cranial nerves. It slows down the heart rate and smooths muscles when the carotid sinus nerve is stimulated (i.e., carotid pressure increases). Likewise, it slows down breathing when sacral parasympathetic fibers are activated (i.e., sacral pressure increases). The vagus nerve also inhibits other organs, including stomach acid secretion, to increase blood flow to the gut in a reflex called vomiting in an attempt to compress the intestines and promote blood flow away from them in a protective mechanism called emesis (from Latin emere "to eat," and ceteris paribus "all other things being equal"). Hence, the fight or flight reaction involves a sudden and dramatic increase in heart rate and blood pressure due to over-activation of the vagus nerve to stimulate the heart and inhibit gastrointestinal activity (inhibit peristalsis).

The vagus nerve response is a stress response we have to varying degrees. It's sometimes called fight or flight. When stressed, the hypothalamus releases corticotropin-releasing hormone (CRH) into the hypophyseal portal system, which goes directly to the anterior lobe of the pituitary, which then releases adrenocorticotropic hormone (ACTH) into the bloodstream, which causes our adrenal glands to secrete cortisol and other glucocorticoid hormones. This "stress response" activates our sympathetic nervous system, or "fight or flight" mode.

When this happens, we may develop an ulcer in our digestive tract that can become very serious. One of the factors that can affect the development and healing of an ulcer is our behavior. Our vagus nerve plays a very important role in this. Under stress, our sympathetic nervous system, fueled exclusively by acetylcholine and norepinephrine, is activated. Norepinephrine inhibits the firing rate of vagal parasympathetic pre-ganglionic fibers; this leads to decreased parasympathetic tone that manifests as arrhythmia (irregular heartbeats) and a reduced heart rate. Norepinephrine also enhances the secretion of adrenocorticotropic hormone (ACTH) via stimulation of the hypothalamic corticotropin-releasing hormone (CRH) receptors. The increase in ACTH increases the secretion of glucocorticoid hormones, especially cortisol. This leads to a reduction in glucose levels and protein breakdown that is used to form amino acids and fatty acids, which are used as fuel for muscles during exertion; this preserves glucose for use by the brain. Cortisol also causes a decrease in blood flow to the digestive tract (by decreasing gut motility), slowing down digestion and nutrient absorption. All these effects aim to provide fuel and energy to the muscles so we can escape a predator.

There's some controversy about how cortisol acts on the gut. One study suggests that cortisol has two effects: it increases mucosal permeability (blood flow to the gut), which leads to inflammation, and it inhibits gastric secretion (reduced acid secretion), which can lead to ulcer formation. Another study found that cortisol did not affect mucosal permeability or gastric acid output; instead, it decreased blood flow by increasing vascular resistance in the hepatic portal system, which slows down food uptake from the gut into circulation.

Characteristics of fight or flight reaction are:

a.   Increased heart rate (tachycardia)

This is due to the sympathetic nervous system driving up heart rate and blood pressure to enhance our ability to run away. Heart rate is increased because the vagus nerve is inhibited by norepinephrine (a neurotransmitter derived from dopamine produced in the locus coeruleus) which decreases the parasympathetic tone of the heart. A reduction in parasympathetic tone leads to an increase in heart rate.

b.   Decreased gut motility

This also occurs due to sympathetic activation; sympathetic stimulation of adrenergic receptors on intestinal musculature leads to decreased gastrointestinal motility and delays stomach emptying, inhibiting gastric acid secretion and reducing blood flow within the gut wall.

c.   Increased blood pressure (tachycardia)

The increase in sympathetic stimulation leads to an increase in arterial pressure by constricting the peripheral veins and arteries.

d.   Decreased ventilation

This occurs by inhibition of inspiratory flow caused by hyperventilation. Lastly, biofeedback techniques can help you control your VN response.

One way to do this is through biofeedback training; during this process, breathing is monitored, and the participant is told when they are breathing too fast or too deeply, which will trigger a response they can consciously control.

Other ways to help control our vagus nerve response include eating more fiber, not eating spicy foods, not eating carbonated drinks and caffeine, getting regular exercise (slow cardio), self-hypnosis, etc...

e.   Increased vagus nerve activity

This occurs when we are in the early stages of an ulcer with inflammation (nodular phase) and necrosis (necrotic tissue). During this time, your vagus nerve will be stimulated at a higher than normal rate causing diarrhea, heartburn, burping, etc... Because this phase is not fully differentiated, there is still some heart and gut motility so that it can be both excreted and recirculated. Once your ulcer is healed, it will decrease to a normal level because the inflammation has been suppressed along with any subsequent damage to the vagal nerves.

f.   Decreased vagus nerve activity

This occurs when your ulcer has healed and is completely differentiated. In this case, no high inflammation or necrosis is causing the vagus nerve to be stimulated to return to normal levels.

The best way to stay healthy and heal your ulcers is to keep your stress levels down and get a restful sleep every night.

These characteristics have been found to affect the development of ulcers. Ulcers are caused by inflammation and increased acid secretion in the lining of the stomach (lower esophageal sphincter), damage to the lining of the stomach or esophagus, or both (called gastric erosions). It is well known that our digestive system functions less efficiently when we are under stress. We experience a reduced ability to digest food, and our stomach secretes less acid. It also has been found that when we are under stressful conditions, the blood flow to the gastrointestinal tract decreases, which contributes to an increase in inflammation, making it more difficult for the body to heal itself from a potentially serious condition. Thus, it is believed that stress can lead to stomach ulcers and make them worse once they develop.

Therefore, it is believed that stress can lead to ulcers and cause them to develop. It is hypothesized that the stress induced by an illness, a divorce, or a death in the family, for example, can lead to gastritis (inflammation of the stomach), which in turn leads to ulcers. According to this hypothesis:

*   Ulcers are genetic-related diseases; they are transmitted from generation to generation via genes.
*   Stress causes gastritis and the development of ulcers; hence stress causes ulcers.

Other factors could contribute to gastric ulcer formation, like personality traits and environment.

*   Stress can cause gastritis, which in turn can lead to ulcers.
*   Stress is responsible for the formation of gastric ulcers.

However, contrary to the hypothesis that stress causes ulcers, stress does not cause the disease; it only worsens the existing disease or prevents it from healing. People who believe that stress causes their gastric ulcers may undergo psychotherapy and medications in modern medicine. Psychotherapy aims to resolve psychological problems such as anxiety and depression by relaxing the person involved so they don't feel so stressed out. Some medications, such as antidepressants and anxiolytics (anti-anxiety medicines), reduce stress levels.

The polyvagal theory's healing power.

The polyvagal theory is a scientific model of the autonomic nervous system introduced by Stephen Porges. It views the vagus nerve as the primary nerve of calming rather than our old-fashioned explanation of adrenaline. It has many similarities to the mammalian fight-or-flight reflex.

Synchronicity is the coherence of meaning between seemingly unrelated events and suggests a meaningful order behind it. In this way, synchronicity can be viewed as a form of physical correspondence concerning time, space, and causality. One very specific kind of synchronicity involves the perception by an organism or human being that one event is relevant to another event that seems entirely disconnected from it by context and time. This perception can be explained as coming about through nonlocal influences or a kind of collective unconscious communication or human instinct or learned behavior.

This theory's healing power is seen in the medical field. It explains how the brain keeps us from putting on weight and can help us with its healing powers. Staying connected to our emotional center, we can forgive ourselves, feel less pain, gain better perspectives, and be closer to peace. Some books cover how to use Nature's system of healing methods to solve problems that may arise.

The polyvagal theory, inspired by the work of Austrian neuroscientist Stephen Porges, is a new view of the autonomic nervous system that proposes two distinct nervous systems in humans—the sympathetic and parasympathetic. Traditionally, these were viewed as two independent systems and have been studied separately. However, the polyvagal theory posits that they can be viewed as two aspects of the same system, with a full spectrum of activation and deactivation between them. The model was developed over decades, starting in the 1980s, by Porges and his colleagues, who studied it as an alternative to traditional views. Early versions of the theory posited that there was a continuum between these two systems. In later versions of the theory, the two systems have been viewed as more distinct from each other and joined by a bridging system.

The polyvagal theory is based on recent neurophysiological discoveries concerning two phylogenetically older autonomic nervous system components, reptilian brain centers associated with defensive reactions and mammalian brain centers associated with social engagement behaviors. The theory proposes that the autonomic nervous system evolved through two major stages (see below). According to Stephen Porges, the polyvagal theory is an integrative theory of social engagement and the fight and flight responses because it proposes that these two systems — which have traditionally been described as separate for each individual — are instead one single phylogenetic system. The notion that mammals have a variety of strategies to deal with threats is not new; however, what is new about this theory is that it proposes that mammals also have a full spectrum of strategies to deal with safety and social engagement.

The Polyvagal Theory, according to Porges (2007), is a relatively recent theory of the autonomic nervous system. "polyvagal" means multiple vagus (i.e., vagus nerve) fibers. However, the Neuro-physiology of Polyvagal Theory proposes that the two types of the vagus nerve are not different entities but instead are components of a single phylogenetically older system that evolved in two major stages: 1) primitive reptilian brain centers that emerged before mammals and 2) mammalian brain centers that emerged after mammals. The theory proposes that mammalian vagal structures are more social because they evolved later to help primates and mammals survive challenges. The basic idea behind the theory is that there is a spectrum of neural circuits ranging from primitive to most evolved. The "newest" circuit evolved first, followed by an intermediate circuit, followed by the "oldest" or most primitive circuit in mammals and other vertebrates.

The polyvagal theory also draws on a wide range of cross-disciplinary research in fields such as neurophysiology, anatomy, linguistics, ethology, communication sciences, audiology, and comparative psychology. It is in many respects an integrative theory because it proposes that the autonomic nervous system can be understood by looking at multiple levels of functioning: the organ level (e.g., heart rate), the visceral level (e.g., visceral organs such as intestines and lungs), the level of structures (e.g., vagus nerve), the behavioral level and finally at the state that integrates these coping strategies into a coherent whole (e.g., variations in state regulation such as distress or social engagement).

The benefits of polyvagal theory's healing power are:

a.   Social Support

Social support is a way to destress the body and mind. We need social support in our everyday life to prevent stress and increase well-being. It is important for healing because it helps keep us healthy and reduces stress through regular exercise, meditation, yoga, or sports.

b.   Emotional Balance

We can do many things to keep our emotions balanced, such as going for a walk-in nature, hiking in the mountains, taking deep breaths, and calming down. The benefits of emotional balance are: feeling more confident and calmer, helping you to overcome problems or conflicts with others or with yourself. Emotional balance improves self-esteem, therefore, keeping us happy and healthy

c.   Self-compassion

Being kind to yourself through eating healthy, exercising, and other good habits helps us to feel good about ourselves. Self-compassion gives us the courage to change bad habits and puts us at ease when we are disappointed and many other things.

d.   Movement

Physical activity is important for our well-being because it keeps our bodies fit and healthy. Physical activities can benefit health if they are balanced with the right amount of physical activity that is not too much or too little, like running a marathon or roller skating on rollerblades without enough physical exercise. Exercise increases endorphins, our natural painkillers. Engaging in physical activities can also help to reduce stress and make you feel calmer.

e.   Mindfulness meditation

Mindful meditation is a practice that helps us to pay attention to the present moment without being distracted by our thoughts or feelings, and it teaches us to observe our thoughts as they come and go in an accepting manner rather than trying to control them through thoughtless criticism or self-criticism. Mindfulness helps us observe how we feel, our body sensations, and what is happening around us in a non-judgmental way. It helps us to be aware of our thoughts and feelings without judging them. It allows us to let go of useless thoughts, emotions, fears, and worries. It brings acceptance and freedom.

f.   Gratitude practice

Reminding yourself of all the things you are thankful for and making lists of them is a great way to increase your well-being and happiness. The benefits of gratitude can be: We can appreciate the simple things, it gives us energy, it helps us to be more present in the moment, and many other things.

g.   Meditation on self-compassion

Meditation on self-compassion is a healing tool because it helps us accept, forgive and love ourselves. It also allows us to accept who we are, with all our flaws and differences, and be comfortable with ourselves.

h.   Meditation on gratitude

Mindfulness meditation is a practice that helps us to pay attention to the present moment without being distracted by our thoughts or feelings, it teaches us to observe our thoughts as they come and go in an accepting manner, rather than trying to control them through thoughtless criticism or self-criticism. Mindfulness helps us observe how we feel, our body sensations, and what is happening around us in a non-judgmental way. It helps us to be aware of our thoughts and feelings without judging them. It allows us to let go of useless thoughts, emotions, fears, and worries. It brings acceptance and freedom. This mindfulness meditation also helps in stress reduction, a meditation on gratitude can help you to feel grateful for all the things you have; that is the beauty of life we all deserve.

i.   Mindfulness at the workplace

Mindfulness is a practice that helps us to pay attention to the present moment without being distracted by our thoughts or feelings, it teaches us to observe our thoughts as they come and go in an accepting manner, rather than trying to control them through thoughtless criticism or self-criticism. Mindfulness helps us observe how we feel, our body sensations, and what is happening around us in a non-judgmental way. It helps us to be aware of our thoughts and feelings without judging them.

Stimulation of the vagal nerve-placebo as an alternative cure to depression.

Stimulation of the vagal nerve-placebo is an alternative cure for depression. It has been known to be an effective treatment and is less expensive than common psychiatric drugs. Moreover, many side effects associated with common psychiatric drugs, such as antidepressants, are absent when using vagus nerve stimulation, while the symptoms of depression are treated more effectively.

Surgical implantation is a non-invasive procedure that requires only a local anesthetic. In this way, the body does not recognize it as a foreign object and rejects it. Vagus nerve stimulation could be an option for those who do not respond to traditional treatment methods, such as anti-depressants and cognitive behavioral therapy.

There are also serious dangers associated with this method of treating depression, some of which were discussed in Sarajevo as a treatable illness. According to the book, people have had a seizure and heart attacks. Although no deaths have been reported, this form of treatment is still new and needs to be studied further.

Since mainstream medicine has yet to acknowledge the positive effects and costs associated with vagus nerve stimulation, many choose to use alternative methods for relieving their depression. The use of vagal nerve stimulation is one alternative method that has proven beneficial for many who suffer from depression.

In many instances, the patient's depression has not only been alleviated but also eliminated with the use of this alternative cure. The cost of this treatment has also proven to be significantly lower than that of traditional psychiatric treatment methods such as drugs and psychotherapy. One issue with vagus nerve stimulation is the fact that an implant is needed, which requires a general anesthetic.

This fact may deter some from trying this alternative treatment method. However, it should be noted that the implant is removable and small (1x1x1 cm). Thus, it would be easy to remove in case of complications or a desire to discontinue the implant.

Vagus nerve stimulation is a non-invasive alternative treatment for depression and has shown to be less expensive as compared to psychiatric drugs. Furthermore, the patients have reported being free of side effects from common psychiatric drugs such as antidepressants. This alternative treatment method has also been more effective in treating depression than standard drug therapy.

Specific nerve blocks may stimulate the vagus nerve by applying electrical current at relatively high frequencies and low voltages to stimulate the brain's hypothalamus or other parts of the central nervous system.

The vagal nerve is a branch of the autonomic nervous system that supplies the viscera (heart, stomach, intestines) and part of the brainstem with parasympathetic regulation, one component of which affects depression or sadness. It also sends branches to many other organs in the body, including two cranial nerves-X, VII-that regulate salivation and swallowing, respectively. Therefore stimulation of the vagal nerve can affect mood states in several ways.

Based on these concepts, vagal nerve stimulation has been investigated as a treatment for depression. Interest in vagus nerve stimulation arose when it was discovered that people with epilepsy, who have epilepsy-related brain damage, were more likely to suffer from depression than otherwise healthy people. This led to the hypothesis that overactivity of the brain area in which this type of seizure started (the mesial temporal lobe) might be responsible for depression and that stimulating the vagus nerve might stop this area from firing so much by sending it inhibitory signals from the parasympathetic nervous system. There is some evidence to support these theories.

Vagus nerve stimulation is a day surgery procedure in a hospital or outpatient clinic. The surgical implantation of the device does not require general anesthetic but only local anesthesia. The last two decades have shown that VNS therapy is feasible and safe in treating depression that has not responded to conventional antidepressant therapies. This non-invasive method has been used in randomized controlled trials and presented at the Neuropsychopharmacology Conference in 2001. Depressed patients who could benefit from vagus nerve stimulation are those with high levels of anxiety, male patients, and patients with more than two failed antidepressant treatments and electroconvulsive therapy (ECT).

Currently, there are two types of vagus nerve stimulation systems: a high-frequency generator with a low-voltage device, and a low-frequency generator with a high-voltage device. These devices must be surgically implanted under general anesthesia with insertion into the vagus nerve approximately 4 cm in length. An electrode that connects to the device is successfully placed at the base of the skull, similar to ECT.

After surgery, patients may experience some dizziness and balance problems. Patients using this form of treatment have reported improvement in depression while on it; levels of depression appear to improve more over time rather than suddenly after treatment has begun. This improvement is also associated with a decrease in anxiety and an increase in mood stabilizers such as lithium.

The actual cause of depression is unknown. Theories include imbalances between the brain chemicals serotonin and dopamine levels, the hypothalamus, and other parts of the central nervous system that transmit motor signals to muscles, organs, or glands. Vagus nerve stimulation has been used as a treatment for depression in patients who have epilepsy found to have or be susceptible to epilepsy-related brain damage, who suffer from depression. Neuroplasticity (which means that neurons can reorganize) may also play a role in mood disorders; areas of the brain responsible for learning and memory may be associated with mood disorders.

Less commonly, the vagus nerve is stimulated by injecting cannulae at the base of the skull and attaching them to the vagus nerve. This involves applying electric impulses at a low frequency with a high voltage for two minutes through a reusable electrode inserted in contact with the vagus nerve stumps. It stimulates the brain's hypothalamus and leads to a reduction of anxiety and improvement in mood if it is effective.

Unfortunately, this technique is invasive and requires general anesthesia, which may not be effective as an alternative therapy to VNS. The technique is also associated with serious risks, including severe headache, discomfort, numbness, or stroke of neck muscles. Another drawback is that the procedure needs to be repeated every year, which decreases its usefulness and convenience.

Therefore, only a few studies have been conducted to assess the effect and safety of this technique on depression. Despite the benefits, this method is considered a potent and alternative therapy but not as good as VNS.

Vagus nerve stimulation has been proposed as a treatment for anxiety disorders. In one study with ten chronically anxious patients, six depressed and four had a generalized anxiety disorder (GAD), vagus nerve stimulation was an effective treatment for improving depression and reducing anxiety levels significantly in individuals with comorbid GAD. However, the effect of vagus nerve stimulation on reducing generalized anxiety disorder in patients with comorbid GAD is unknown. Therefore, currently, there is no evidence supporting the use of VNS for generalized anxiety disorder.

Although this method shows promise as an alternative therapy for depression, the procedure has some limitations. The procedure's effectiveness has not been proven as first-line therapy for major depression. Since the surgery is invasive and has some risks attached to it, to make sure that this is an effective treatment, further studies need to be conducted using randomized controlled trials with a large number of patients who have major depression and comorbid generalized anxiety disorder (GAD). To finalize its effectiveness in the treatment of comorbid GAD and major depression, further studies should be conducted in the future.

Diaphragmatic Breathing

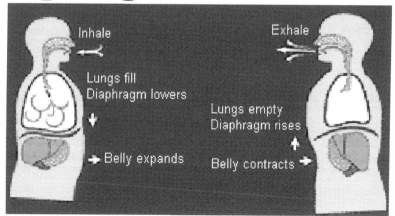

Benefits of diaphragmatic breathing.

At the base of the lungs, a thin sheet of muscles called the diaphragm is responsible for breathing. When you inhale, this muscle contracts and moves downward, which allows your lungs to expand. When you exhale, this muscle relaxes and returns to its original position. Diaphragmatic breathing can make it easier for these contractions to occur with every breath.

When doctors first started learning about diaphragmatic breathing in medical school, many experienced immediate reliefs from their asthma symptoms and allergies when they practiced it regularly at home as prescribed by their instructors. Following this procedure quickly improved the quality of a patient's life and increased the effectiveness of their medical care.

The beneficial effects of diaphragmatic breathing extend beyond the respiratory system. It's been shown to improve the health and wellness of people who suffer from allergies, physical disorders that cause pain, various digestive problems, and other conditions.

The function and purpose of the diaphragm have been known for thousands of years. Even though it was called the "windpipe," it didn't work like a windpipe. Even though you can see the diaphragm at rest, there is no way to tell from looking at it that it's in use. Only when you press on its surface and feel it contract is this layer of muscle able to do something.

Diaphragmatic breathing may seem easy enough as there are only two steps involved:

1) Before starting any exercise program, learn to breathe without tensing your abdominal muscles or tightening your throat or jaw.

2) After you learn to breathe naturally, learn to breathe from your diaphragm.

Once a person becomes familiar with their diaphragm, they often find that it helps them in daily life and exercise.

Diaphragmatic breathing is:

- More efficient than other methods of breathing
- Easier and more comfortable than breathing through the mouth or nose (directly into your lungs)
- Can be practiced anywhere and anytime
- Can be practiced by anyone, regardless of age or health condition
- Helps people with stress and asthma conditions

Diaphragmatic breathing is one of the easiest breathing methods to learn. There are no special exercises or equipment required.

Here are some tips for learning how to breathe from the diaphragm:

1) Keep your stomach tight so the diaphragm feels safe, like a pillow.

2) Exhale through your lips by pursing them slightly, keeping them pressed lightly around your lower teeth (like you might do when saying "ooh!").

3) Inhale through the nose (keeping it relaxed, like inhaling into your mouth). Try not to cough during this step.

4) Raise your shoulders and gently pull them down toward your ears.

5) Continue breathing into your lungs for the rest of the exercise.

6) The more you practice, the easier it becomes to feel the muscles in your chest working together with the diaphragm. Try to find a comfortable breathing rhythm that feels relaxed, peaceful, and empowering.

A person who suffers from allergies or other conditions that cause pain are often told by their doctors or physio-therapists to do deep breathing exercises through their mouth as they lie in bed or on a treatment table, which doesn't work very well as most people can't take much pressure on their necks and heads with their arms bent at the elbows.

Diaphragmatic breathing is much easier for these men and women to manage, as they can relax the muscles in their necks and heads during the exercise. This type of breathing also encourages people to breathe better overall.

The diaphragm has been known for thousands of years as the "windpipe" or the "heart-lung" because it is responsible for breathing. It is located in the lower abdomen, just above the stomach. The diaphragm is a thin, yellow-white muscle about 8 inches in diameter that separates the chest from the abdomen. The diaphragm contracts and relaxes with every breath, moving down with inhalation and up with exhalation. Though you can't see your diaphragm at rest because it's inside your body, you can feel its motions by placing your fingers on top of your belly (in line with your navel). The stomach muscles stay relatively still during breathing; they move only enough to allow the diaphragm to contract and relax.

When you breathe, first inhale through your nose, then fill your stomach with air and hold it there. Next, gently exhale through pursed lips by pressing gently on your abdomen (lower belly) to feel the diaphragm move downward and relax. Hold this position for a few moments, then inhale again through your nose. Release the air from your belly in tiny puffs as you allow the diaphragm to rise into its original position.

Start by practicing anytime, anywhere, for about 5-10 minutes. Try to focus on gentle inhalation and exhalation of breath. If you focus on counting the breaths, this is normal; try to let go of the numbers and return your attention to the diaphragm and its movement. As your breathing becomes more balanced, you may count your breaths again or not at all.

The body's nervous system is designed to send messages from one part of your body (or even in mind) to another part of your body so that both parts respond at once. This is called reflex action or a reflexive response. When a signal reaches the brain or nervous system, its response is automatic, without requiring conscious thought.

When you detect any warning signs of breathing problems (such as unexplained chest pain), do not wait for the chest pain to occur before beginning diaphragmatic breathing.

Diaphragmatic breathing can be used alone to reduce or eliminate the symptoms of several respiratory ailments, including asthma, emphysema, and chronic bronchitis. As with asthma, this technique has been shown to reduce or eliminate the frequency and severity of attacks in people suffering from emphysema. Diaphragmatic breathing is also a very effective tool for relieving symptoms of chronic bronchitis.

Diaphragmatic breathing exercises can treat reflux, GERD (gastroesophageal reflux disease), and many other gastrointestinal problems.

One researcher said that diaphragmatic breathing is "the most powerful and simple technique for treating many common illnesses." He concluded, "It is a wonderful, simple technique that can help people who suffer from not just one but many disorders. Once you learn how to breathe with the diaphragm and practice it, you can breathe better most of the time and even enjoy new health benefits."

Diaphragmatic breathing is especially helpful for reducing stress, alleviating pain, strengthening your lungs and muscles, and improving sleep. There are a variety of diaphragmatic breathing exercises you can practice.

Diaphragmatic breathing is one of the easiest, most natural breathing techniques to learn and practice. It is also a very inexpensive, simple, and practical method of health care that is easy to learn and understand.

Therefore, it's worth a try if you or anyone you know suffers from asthma, tension headaches, allergies, asthma, and many other problems.

- Diaphragmatic breathing reduces stress, improves your ability to deal with pain, and lowers blood pressure. It also strengthens your diaphragm.
- People with asthma who practice deep breathing frequently find that their symptoms disappear or become less severe.
- Some patients who suffer from chronic bronchitis report easing symptoms just two weeks after they begin practicing deep breathing exercises.
- The deep abdominal breaths that help relieve stress create a "reset" button in your brain that helps you return to normal after reacting to stressful situations.
- People who suffer from reflux and gastroesophageal reflux disease (GERD) usually have the most success with breathing exercises.
- Many people who practice deep breathing regularly can reduce or eliminate their dependence on drugs for treating allergies.

If you frequently suffer from stress, anxiety attacks, or symptoms of chronic bronchitis, it's worth a try. Do your research, find a place and time when you will be free from distractions and interruptions for about ten minutes each day for your practice sessions, and learn the art of deep abdominal breathing.

The next chapter will discuss exercises. Exercising is important since exercise strengthens the body and gives it a feeling of wellness. Exercise is one thing that can help to improve your body. What you do for yourself counts because, with exercise, you can strengthen your body and have better health.

There are many things that you can do that will benefit your body. Having a formal workout routine provides the greatest benefits for your physical well-being, but it's important to remember that exercise isn't only about physical fitness; it's also about emotional fitness. Exercise helps boost self-esteem and feelings of self-worth, which are crucial components of emotional health. The more energy you have, the better you feel about yourself, improving your confidence level. Exercise can give you a new lease on life. Start by finding an exercise program you enjoy and will stick to, then set realistic goals. Observe your progress by measuring and weighing yourself regularly.

EXERCISES EXERCISE ON RESTORING MUTUAL COMMITMENT.

Mutual commitment is not given or taken but is mutually created by both parties.

To restore mutual commitment, you should look for opportunities to do things together in which you can experience a sense of satisfaction and accomplishment.

As with anything valuable, it takes some work and effort to maintain the beauty and quality of this "mutual commitment." It might take a little more time, but the rewards are well worth the effort. You may have to sacrifice your pursuits for a while, but soon enough, the road ahead will be clear and open with no surprises waiting around the corners.

You deserve an energetic partner who feels fortunate to walk down it with you. Therefore, exercising mutual commitment is a great way to find that partner. Moreover, restoring mutual commitment will keep your relationship healthy and vital in the years to come.

Exercising mutual commitment is something that you and your partner can do together. This is a step toward gaining more appreciation and meaning in the marriage. However, it is not so much of a commitment where you will be required to give up all your other interests or activities. It requires a little work to keep a warm, happy relationship with each other over the years.

There are several exercises that you can use to restore mutual commitment between each other. The most effective exercise for bringing about this end will be for every partner to make time for at least one hour each day to be alone on purpose. Extend the time with each other to an hour or two if you can. This alone should begin a mutual process of commitment for each other.

Therefore, exercises that can restore mutual commitment are:

a. Exercising together - you can take up a sport such as joining a gym or going for walks together, taking a dance class, or hiking. Just find something that interests both of you and do it.

b. Talking about the future - discussing the children, your dreams and goals for the future, and your financial plans for saving money and buying a home will also strengthen the commitment to each other.

c. Having friends over for dinner - having friends over for dinner on occasion will let your partner know that his/her company is valuable to you and worth investing in by making time for him/her.

d. Making Life Choices Together - making decisions, such as what to eat, what clothes to wear, and where to go will help you feel more connected and responsible for each other. This is especially challenging when choosing what to wear.

e. Using your talents together - using talents such as music, art, sports, and dance together in a manner that enforces cooperation and unity will also build you up emotionally and strengthen mutual commitment.

f. Making time - making time for each other can be very frustrating. It is not as simple as it sounds. This exercise requires you and your partner to overcome the difficulty of setting aside personal agendas, schedules, and individual interests to focus on each other for a few hours each day. By making time for each other in this exercise, you will develop a bond of appreciation for your partner's value in your life.

g. Celebrating the good times - a great way to strengthen mutual commitment is to celebrate the good things that have happened during the day or at the end of each week. This can be as simple as sharing a meal or going out for ice cream.

h. Having shared interests - finding common interests with your partner will make it easier to create a sense of mutual commitment. Whether it be cooking, collecting artwork, or gardening, these shared interests will help you appreciate each other's values and what is important to one another in life.

i. Visiting with friends - this is not always possible, but going out in public together will help you feel more connected and help build commitment between you over time.

j. Showing appreciation is a great way to strengthen your commitment to one another. It does not take much time or effort, but it could make all the difference in the long run.

k. Reading to your partner - reading books will help you gain insight into others' experiences, which helps you appreciate life in general and each other as individuals and as a couple.

l. Building a family history together - working together as a family to write down your family history, stories of how you came together, and how your children were born will help strengthen commitment between generations and generations of parents and children.

The neurofascial release technique.

This therapy improves one's quality of life through self-manipulation and exercises.

The neurofascial release technique is the therapeutic use of manual therapies and techniques that release restrictions in body tissues, reduce pain, create motion, and increase function.

Therapies such as massage can re-establish fluidity in muscles that may have become "knots." Once muscles are more relaxed and distended, they are better able to expand and contract as needed. Massage techniques often include kneading the muscle with the thumb or fingers or using a stationary pressure point such as a particular tender spot on the back.

Physical exercise is also used for treating and managing musculoskeletal pain and may include stretching, isometric exercises, resistance training, cardiovascular exercise, and aerobic exercise. However, ensuring that an individual has warmed up first is important, as this reduces the risk of injury. Special types of exercises are designed to be gentle on the body but still provide a good workout, such as Pilates.

Aerobic exercise has been found to decrease muscle tension in women with fibromyalgia (FM).

Massage therapy is a profession that has been around for many years. Its use has spread from medical specialists to the general public. The popularity of massage has increased tremendously in recent years due to the rising number of massage therapists and schools which offer training.

For therapy to be effective, certain variables need to be in play; these variables include the therapist having proper qualifications and experience, a client having an understanding of what he wants from therapy, having an open mind and being relaxed, as well as therapist's willingness to work with client's individual needs.

The number of people with musculoskeletal pain and discomfort increases yearly due to increased working hours, stress, poor diet, and sedentary lifestyles. This has led to a demand for a massage therapy as an effective treatment alternative.

A therapist can improve a client's quality of life by teaching him how to self-manipulate certain structures in his body and then using techniques that release tension, reduce pain and create motion.

With the increasing use of massage therapy, it has also become a popular field of study. It is now possible to find schools that offer certification and continuing education units for practicing therapists.

Massage therapy is very effective because it allows one to focus on particular areas causing discomfort and then provides relief through manipulation of the soft tissue.

Scapula and Upper Back: By massaging the upper trapezius, upper trapezius, rhomboid, and levator scapulae, the practitioner can enhance the range of motion in the scapula and improve the function of the deltoid muscles.

Shoulder: The cross-side stretch is excellent for a client who experiences pain when they are asked to do overhead work. Also, this movement will stretch out the scapulothoracic fascia and loosens tight muscles in the anterior shoulder.

Forearm: Hand massage will reduce muscle spasms and increase circulation at a point very close to nerve fibers. Also, this is a great move if you have been hurting with strained hand muscles.

When to use neurofascial release technique:

* Enhance quality of life through self-manipulation and exercises.
* Treat pain and discomfort.
* Open up restricted tissues in the body.
* Treat frozen shoulder.
* Reduce pain during recovery from surgery.
* Reduce fibromyalgia symptoms and improve sleep quality.
* Rehabilitation of injuries.
* Reduce tension and increase flexibility in the body.
* Restore range of motion at joints.
* Increase blood circulation to the musculature.
* Improve function and reduce symptoms associated with RSI (repetitive strain injury).

The neurofascial release technique can be used on itself, but it can also be used in conjunction with other techniques, such as manipulation, massage, or exercise. The objective is always to improve quality of life through self-manipulation and exercises.

How to use neurofascial release technique for social engagement:

* To be successful with this technique, you need to have a positive and open mind.
* To get the best results, you must desire to change.
* During this process, you must always be committed and ready to learn new techniques and exercises.
* Neurofascial Release Technique can be introduced to complement other techniques that may help shyness or social discomfort, such as cognitive behavioral therapy.

The neurofascial release technique helps clients manage anxiety, social anxiety, or shyness by promoting normalization behavior that is acceptable in different situations.

The salamander exercises.

Salamander exercises are essential since they strengthen the muscles of the heart and lungs, which can protect against heart disease and lung diseases. Generally, they are performed by exhaling while sitting up straight.

They can be done at home, but it is preferable to do them in a special room.

Though these exercises are beneficial, it is a good idea to ask your doctor or another health professional beforehand if you are depressed or have any other preexisting medical conditions. Moreover, ask if the exercises are right for you or if there is a better alternative.

The following steps guide you through the regimen of salamander exercises:

(1) Grip bar. Stand up straight, with your eyes closed. Place your hands onto a bar held tightly at shoulder height, with your arms extended out from your body; palms down. Then lean back until you feel like you are about to fall backward. When this happens, let go of the bar and gently sit down on the floor, landing on your feet with legs and knees slightly bent.

(2) Lay-back on inclined board. Lie down on an inclined board; your head should be folded over your hands, with your elbows tucked into your side. Tip: Your head should be positioned so that the curve of the board forms a gentle S-shape when you're lying on it.

(3) Hanging with elbows and hands. Enter a hanging position with your arms extended out from the sides of your body, elbows down, and fingers touching next to the head. Tuck in the toes and rotate one arm downward at a time; then rotate them both inward again until you reach a vertical position, elbow tips touching the sides of your waist.

(4) Lay back up against a wall. Lie down on your back, with your arms stretched over your head and your hands clasped. Then slowly lift your head off the floor until it's perpendicular to the floor. Keep your elbows bent and slightly tucked in at your waist's sides while doing this.

(5) Lay back on an inclined board so that neck is straight up and down. Lie on an inclined board with a slight curve at the neck, facing away from the wall. Keep both arms extended out from the sides of your body, elbows down, and fingers touching next to the head; then rotate one arm downward at a time; then rotate them both inward again until you reach a vertical position, elbow tips touching next to the side of your waist.

Your joints, muscles, and ligaments are your body's natural shock absorbers. They can be a major factor in how you feel throughout the day. Joints and ligaments provide stability for the bones that make up our frames so that we can move about without being in pain or suffering injury. Muscles are what allow us to move around, from running down the street to writing our thoughts on paper.

There are two types of salamander exercises:

* Half salamander

This is when you raise your head and shoulders off the surface of the ground but continue to push your lower body away from the ground. In addition, tip: keep the head and shoulder raised, so the back of your head doesn't touch anything other than the ground.

This exercise helps strengthen the neck and abdominal muscles, so they don't become weak and lifeless.

- Full salamander

This involves raising your entire body off the floor, with your hips, knee, and toes still on the ground. In addition, tip: keep your head, shoulders, and hips raised off of the floor to maintain a balanced position.

This exercise helps strengthen the back muscles and improves spinal flexibility; it also strengthens the chest and abdominal muscles for optimal breathing capacity.

Here is an example of a full salamander exercise: Place hands on a bar behind you with your arms extended out from your body; palms down. Then lean back until you feel like you are about to fall backward. When this happens, let go of the bar and gently sit down on the floor, landing on your feet with legs and knees slightly bent.

There are no contraindications for salamander exercises; however, if you feel light-headed or nauseous while doing them, tip: put your hands on a sturdy surface by your side until you feel better.

Salamander exercises are not very expensive, as most of the equipment can be found at home or bought for a low cost. Moreover, there is no need for specialist physicians or therapists to perform them. Therefore, they are widely used and practiced in countries where health insurance is not widely available.

Massage for neck tension release.

Neck tension can lead to neck and shoulder pain, headaches, and even injury. This exercise can help release tension in the neck and relieve fatigue.

The goal is to release pressure in the muscles of the neck. The best way to do this is by massaging with your fingers (or a tennis ball).

1. Sit in a chair and put a tennis ball under your neck, wedging it between the floor and the top of your back.
2. Slowly roll from side to side, letting gravity work—this will take some time as you are not moving much just yet.
3. Once you feel you have released the muscle enough, move your neck in a circular motion to stretch and twist the muscles.
4. Move your neck in a back-and-forth motion to loosen up the neck muscles even more. You might feel like you are dizzy, but that is normal! This means that you are releasing tension in the muscles of your neck.
5. Roll around on the floor some more, as this will help eliminate any aches and pains. After a while, you may feel more relaxed and refreshed.

This exercise is essential since neck tension can cause neck and shoulder pain, headaches, and even neck injury.

Lie down on the floor with your back on the ground and your head resting at a 45-degree angle. Place a small towel under your forehead to prevent it from getting dirty. Grasp the area close to your neck and pull gently towards you in an upside-down U shape. Do this 10 times and switch to the other side of your neck for 20 reps for optimal results.

Exercise: Neck Tension Release

Do this massage 10 times, alternating between the sides of the neck. This will help relieve tension from around the level of the thyroid cartilage, giving you relief from pain or pressure caused by muscular tension around it (elevated hairline).

Neck tension release can enable people to:

a. Reduce pain and pressure around the level of the thyroid cartilage, which is frequently caused by muscular tension.
b. Relieve head and muscle tension (reduces pain and tightness).
c. Relax your shoulders, making it feel easier to turn your head.
d. Feel more relaxed; feel your body's natural healing process kick in faster to heal tension/pain/discomfort related to neck or thyroid cartilage level.

Repeat 10 times on each side.

If you are prone to headaches, make sure you do this exercise daily because it will help to release the body's natural healing process and help prevent headaches in the first place.

Step 1: Sit up straight with your feet flat on the ground just above your knees, feet relaxed and shoulder-width apart.

Step 2: Cross your arms at chest level in front of you. Fingers should be together, palms facing down. Keep elbows tucked close to body as shown in the photo.

Step 3: Lift your arms overhead to make a right angle between your torso and arms (as if you were hugging a tree). Lower your arms back down to the starting position. Repeat 10-20 times.

Repeat 3-5 times daily until tension is relieved. If you experience pain, continue doing the exercise until you feel relief from the pain.

(Remember this exercise if you want relief from tension when driving & difficulty turning your head)

This exercise helps to relax and stretch the tight neck, shoulders, and upper back muscles caused by muscle tension or stress in other body parts. For example, tightness in the lower abdomen can affect tension around the neck or thyroid cartilage level. Also, tightness in the back can affect tension around the neck or thyroid cartilage level.

It also helps stretch and loosen muscles around the neck and thyroid cartilage level, allowing it to turn more freely, alleviating tension in this area. Suppose you don't regularly do this exercise and are experiencing tension in your neck, shoulders, or upper back. In that case, it is a good idea to start doing this exercise daily to loosen up stiff muscles around your neck and thyroid cartilage level. This exercise is also great if you have frequent upper back or neck headaches. It will help to release tension in these areas, helping to prevent headaches.

SCM sore neck exercise.

The winter months often bring a decrease in the amount of physical activity. This can lead to muscle stiffness and soreness. The neck is one area that can be affected by prolonged periods of bad posture from hunched shoulders, tense muscles, and poor sleep habits. It can cause pain at the base of the skull, migraines, difficulty swallowing or speaking, headaches, sinus pressure, congestion, and other symptoms. The intense pain often leads to stiff necks, chronic headaches, and sleep disturbances that can impair our daily activities. It is recommended that anyone experiencing neck pain should seek professional medical advice to prevent any serious complications. This can sometimes be done at home by performing the following exercise.

Sitting in a reclined upright position, place the palm of one hand on your head, and squeeze your neck muscles in a circular motion with your other hand. To make sure you are using as much of your neck muscles as possible, contract them slightly upwards. It is advisable to stretch these muscles after you have finished this exercise.

To help prevent a stiff neck from occurring again, it is recommended that the following tips be applied:

a. Maintain good posture, especially when sitting and standing.
b. Avoid slouching, which can lead to muscle stiffness.
c. Stretch the neck muscles before bedtime to maintain the range of motion in your neck and avoid stiffness while sleeping.
d. Get a good night's sleep regularly, as having poor quality sleep can lead to pain and other problems associated with the neck area.
e. Pay attention to your posture when using electronic equipment such as phones or computers so that you do not become slouched over them.

The SCM muscle consists of a long band of skeletal muscle extending from the neck's front and side to the upper back. It is located in front of the scalene muscles and on the sides of the trapezius. This muscle plays an important role in turning our head, moving it sideways, and tilting it downwards towards our shoulders, such as when we look at something below us, such as when getting out of bed. The main role of this muscle is to keep our heads steady to help prevent dizziness and weakness, which can occur after prolonged periods of poor posture or due to other factors such as stress or fatigue.

Avoid any posture causing the problem (e.g., sitting or driving while sitting), and don't rest against a car seat when driving. Do not turn your head too far sideways, leading to pain and muscle stiffness.

Always look straight ahead and keep your eyes level with the horizon. Make sure the top of your head is not tilted downwards, which can cause dizziness or neck pain if you lean forward too far.

A good way to test the strength of your muscle is to hold a pencil between the fingers of one hand and observe how much pressure it takes to hold it steady in front of your face. Try holding this pencil level with a fingertip tip against the middle finger (not touching it), then try holding it firmly against your forehead so that both fingertips are touching. This should be hard enough to maintain it in position without dropping it but not too strong as to hurt afterward.

SCM sore neck exercise: Stand with your head backward and shoulders back while keeping your eye focused on a point between the floor and ceiling. Let your arms hang at your sides and bend your torso forward, keeping your chin down and looking straight ahead (a). Slowly contract your sternocleidomastoid muscle until you feel the tension in the neck region. Maintain this contraction as long as you can. Avoid bouncing up and down, as this will increase potential strain on the SCM muscle. Repeat 10 times with a 2-minute rest after each exercise.

This exercise, if regularly practiced, will help control headaches, migraines, and muscle spasms. Also, it will strengthen the sternocleidomastoid muscle. This exercise is essential since it strengthens the muscle and relieves pain. Moreover, exercise can prevent chronic headaches and migraines.

Proper posture is important in maintaining health and reducing the frequency of headaches. You can maintain proper posture and reduce lower back pain by performing these exercises. The exercises can be done while sitting in a chair or lying down.

Twist and turn exercise.

Twist and turn exercises are verticle exercises you can do at home. All you need is space with enough floor space for jumping and a chair or bench.

It helps to have someone that can spot you while doing this exercise.

Start the jumping portion by standing on the floor before your jumpable surface. Twist your body to the right so that your right arm is over your head and your left leg is straight out behind you, making a 90-degree angle. Jump as high as possible and afterward land on the straight leg without letting either foot touch down first. Switch legs before twisting back to jump, and keep alternating until time runs out. The more twisted you are, the harder it will be, but the better your oblique muscles will get.

If you don't have a jumpable surface, use a chair or bench instead and start standing on it.

This exercise can be performed with one or two legs. The two-leg version is usually harder than the single-leg version because of the added weight on one foot simultaneously when landing, so it's preferable to start with one leg before trying to do both.

Start this exercise by standing with both feet on either side of a bench in front of you. Put both hands on your hips, and bend forward at the waist, so your torso is parallel with the floor. Simultaneously extend all four limbs before you, ensuring your knees are bent, and your ankles keep their pivoting points. If you notice one leg is going out of the "legs" line, straighten it while remaining in a leaning position as if doing a two-legged twist and turn. Land on the same foot if it's still out of place when alternating legs next time.

Once you can do this exercise without any issues, start doing it without touching any surface, just standing still on both feet. The only thing you'll use is your balance.

This exercise mainly works on your abdomen, and starting with one leg is easier before trying to do both.

Start this exercise by sitting on the floor with your legs straight out in front of you. Have knees bent so they are at a 90-degree angle, and hands are placed palms down on either side of your body. Keep back and spine straight, not leaning forward or backward.

When lifting, try to rotate your torso as close to 90 degrees as possible before moving it up further by extending at the knees. When lowering down, also do this in a controlled manner where every part of the body moves at once while keeping the back and neck straight.

Jumping jacks on the bench.

If you can't quite reach the floor with your feet during the twist and turn exercises, you can also do this exercise seated. Just be careful not to jump too carried away and miss the bench. All you need is a bench or chair and a place to jump from.

Start by sitting on the edge of the bench with your feet facing forwards. Start reverse jogging (backward) off of the bench. When one foot reaches the floor start jumping jack style, stomping down hard on the floor for maximum jumping height, then switch feet before landing on the bench again.

Explosive jumping.

Some people find getting more power in their jump easier if they start with a small leap, then launch themselves into the air as high as possible.

This exercise is also great for developing quick bursts of power. All you need is a floor wide enough to give you a good running start and enough room to jump around when you land. Start by gradually speeding up your running speed until you have a good head of steam, then take off into the air with both feet as high as possible, alternating legs on each jump without touching down first. If you're jumping onto a hard floor you can add more power by holding your hands above your head with the thumbs touching each other.

Start standing on the floor in front of your jumpable surface. Jump up as high as possible, land on that same leg, then switch legs before landing on that same side; keep alternating until time runs out. If you're having difficulty keeping up with this exercise, it can help to hold onto something above you so that you can reach higher. 5-minute workout. Do 60 jumping jacks, 30 twists and turns, and 15 explosive jumps.

12 vagus nerve stimulation techniques.

1. Set up your vagus nerve stimulator before going to sleep by keeping it plugged in and turned on all night.
2. Set your timer to go off every hour throughout the day, and then turn it off instantly when the alarm goes off without moving or making any noise at all.
3. Spend an entire day without talking except when necessary (i.e., ordering a menu item).
4. Wear a fake mustache or other false facial hair throughout the day and avoid speaking with people as much as possible, so you don't have to remove it if necessary
5. Don't speak at all during a movie or TV program
6. At the end of a movie or TV program, turn down your hearing aid or cochlear implant to the lowest volume setting and keep it turned that way for an hour.
7. Sit in front of the TV and don't turn it on. If you get bored, go occupy yourself with another activity before turning it on again after one full hour.
8. Whenever you go anywhere, take a walk before you get there instead of driving, and then determine whether your destination is more than 10 minutes away from where you are standing (or walking).
9. Lie down on your back in bed and then stand up again using only your willpower.
10. Whenever you are tempted to speak, count silently in your head for 15 seconds instead.
11. If you start to feel the urge to speak out of the blue, walk away from any people around you and make sure your hands are occupied with something (e.g., fidget toys).
12. Instead of saying anything whenever someone asks you a question, just shrug both shoulders instead (i.e., make a non-word sound with both shoulders).

Vagus nerve stimulation techniques are essential since people who use them can maintain a higher level of control over their tinnitus and other misophonia symptoms than those who do not. However, they must be used carefully since over-exercising can cause more harm than good. Moreover, there are several ways to increase the activity of the vagus nerve naturally, so it's a good idea to explore them first.

This stimulation forces your body to be more active and thus more alive. The most common vagus nerve stimulation exercises involve physical activities such as walking, jogging, weight lifting, etc.

To get the most out of your vagus nerve stimulation exercises, you need to keep them simple and repetitive so that you can stick with them long enough for your body to get used to them. Repetition is important because it helps your mind learn to accept certain tinnitus symptoms as "normal."

Walking is one of the best forms of vagus nerve stimulation exercises since it involves physical and mental activity. It also doesn't involve talking, so you won't have to worry about breaking your silence rules.

Another great thing about walking is that it can be done anywhere, at any time. All you need to do is lace up your shoes and step out the door.

If you want to walk in your home, go ahead and do that; however, if you want to take a walk outside, then make sure you're near some other people. This helps make sure that your tinnitus symptoms don't get worse. Some people also find it helpful to listen to white noise or similar sounds by walking near a running car or along a busy street.

One important vagus nerve stimulation exercise I often do is called the "shoulder shrug." The premise is that you're trying to shake off all your tinnitus symptoms. In this case, the shoulder shrug is a visual trick that forces you to shrug your shoulders.

First, imagine a weight hanging from each shoulder, and then try to raise them in one fluid motion before you shrug your shoulders. This exercise should be done first and then gradually speed up until it becomes difficult for you to keep it going for any length because of how easy it becomes.

Another incredibly useful form of vagus nerve stimulation exercise involves prayer. Prayer is simply speaking out loud and wishing for your tinnitus, hyperacusis, and misophonia symptoms to disappear. You can do this exercise daily or whenever you feel the urge.

The idea behind prayer is that if you keep it up long enough, your mind will eventually start accepting that your tinnitus, hyperacusis, and misophonia symptoms aren't going away by themselves. One of the best vagus nerve stimulation exercises involves music. Music has a very strong effect on our emotions and thus has a powerful impact on our moods.

The next chapter will discuss useful tools that can assist in putting the therapies into practice. These tools include tinnitus maskers, sound generators, and hearing aids. Therefore, knowing what these tools are and how to incorporate them into your tinnitus management strategy is essential.

The chapter, will discuss the most common tools used to manage tinnitus. You will learn all the basics and how to incorporate them into your treatment program. For example, Tinnitus management is not easy and requires a lot of work, but at least now you can have some help with the basics of tinnitus therapy.

These tools make it possible to reduce stress and control the severity of symptoms. In addition, hearing aids can provide better outcomes for people with hyperacusis by allowing them to hear better than they could without a hearing aid.

Although acupuncture is not a method for treating tinnitus itself, it can help you cope with your symptoms by reducing stress and helping you relax your body to fall asleep at night. This can be very useful for people who have problems getting rest at night because of their tinnitus symptoms.

USEFUL TOOLS
TOOLS THAT HELP PUT THE THERAPIES INTO PRACTICE;

These tools are very useful in managing both early-onset and late-onset cases. Therefore, psychotherapists should use them in their practice.

These tools include:

a. Clinical interview schedule (CIS)

This tool is very useful tool in evaluating various kinds of OCD. It determines the nature, content, obsessive and distressing thoughts. This tool will help the psychotherapist understand the patient's symptoms better and find out if there is any connection between them.

b. SET and IST

This tool can determine the severity of the patient's symptoms and whether any psychological problem exists. This tool also helps to determine whether the patient is impulsive, whether he has more obsessions or fewer obsessions, etc.

c. Cognitive Behavioural Therapy (CBT)

This tool helps eliminate OCD from the patient's life by altering how he thinks about himself and his fears. The psychotherapist will have to guide the direction after evaluating information about a particular anxiety problem. CBT commonly uses ideas such as "positive" thought, "self-statements," and "self-control."

d. Exposure and Response Prevention (ERP)

Once the obsessions are identified, the psychotherapist will help the patient to face his fears. This tool involves "exposing" the patient to the feared situation, idea, or activity in a safe and controlled manner. The treatment continues until the patient is able to face his fear for an extended period without responding with compulsions (for example: wash, check, re-check, avoid, etc.). This is called "exposure," and once these fears are no longer causing distress or anxiety, they are referred to as "no-longer-feared." Finally, once patients can abstain from performing compulsive behaviors, they are referred to as being in "response prevention."

e. CBT-F

Cognitive Behavior Therapy-f is a manual of cognitive behavioral therapy that effectively treats OCD in children and adolescents. This therapy helps to build "self-efficacy," which is a person's belief that he/she can cope with life's problems. The treatment comprises four stages:

1. Awareness (includes information about OCD)- developing an understanding of what OCD is, who suffers from it, and how serious it can be;

2. Education (this encourages children to talk about their fears);
3. Mental strategies (the necessary skills for managing their fears) and;
4. Cognitive restructuring (their belief about themselves).

f.   Response prevention

Response prevention is an approach to preventing anxiety-provoking behaviors by avoiding the situations that generate them. In OCD, this can be as simple as telling a person to avoid doing an activity instead of performing it compulsively. For example, a patient who is obsessed with germs could be asked to wash their hands and not wash again, or they could be asked not to wash and not touch anything. Or if they touch something, they could be asked to touch a clean part of their body, such as their tongue, without touching the rest.

g.   Comprehensive assessment and referral tool (CART)

This tool is used to help identify the most appropriate treatment for a particular patient. This helps in identifying the best treatment to be used first and middle-wisely. The assessment also helps identify any comorbidity with other disorders, like substance use, depression or anxiety disorders, etc.

h.   Measure of the severity of obsessions and compulsions (MOS-OC)

This tool helps in helping to assess the severity of OCD symptoms by performing a checklist that measures the degree of obsessions, rituals, and compulsions in a patient's life.

i.   Yale-Brown Obsessive Compulsive Scale (Y-BOCS)

This tool helps assess the severity of OCD by observing the urge the patient has to perform a certain task, the time it takes to complete it, how much distress there is from doing them, and if he can control them.

j.   Overt Response Counting (ORC)

This is an effective tool for identifying and tracking compulsions by counting overt activities such as hand washing or hoarding. Obsessions are also recorded on a 10-point scale, which helps determine whether there is an obsession.

k.   The Coping Strategies Questionnaire (CSQ)

This questionnaire can be used to document the coping strategies of a patient, and it is a good screening tool. This tool helps identify the problem, monitor changes, and give feedback. The patient and therapist can use it to give feedback to each other.

l.   Yale-Brown Obsessive Compulsive Scale for Children (Y-BOCS-C)

This tool helps assess the severity of OCD by observing the patient's urge to perform a certain task, the time it takes to complete it, how much distress there is from doing them, and if he can control them.

m.   Perceived Competence Questionnaire (PCQ)

This tool obtains information about a patient's perception of competence. The tool helps the psychotherapist to determine if the patient has a high or low level of competence; it helps in understanding if they can cope with life's problems.

n.   Obsessive-Compulsive Inventory for Children and Adolescents (OCI-A)

This questionnaire is used for children between the age of 8 and 18. It helps assess their symptoms in terms of time spent on their obsessions, number and severity of rituals, amount of distress experienced from performing compulsions, insight into OCD through rating scales, and quality of life.

Many pharmacological, psychological, and alternative methods are available to treat OCD. Medication is usually the first line of treatment for patients with OCD. The two most common medications used to treat OCD patients include serotonin reuptake inhibitors (SRIs) and selective serotonin receptor inhibitors (SSRIs). Some commonly prescribed medications are; clomipramine, paroxetine, fluvoxamine, sertraline, citalopram, and escitalopram.

Clomipramine is a tricyclic antidepressant that helps improve obsessive thoughts and compulsions by increasing serotonin levels in patient's brains. The medication at lower doses gives a modest response, while at higher doses, it achieves a much better response. Common side effects include drowsiness, constipation, dry mouth, and weight gain.

Paroxetine is the only antidepressant that inhibits both serotonin and norepinephrine uptake. Paroxetine is effective in treating OCD in children. The medication can lead to mild side effects, including insomnia and anorexia nervosa.

SSRIs are derived from tricyclic antidepressants but are less risky for side effects since they act primarily on serotonin receptors on nerve cells rather than affecting neurotransmitters like norepinephrine. SSRIs are not effective in treating childhood-onset OCD. Studies have shown that SSRIs can help reduce the time of onset, frequency, and severity of OCD symptoms if taken regularly. Some common side effects may include nausea, sexual dysfunction, headaches, agitation, and insomnia.

Selective serotonin receptor inhibitors work by inhibiting the reuptake of serotonin and other neurotransmitters from the synaptic cleft; these effects manifest with a delay of up to one to three weeks after administration. They are effective in treating adults with OCD but are less effective for children; these medications also pose a higher risk for side effects which is why they should be taken cautiously.

Alternative treatment options are also available to treat patients with OCD. Cognitive behavioral therapy (CBT) is a common psychological intervention method that helps patients with distorted thoughts and negative feelings about their obsessions and compulsions. CBT helps the patient understand their problems and find out reasons for behaving obsessively.

Another alternative to medication is deep-brain stimulation (DBS), which can effectively reduce the severity of OCD symptoms by making the treatment permanent.

In terms of prognosis, research shows that OCD has a higher relapse rate after treatment than other psychiatric disorders; this may be caused by continued exposure to compulsions and obsessions (not performing them can lead to more anxiety).

The next chapter will discuss anxiety, fear, and rewinding the mind. These three topics have been known to affect many people. Anxiety can be physical or psychological. Anxiety can also be brought on by stressors or situational factors, even in daily life. Examples include a bad day at work, a traffic jam and long line of cars, a tornado warning, animal attacks, and medical emergencies. Fear is often associated with anxiety; however, it has nothing to do with anxiety. Fear is a form of protection that helps keep you safe from danger and threats. Many things can cause one to be fearful such as if they see other people being attacked by animals or if there is a tornado rolling into their town. When one is fearful, one may be aware of the danger but not know why. The body produces the fight or flight response, and then the body goes into a state of fear. This can result in many physical symptoms such as; sweating, trembling, raised heartbeat, excessive salivation, and even vomiting. When it comes to rewinding the mind, it is where someone tends to replay past events repeatedly. Some common examples include when someone goes over things they said or did that they later regret or can't undo or if they simply want to relive an event just because it was a good time.

BONUS
HOW TO PREVENT ANXIETY, FEARS, DEPRESSION, AND ANGER FROM COMING BACK.

When you learn how to treat your brain, it will be easier for you to handle stresses in life and not give into the common traps that cause anxiety, depression, and anger. It is depressingly easy for our brains to spiral downward even when we have the slightest bit of trouble with our lives.

Treat these stressors quickly and effectively before they consume your thoughts and make you feel out of control again. You can prevent these feelings from returning by trying simple techniques that focus on the basics.

* Start with a warm and supportive environment.

If you feel sad, seek out someone with whom you can express your emotions and be open about what's going on in your life. If you are feeling depressed, love yourself and realize that it's okay not to be okay. Don't overthink what has happened because it will just make everything harder to deal with. Don't try to move on until you have dealt with the problem hasn't let go of. This is the first thing to focus on when dealing with anxiety, depression, and anger.

* Treat your sleep and diet.

When you struggle with anxiety, depression, and anger, it is common to experience sleep disorders that keep you from getting a good night's rest. Besides being fatigued because of this lack of sleep, you will also be more anxious, depressed, and angry than normal. The same goes for not eating right or consistently (this can cause many other issues as well). Not only is it important to take care of these things for the sake of your mental health but also your physical health.

Your body needs all the energy it can get to function properly. You will have issues later in life if you don't exercise regularly and eat well. Your body is your temple, and who will if you don't take care of it?

* Relax and meditate.

This is always a good thing to do. When you relax, your brain can then better process everything around you. It will also help you focus on what's happening in the present moment so that you won't be worrying about the past or obsessing over the future. Many studies have proven that meditation can help ease anxiety, depression, and anger, so why not try it out?

* Read or listen to something that makes you think.

This applies to any kind of reading, listening, or learning experience (even watching a show. Just make sure it makes you think and doesn't make you scared of the unknown). When we are worried, angry, or sad, our minds will work overtime to figure everything out. This can lead to depression, anxiety, and anger. It is your mind's way of trying to protect you from the bad things that have happened in life. This causes us to react when we don't like what's happening around us because it is all our brain's fault. You don't have to be sad all the time just because your mind controls that way of thinking.

* Don't try to solve a problem quickly when it first shows up (or even later).

As I said before, our brains will work overtime when we are anxious, depressed, or angry. They are trying to protect us from worrying, stress, and scared. This means you are more likely to get upset than you normally would have had you not reacted the first time.

* Find healthy hobbies and outlets.

To deal with anxiety, depression, and anger, we must do something to reduce our stress levels. We must have healthy outlets for our feelings because they will build up over time.

* Don't cast judgment on yourself.

When we judge ourselves, we place ourselves in a situation where we feel bad about ourselves. It is amazing how the human mind works. All it takes is one judgmental thought to completely ruin your mood. Don't tell yourself that you are not good enough or capable of something just because you feel like you can't do it. Telling ourselves that we can't do something right away creates stress and anxiety because the brain thinks that if it did attempt to do what was asked, life would be worse off in the end. You will have sooner or later realized this is not true after dealing with anxiety, depression, and anger for a time (I'm sure).

* Don't beat yourself up.

When we feel guilty or deem ourselves worse than we are, we are going to make bad things happen to us. For example, if you feel angry and put yourself down because of it, the next time something goes wrong, you will be angry at yourself for being so stupid. We have all done this for one reason or another, and it is important not to do it anymore because of the potential negative effects on our mental health.

* Learn from your mistakes, but don't dwell on them.

It can help to learn from past mistakes and then move on but don't let those past mistakes destroy your present happiness or work towards the future. Don't think about how things could have been different because you will only get upset. Instead, think about how you can do the same thing differently in the future to work out better for you.

So there you have it; these are some of the best tips for dealing with anxiety, depression, and anger. It does take some work, but once you get used to not letting these things affect your life and taking steps to fix them, they will no longer control your life. Treating these issues is very important and should always be a top priority because if we don't, they will only worsen over time. You must talk to someone if you have difficulty dealing with these emotions. You must open up and share your emotions with the people around you. If they do not understand what you are talking about, find another person that can help. There are many places to get help with emotional issues so don't be afraid to reach out and grab that life-saving help that could be right in front of your face. With this new information at your disposal, I'm sure you will have no problem getting rid of anxiety, depression, and anger.

There are a lot of people out there who have been victims of emotional abuse or bullying. It can be devastating to our emotional stability if we don't know how to deal with it. Knowing how to deal with emotional abuse and bullying is the only way you can move on and not let it affect the rest of your life.

One of the best ways to deal with emotional abuse or bullying is to avoid it. This doesn't mean walking around afraid all day because that will negatively affect your mental health, but it does mean that you should have an escape plan in case something happens so that you are not stuck in that situation for too long.

By having a plan of action or knowing what to do, you are already taking steps toward dealing with this type of abuse effectively. If you are currently dealing with emotional abuse or bullying, I recommend you talk to your parents or teacher about it. You must let someone know what is going on in case it happens again for some reason. Talking about things like this can help the problems go away faster because of what you tell them. You will also get the help you need if they want to give it to you.

After speaking with your parents or teacher (or sometimes both), your next step is to make sure that they do not allow this type of thing to happen again and if they know who did it, make sure that s/he is being punished for doing so. If your parents or teacher do not do something about it and you feel like nothing is changing, you can always go to a different adult that you know would be able to help you.

Another step toward dealing with emotional abuse or bullying is to avoid the person doing it if possible. If they are just bullying you in school, try sitting away from them, standing where they can't get to you easily, or even sitting with another friend. These steps will keep them from bothering you; this way, they don't have any power over what happens to you anymore.

If the emotional abuse or bullying continues, talk with someone after school instead of going straight home, so the bully doesn't see what happens to you afterward.

How to overcome fear through self-management techniques.

Overcoming your fear is not easy – it takes the right set of skills. This is where emotional self-management comes in. This technique takes some time to master, but the benefits can be huge.

If I could give one tip for managing your emotions, it would be to try putting yourself in a positive space every day. Maintenance work like this can help keep negative thoughts at bay so that they don't consume your whole day! Plus, finding happiness in the little things makes coping with other obstacles a lot easier when they come along.

Self-management techniques can be used for anything that affects your emotions.

One of the most common benefits of emotional self-management is learning to ignore negative thoughts and turning them into part of your positive routine.

Therefore, these tips can enable you to overcome fear through self-management techniques:

1. Identify the source of your fear and talk to it

The best way to overcome your fear is to know what it is. Start by identifying what your fears are the most. Identifying your fear will enable you to find ways to manage them.

2. Identify sources of support

A good way to overcome fear through self-management techniques is to identify your sources of support.

You can find sources of support in your family, friends, and other people you trust. Surrounding yourself with people that care about you will help you overcome fear through self-management techniques.

3. Get rid of negativity

Because fear is a negative emotion, an effective way to overcome fear through self-management techniques is to get rid of negativity in your life. Being around negative people or things that bring you down will only lead to more fear. You need to find methods for getting your mind off of whatever is causing your fear that you can practice every day.

4. Remove any safety measures

Part of overcoming your fear through self-management techniques is taking away any safety measures you have put in place because of the fear. If you have a phobia of spiders, talking yourself into confronting one won't work unless you are willing to do so without safety measures like running away or calling other people for help.

5. Face your fears

The best way to overcome your fear is to face them. This can be done by confronting the object of your fear, telling yourself that you will no longer be afraid of it, and not letting yourself retreat into fear due to the discomfort that this causes.

6. Focus on the positive aspects of things

A good way to overcome fear through self-management techniques is simple: just look at things that you are curious about and think only positive thoughts about them. If you're curious about snakes, don't think about what will happen if one bites you; just think about how cool they are. Ending up in the ER will not likely make you less fearful of snakes!

7. Think of the worst-case scenario

Remember that the worst-case scenario is not always as bad as you think. The next time you are afraid of something, think about what will happen if your fear is realized. Chances are, it's not going to be as bad as you think; if it is, there may be a way around it or someone who can lend a hand.

8. Change your perspective

One of the best ways to overcome fear through self-management techniques is to change your perspective. It's natural for the mind to focus on the worst possible outcomes of a situation, but you can't change what happens in reality by focusing on it.

9. Don't let fear dictate your life

Fear can take over a person's life if they let it, so don't let that happen to you! If one of your fears keeps you from doing something you want to do, make sure that there is another way around it or find a way to remove that fear entirely.

10. Focus on the present

One of the best ways to overcome fear through self-management techniques is to focus on what is currently happening. Doing this will take your mind off whatever could go wrong in the future. You may be afraid of flying, but instead of dwelling on the past or worrying about a potential future flight, just focus on your current situation.

356 – CBT, DBT, ACT, HSE AND VAGUS NERVE THERAPIES

11. Think about something that you can control

Another great tip for overcoming fear through self-management techniques is to focus on something you can control in front of you – your hands or feet, for instance. Focusing on something you can control will help your mind focus on positive things rather than the fear you are feeling.

12. Don't waste your energy thinking about things you can't control

One of the best ways to overcome fear through self-management techniques is not wasting your energy worrying about things you have no control over. It's highly unlikely that worrying about something your boss might say will make them like you more, so don't waste your energy thinking about it.

13. Keep doing what makes you happy

A good way to overcome fear through self-management techniques is to keep doing things that make you happy – even if it's something as simple as watching funny cat videos online.

14. Put your fears in perspective

A great way to overcome fear through self-management techniques is to put your fears in perspective. Think about what you have sacrificed because of your fear and whether or not it was worth it. If it wasn't, confront that fear the next time you have the opportunity.

15. Use positive self-talk

Another great way to overcome fear through self-management techniques is to use positive self-talk when facing a tough situation or a fear that keeps you from doing something you want to do. Tell yourself that you can do this, and if things don't work out right away, just keep trying until they do.

16. Make plans for the future

You may think that your worst fear is bugging you right now, but what if it's not? What if your fear is something that is happening in the future? Making plans for the future can help build up positive expectations and make you less afraid of things that will happen.

17. Don't focus on negative events in your life

If you're focusing too much on bad things that have happened in your life, relive those memories and spend all of your time worrying about them instead of making new memories that are more positive. Instead, focus on the future and the things that you want to do.

18. Look at the bright side of things

Using positive self-talk is another great way to overcome fear through self-management techniques, but there's no reason why you can't take this idea one step further and look at the bright side of everything. Even if something bad happened in the past, there's a good chance it won't happen again.

19. Imagine what you're afraid of

If you fear something like public speaking, for example, imagine yourself in the situation. If your fear is that bad, you will find that your fear does not come true, even though your imagination may have gone into overdrive.

20. Practice!

Practice makes perfect! Remember learning to ride a bike? Now, how many of you are nervous when riding a bike now? The more you do something that makes you afraid, the less frightening it becomes. So practice everything from public speaking to your favorite sport if it helps to make it less stressful.

21. Don't make it a big deal

One of the best ways to overcome fear through self-management techniques is to pretend nothing is wrong. If someone is afraid of something, smile and say, "Hey! You don't have to be afraid of that – I'm here with you!". This way, you can encourage your friend that there's nothing to worry about.

22. Take deep breaths

Deep breaths are the perfect way to keep yourself from panicking and showing any signs of stress when facing a tough situation. Deep breathing has numerous health benefits, including long-term stress reduction.

How to rewire your mind to experience the benefits of a more positive and emotionally-stable life.

For most people, negative thoughts run rampant - and that's not a good thing. We've created a list of the most popular online websites where you can find like-minded folks who are working diligently to break free from these negative patterns in their lives.

The majority of us would have become resigned to – and oftentimes even comfortable with – our negative thoughts. Many of us allow them to drive our every waking moment and are rarely surprised by their influence. The result is that we spend most of our lives feeling frustrated, sad, angry, or disappointed.

Rewinding your mind to a more positive slant can be an arduous and often challenging process. But it's a process that can be very rewarding and is essential for anyone wishing to live a more balanced, present, and happy life.

There are many jargons used today – such as mindfulness, self-help, and New Age techniques – but what they all have in common is a focus on the mind or your ability to change it. This book will take you through some of the many systems and techniques that have been developed over the past few decades to do just that.

There are many different ways to live a more balanced and present life, but here's a great starting point for anyone looking for ways to change their mindset.

Mindfulness and Mindfulness-Based Cognitive Therapy: The practice of mindfulness is simply being aware of one's current thoughts and feelings, including any painful emotions while not judging them as good or bad. It is accepting your experiences and observing them with non-judgmental awareness – thereby creating an inner space that is calm and stable.

The practice of mindfulness has been shown to help reduce stress, anxiety, and depression. It also helps control impulsiveness and negative emotions – such as anger, hatred, resentment, and fear – which cause many problems in our lives.

One of the most popular programs for mindfulness is Mindfulness-Based Cognitive Therapy (MBCT). It combines cognitive therapy and mindfulness training to assist people who are at risk of relapse during times of stress.

While there are many other ways to learn about mindfulness and MBCT, these websites offer a good starting point for anyone wishing to learn more:

The benefits of learning MBCT include the ability to cope with daily stresses, live in the present moment, and let go of negative emotions such as fear, anxiety, and depression.

Self-Awareness: Being self-aware is a very important skill that can be learned through various techniques used by psychologists. Self-awareness is knowing yourself, understanding yourself, and accepting yourself. We all have things that make us unique and interesting – but it is the difference between being aware of them and being self-absorbed.

Self-awareness can be directly related to improving your life. This skill allows you to understand your emotions and give you a chance to achieve more in life by taking into consideration what makes you happy.

The benefits of learning how to be more self-aware include creating a better understanding and appreciation for all of your experiences. This, in turn, allows you to live a more balanced life and make better decisions.

As the saying goes – knowledge is power, but freedom is mightier still. This is especially true when it comes to living a happy, balanced, and present life – which can only be achieved by using many different tools and techniques. Due to the nature of these tools, they can often help provide you with freedom from the mental prisons that you find yourself locked in on a daily basis.

Freedom from the many negative emotions that you experience on a regular basis.

To use our previous example – freedom from thinking about the past and future. Many of us spend a huge portion of our lives thinking about things that haven't even happened yet – while ignoring what's going on right now.

Learning how to be more self-aware and live in the present moment can be challenging, but it's also one of the most liberating things you'll ever do.

Access Consciousness: Access Consciousness is yet another method used to get in touch with your inner self and gain more control over your life and happiness.

Like many other philosophies and techniques, this system holds that you can change your life by changing your underlying beliefs. And it works within the premise that you are already perfect in every way, but that you often don't realize it.

So how do you access your inner self? You don't train yourself to be conscious – you train your unconscious mind to become conscious through the use of autosuggestion, visualization, affirmation, and self-hypnosis.

This process is designed to allow you to create a new level of awareness in yourself with the help of specially trained coaches. This, in turn, allows you to gain more control over your life and your emotions.

The techniques involved in accessing consciousness are very similar to those used for traditional alternative therapy; however, it also includes modern techniques that have been developed by psychologists over the past 50 years or so.

This is a great resource for anyone interested in learning more about this system:

The benefits of accessing consciousness include being able to:

* Separate yourself from your emotions and control the situations you find yourself in.
* Understand what you want and what you don't want in your life.
* Create specific goals for yourself that will make you happy.
* Become mentally stronger and happier.

We all have the power to change our lives – by changing the way we perceive the world around us. In some cases, this may require a different approach than using traditional therapy – but if it works, it can be very rewarding in the long run.

Emotions or Emotional Freedom Techniques: These techniques are based on the principles of hypnosis, but are different from other systems because they don't involve any kind of traditional training. They work by opening up a mental and emotional channel for you to release your feelings.

This process is effective in allowing you to let go of unwanted emotions and move on with your life.

With emotions, you're not going to experience any kind of trance-like state – but it still allows you to gain access to your unconscious mind which can help create a new mindset – one that's more aware and happier.

It also helps in eliminating some negative emotions such as anxiety and depression caused by past experiences.

The next chapter will discuss Frequently Asked Questions. These questions cover a variety of topics that are important to understand when considering the use of alternative therapy and self-help methods. Moreover, they will also answer many of the most common questions that people ask. Therefore, the chapter will cover a variety of questions that commonly arise when considering the use of alternative therapy methods.

FAQ

Q: How will these therapies help me or my patients?

A: With the tried-and-true listening skills, deep empathy, and strong focus on safety and trust, these therapies are perfect for patients who may require a helping hand to recover from trauma from their past or who have a difficult time expressing themselves verbally.

Q: Is this good for beginners?

A: Definitely! The highly-trained therapists behind these programs are experts in their field and provide an extremely gentle and supportive introduction to hypnosis and NLP. Often, patients find that these introductory sessions are enough to provide a lasting positive impact on the issues that brought them in the door.

Q: Why are these therapies different from other treatments?

A: This series of programs offers the real, tangible help you need to make positive changes in your life, no matter what the issue. Whether it's managing pain and stress, overcoming negative habits or emotions, changing unhelpful perceptions and reactions, or building rapport with other people, these therapies will provide you with the tools to do it all.

CONCLUSION

The vagal nerve communicates with the brain stem, which controls the heart and lungs, and can thus decrease heart rate. It also connects to various other organs in the body. Essentially, it influences every part of your body so that you can focus on what's happening in your mind.

Several therapies reverse many mental issues by using the vagus nerve to create a new connection between parts of the brain - like when your smartphone connects to a wireless network. In this case, not only is there no need for drugs or surgery, but it could be an improvement on traditional therapies.

This will come as a surprise to many, but it was thought that the vagus nerve led to brain death for a long time. However, there is no evidence that this is the case, and these days, you can have many operations with barely any pain and return to normal life. In addition, your well-being will improve significantly.

Nevertheless, a lot of people are still unaware of these breakthroughs. In fact, in the past few years, many new studies and medical reports have shown just how safe and effective this nerve therapy is. So, whether you are an individual or a representative of the medical field, you can learn much from this information.

These medications are available in most pharmacies, and they work by creating new fibers in the brain through an electrical current passing through it. Normally they break down fiber signals before they can pass through brain cells, but this new way of operating increases them over time so that they can stay alive longer without their fibers breaking down.

CBT is the most effective therapy used to reverse abnormal brain signals in people who develop dementia. The treatment for this condition involves sending an electrical current through the vagus nerve to the brain stem, which is located at the base of the skull. Through electrical impulses, this new method works on communication between different parts of the brain and effectively reverses negative thoughts or actions.

DBT is a less invasive approach than CBT and sends direct impulses into your abdominal region. However, it still sends electrical signals through the vagus nerve to create new connections between different parts of your body and mind. This therapy works especially well on mood disorders, including depression and addiction.

ACT is a treatment that involves creating new neural pathways in the brain. Essentially, you can use breathing techniques along with muscle exercises to stimulate your vagus nerve. The best part of this method is that it's completely non-invasive, so there aren't any drugs or surgery involved. Instead, you can send signals directly to your brain to help you relax and clear your mind.

HSE uses an electrical current to stimulate your vagus nerve for therapeutic use. An implanted stimulator sends signals through the nerve so that they can pass through your body and stimulate different brain areas. For example, an implant in the ear could help with pain management, while one in the neck could serve as a form of treatment for depression or post-traumatic stress disorder. Essentially, this method works to treat a variety of conditions, including anxiety and even weight loss or smoking cessation.

When you begin working on treating any mental health-related issues, it's important to know just what type of therapy is best for you. For example, if you have chronic depression, you could opt for vagus nerve therapy to get better sleep and feel more positive about your life. Another option for depression is VNS Therapy which involves sending electrical impulses through the nerve to control your brain and heart.

While the vagus nerve is used mostly nowadays to treat pain, it's also commonly used to treat heart conditions by slowing down the heart rate. This method is called a VNS pacemaker or implant, and it works by creating a new neural pathway between your body and mind. Essentially, this treatment can help patients with issues like migraines or those who've had a stroke by stimulating their vagus nerve to regulate their heartbeat.

HSE helps reverse chronic pain by sending electrical currents through the vagus nerve, which connects to the same brain area where a migraine originates. This treatment is performed on an outpatient basis and has few side effects, unlike many other therapies.

Ultimately, all of these approaches help to create new connections between parts of your body and mind, which are created through electrical currents passing through your vagus nerve. The more you use this method, the better you'll feel, so be sure to spread this information and continue your research.

Highly Sensitive Empaths have both heart and head wired together, whereas others mostly have heads wired to the heart.

The result is that Highly Sensitive Empaths can feel what others feel. Another word for this is "high empathy." But what is empathy? Empathy is the ability to understand others' feelings and emotions, and it turns out that Highly Sensitive Empaths are very good at it. So much so that they often find themselves overwhelmed by other people's feelings.

Most empaths go through a stage of suffering because they experience too much of how others feel (and think). And for some empaths, this suffering mostly comes from thinking about other people's feelings. Suffering from too much of someone else's emotion is called "transference."

Empaths undergo a period of Transference when they suffer because of other people's emotions. Empathy is a process that happens in healthy empaths and empaths suffering from too much transference. If you are an empath, you can learn how your brain works and take steps to stop being overwhelmed by other people's feelings.

Some suggest a two-step process of understanding another person's feelings – firstly, you need to understand that they feel what they feel (high empathy/high empathy).

Therefore, these therapies can be used to help you develop your natural healing energy. The feeling of extra energy is called "heart energy," It creates a connection between your heart and mind, like when someone has the privilege of connecting to a wireless internet network.

Highly Sensitive Empaths, or HSE, are people who are very sensitive to all types of things. This can be compared to being wired in two different ways. If you compare this with others who have "more head wiring," one way is that they can feel what others feel (high empathy). The other is that they are very sensitive (head wired) to situations and events.

Highly Sensitive Empaths, or HSE, are extremely sensitive and can easily pick up on other people's feelings (emotions, thoughts, and intentions).

This is why most empaths suffer from being overwhelmed by other people's emotions. This happens because an empath has both heart and head wired together.

The result of this is that empaths can feel what others feel - this is called being sensitive. Another word for this is "high empathy." But what is empathy? Empathy is the ability to understand others' feelings and emotions. It turns out that Highly Sensitive Empaths are very good at it. So much so that they often find themselves overwhelmed by other people's feelings.

GLOSSARY

CBT: a form of psychotherapy that aims to help people with a range of mental health disorders (e.g., anxiety, depression)

DBT: a combination of cognitive-behavioral therapy and dialectical behavior therapy. It is used in the treatment of individuals who have bipolar disorder as well as other mood disorders

ACT: an acronym referring to acceptance and commitment therapy, it is often employed in conjunction with other forms of complementary behavioral therapies

HSE: stands for Highly Sensitive Empath

Vagus nerve stimulation: is an invasive technique that stimulates the vagus nerve by implanting small electrodes under your skin. This procedure is often used in clinical trials to test new psychiatric drugs and treatments.

Neurological disorders: disorders that involve the nervous system (brain, nerves, and spinal cord)

Neuropsychiatric disorders: psychiatric disorders that involve the brain and nervous system. These include anxiety, depression, bipolar disorder, schizophrenia, and psychosis.

Mind-body medicine: a form of complementary medicine that involves exercise, meditation, yoga, and other healing techniques within a holistic framework. Mind-body medicine is integrative. It treats mental, physical, and spiritual well-being together.

Emotional triggers: a feeling, occurrence, or event that causes you to feel anxious or upset.

Neuroplasticity: a form of plasticity that refers to the ability of the nervous system to change.

Highly Sensitive Empaths (HSEs): HSEs are people who experience their emotions so intensely that their bodies and brains routinely respond to events and other stimuli in an over-reactive way. This often makes them ill with anxiety, depression, and other mood disorders. It is estimated that one in every thirty-five people in the U.S.

Post-traumatic stress disorder: is a psychological disorder associated with exposure to trauma, violence, and disaster.

Victim mentality: is a distorted pattern of thinking where you blame yourself for events and experiences in your life.

Cognitive distortions: distorted thoughts that cause you to misperceive situations or believe wrong things about yourself, others, or the world. Cognitive distortions are one of the main elements of CBT, DBT, and ACT.

Prolonged exposure therapy: a type of CBT wherein you face your fears so that they gently become less frightening with time. This method is very effective at treating Post-traumatic stress disorder (PTSD).

Dialectical stance: a therapeutic approach in which you view and confront your emotions and the situations or circumstances that cause them, with a willingness to accept rather than fight or escape them.

Empathy: a psychological process whereby you identify with someone else's feelings and experiences. Empathy is an important part of DBT.

Risk factors: factors that increase your likelihood of developing certain health conditions. In the context of mental illness, it refers to factors such as genetics, environment, lifestyle, and relationships with family members that make you more susceptible to developing a mental illness or disorder.

Autonomic nervous system: the part of the nervous system that controls your body's automatic processes. These include blood pressure, heart rate, respiration, digestion, urination, etc.

Neurotransmitters: chemical compounds released by one nerve cell and travel to another nerve cell via the synapses. Neurotransmitters may affect how you feel (positively or negatively) in certain situations or circumstances. Certain neurotransmitters such as dopamine and adrenaline increase excitement and excitement while others like serotonin allow you to feel emotions like sadness and anger.

Cognitive neuroscience: is the branch of psychology concerned with understanding how the brain works biologically.

Parasympathetic nervous system: one of the two major divisions of the autonomic nervous system. The parasympathetic nervous system is responsible for slowing down your heart rate, decreasing blood pressure, and relaxing muscles.

Somatic: relating to the body

Psychosomatic: relating to both the mind and body

De-sensitization (unlearning fear): a common treatment approach in CBT in which you gradually expose yourself to situations or things that cause you anxiety to "habituate" yourself to them, so they no longer cause anxiety. Habituating is when you become less sensitive or respond less strongly with time.

The polyvagal theory: is the view that humans have both sympathetic and parasympathetic nervous systems. The idea is that we can sometimes experience both states simultaneously (is this you right now?), which explains why sometimes we feel really upset and, in other situations, feel calm and peaceful.

Interoceptive: related to your body

Exteroceptive: related to your surroundings

Focus on the present moment: a form of mindfulness that teaches you to live in the moment by focusing on what is happening right now rather than worrying about the past or thinking about things that might happen in the future.

Neurofascial release technique: type of bodywork used to treat tension and muscle pain in the body by releasing tight muscles, connective tissue, and scar tissue in your body.

Freeze response: an initial response to a threat, which allows you to remain motionless so that you are less likely to be detected by a predator. In modern times it refers to a physiological state where your heart rate, blood pressure, and breathing can either decrease or increase dramatically depending on the situation.

Sympathetic nervous system: one of the two major divisions of our autonomic nervous system. The sympathetic nervous system is responsible for increasing your heart rate, mobilizing energy, and increasing feelings of excitement.

Emotional regulation: the ability to appropriately identify, express, control, and manage your emotions to feel happy, sad, angry or calm, etc.

The influence of blood vessels: the idea that blood vessels may help to regulate your body temperature and keep it within certain ranges (e.g., if you go outside without a coat on when it's very cold outside, your blood vessels constrict so that less blood flows to your skin which helps to keep you warm).

Reciprocal inhibition: learning between two behaviors whereby the less dynamic behavior (e.g., social withdrawal) becomes more active if another behavior (e.g., talking) becomes more active.

Self-injurious behavior: excessive and deliberate behaviors that harm you or others. Self-injurious behavior usually results from an inability to cope with emotional pain, stress, trauma, etc.

Reference

Harris, R., & PhD, S. H. C. (2019, May 1). *ACT Made Simple: An Easy-to-Read Primer on Acceptance and Commitment Therapy (The New Harbinger Made Simple Series)* (Second Edition, Revised). New Harbinger Publications.

Lcsw, M. V. D. (2022, May 10). *The 12-Week DBT Workbook: Practical Dialectical Behavior Therapy Skills to Regain Emotional Stability* (Workbook). Rockridge Press.

Psy.D., L. T. (2022, March 1). *CBT Workbook for Therapists: Essential Cognitive Behavioral Therapy Strategies to Treat Mental Health* (Workbook). Rockridge Press.

Torres, E. (2021, November 20). *CBT + DBT + ACT: 7 Books: Cognitive Behavioral Therapy, Dialectical Behavior Therapy, Acceptance and Commitment Therapy. Includes: PTSD, Vagus Nerve, Polyvagal Theory, EMDR and Somatic Psychotherapy.* Independently published.

Made in the USA
Las Vegas, NV
29 October 2023

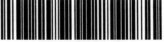

79911686R00203